Dedication

To
parents, my nurturers
patients, my inspiration
Meenakshi and Prateek, my supporters

Foreword

Managing Heart Problems is a very educative compilation on several aspects of cardiovascular health. The write up is very topical and assumes special importance in view of the magnitude of the problem of heart ailments in our country and region. Dr P. R. Sinha has gone into great details to explain its importance and the preventive measures which are urgently required to combat heart ailments.

According to conservative estimates, we have approximately 5.5 crore patients with heart diseases secondary to coronary atherosclerosis. A large body of data including the studies carried out on South Asian population has identified 9 risk factors which can account for 90 % of the heart attacks seen in our population. Six among them lead to adverse outcomes, these are—smoking and tobacco use, high blood pressure, diabetes mellitus, obesity especially truncal type, high levels of bad cholesterol in blood and stress. The importance of stress as an independent risk factor till recently had been debated but hard scientific data from the INTERHEART study has, beyond a doubt, demonstrated that stress is indeed one of the key risk factors leading to heart disease. The three protective risk factors to be taken into account are regular exercise, consuming plenty of fresh fruits and vegetables and alcohol in moderation.

The benefits of alcohol are very modest and are controversial, since it has many downsides which include psychosocial problems and liver diseases. However, when it is consumed in excess it causes depression of the heart itself and increases problems like high blood pressure. For this reason alcohol is never promoted as a protective measure.

The gist of Dr Sinha's hard work can be summed in the form of ten tips for a healthy heart:

1. Exercise for at least 30 minutes every day, at least 5 times a week.
2. Abstain from tobacco use.
3. Eat a healthy diet (consisting of 4 to 5 servings of seasonal fruits and green leafy vegetables per day).
4. Maintain ideal body weight for your height.
5. Have a yearly medical check-up after the age of 30 years. The medical checkup consists of general examination, blood pressure measurement, estimation of blood sugar and blood cholesterol levels.
6. Avoid anger, hostility and greediness.
7. Avoid a high fat diet (full cream milk products, excessive consumption of red meat, etc.).
8. Regular intake of almonds and nuts (6 to 8 per day).
9. Regular yoga and meditation to de-stress yourself.
10. Stick to the rule of 100. Keep your fasting sugar less than 100 mgs, maintain your blood pressure around 100 mm Hg (at least less than 120 mm), keep your bad cholesterol that is, LDL cholesterol less than 100 and triglycerides close to 100 (at least below 150 mgs)

I am sure the book *Managing Heart Problems* is going to be an enlightening reading for all the country men who are interested in keeping their hearts healthy. A billion healthy hearts would go a long way in keeping the nation healthy. Dr P. R. Sinha needs to be congratulated for writing this book in a very simple and lucid style.

Prof Upendra Kaul, *MD, DM, FCSI, FAMS, FACC, FSCAI*
Awarded Padmashri and Dr B C Roy Award
Executive Director and Dean Cardiology
Escorts Heart Institute and Research Centre, New Delhi
and Fortis Hospital Vasant Kunj, New Delhi

Preface

With each passing year the magnitude of people affected by heart attack and stroke is on the rise. Heart attack and related heart problems are primary factors leading to death all across the globe. A vast majority of those affected by these factors are in developing countries with an exception to the sub-Sahara region. The need to keep a check on heart disease is of utmost importance because it is growing at a fast pace. Enough scientific data is available which suggests that heart attack and stroke represent an urgent international issue and are more prevalent than previously thought of. The death and disability caused by the disease is causing immense financial burden to the low and middle classes of the developing countries. Currently, East Europe and Middle East are greatly affected by heart disease and the same trend can be witnessed in other parts of the world as well. It is more prevalent in the developing countries including China, India, Brazil, Mexico, Indonesia and North African countries. South Asian countries and China contribute to a large chunk of global population and in the near future, the maximum number of people afflicted by this disease may be witnessed in this region.

We should understand that the South Asian population is different from the western population. The South Asian population is represented less in clinical trials which are mainly conducted by the Western World. These clinical trials are used to formulate treatment guidelines for various heart problems. However, considering this limitation of non-representation, the proposed guidelines for West may not be totally applicable for the South Asians. Among the South Asian countries, India followed by Pakistan, Sri Lanka and Bangladesh have been found to have the highest death rate due to heart diseases amongst all ethnic groups studied so far. As applicable to all developing countries, including South Asia, heart disease develops at an early age, have more extensive and severe presentation with high death rates than their western counterparts. The disease has struck the most productive age group thus it has adversely affected the prosperity and progress of the nation. It has reached an alarming magnitude and in the near future it can be classified as endemic to the Indian sub-continent. The disease is four times more prevalent amongst urban Indians as compared to rural Indians and it is projected that by 2040, 40 % of Indians will live in the urban area due to rapid industrialization and urbanization. WHO has already warned that India will become the capital of heart diseases and diabetes by 2025. There is an urgent and crucial need to understand the disease process and to have awareness for preventing the disease before it manifests itself. Considering the magnitude of the problem, limited resources and costly treatment options in developing countries, the power of prevention cannot be undermined. Based on the future projections of heart disease spreading as an epidemic, it will be most wise and economical to nip the problem before it begins rather than cure it. Therefore, understanding the disease along with the preventive measures proposed is extremely essential.

Awareness is the key for successful prevention of any disease and unfortunately it is almost negligible in developing countries including India. One can blame government agencies, medical fraternity, media personnel and society as a whole but no amount of blame game is going to solve the problem. Health is an individual entity and one should take the responsibility urgently regarding his own health. Awareness can be started on an individual basis and can be spread to the society and nation as a whole.

Awareness and action requires no financial liabilities and is the cheapest option to tackle any problem. Awareness helps in detection of the disease at the earliest and hence suffering and complications can be prevented. Modification of lifestyle is almost always required and mandatory, the saying that man does not die as a result of his disease but of his character is true for heart disease also.

However, the book is not meant to be a detailed reference textbook. The main aim of this book is to be guiding material for the common man to have better cardiac health based upon modern scientific approach. The readership will include common individuals, patients, nurses, internist, primary care physicians along with other interested heath conscious and careful people. The text is directed towards the most basic aspects of care and prevention. The various indications and modalities of therapy – especially, the use of drugs have been deliberately not included to avoid confusions and controversies as treatment of a specific disease is an individualized approach and the treating physician is the best guide. This book is mainly meant to make people aware of the perils of heart disease and of the risk factors which can make them prone to heart disease. It also includes the various lifestyle changes which can help you to have a healthy heart. The book is mainly focussing on the developing world and especially on Indian statistics and lifestyle which are not a part of standard text books.

The heart is the seat of gentleness, joy, sorrow, grace, admiration, sympathy, harmony, warmth, and also the lifeline of an individual's life. The book is the genesis of various extraordinary experiences felt during the treatment of patients of heart disease. The inspiration of writing this book came from various queries, confusions and myths prevalent among heart patients. Today, patients get all types of advice from the sources which are ill-informed or based on personal experiences. In India, health is the only subject where one can get interference and ample advice from all walks of life. Illiteracy, poverty, ignorance, confusion, false belief and inability to accept the disease encourages the patients to follow these advises. One should realize that the body is a precious gift and it is not meant to be experimented on. The inability of the patient to accept that they are suffering from heart disease causes more harm than benefit. One should understand that heart disease develops slowly and gives an individual ample time to change its course. Ignoring it, may lead to catastrophic events such as a heart attack and/or even death. In India as well as in other parts of the world obesity is perceived as a cosmetic problem, physical activity as a waste of time, and tobacco consumption is assumed as harmful but not dangerous to life. All these are considered lifestyle choices and are not covered by insurance. A majority of premature deaths due to heart attacks can be avoided if we would simply change our lifestyles. If these common public issues are not addressed urgently then it is quite possible that the incidence of coronary heart disease (CHD) will continue to rise.

This casual approach towards our heart may be dangerous and may cost an individual his life and may change the life of an individual's family. The disease which was prevalent among the rich few decades earlier is now affecting the poor as well, due to unhealthy food habits and sedentary lifestyle. This all is due to the fact that we are drifting away from nature and have become part of the industrialized and urbanized culture. When we are young we have different goals and in the race to make our career and financial objectives we often neglect our health. Good health should be a priority for all so that one can enjoy his/her life to the fullest. Hence the aim of this book is, 'Today's care is tomorrow's cure'.

I need to acknowledge all my patients who had not only provided the questions but shared their experiences with me. I am indebted to Prof. Upendra Kaul who has gone through the book and accepted to write the foreword for the same. I am grateful to Prof. Nakul Sinha, Prof. Aditya Kapoor and Dr S.J. Singh for giving the inspiration and encouragement for writing the book. I would like to thank my colleagues, especially Dr Amitabh Hatwal and Prof. S.K. Singh, who provided extremely helpful suggestions and encouraged me at each and every step of this book especially in the chapters of Diabetes Mellitus and Metabolic Syndrome. My sincere thanks to Mr Christopher, Dr Rajeev Kumar and Mr Ashutosh Mishra for providing critical comments and corrections at various levels. The efforts, guidance and criticism from Dr Geeta Arora, Head of the Pharmaceutical Wing, B. Jain Publishers are also worth mentioning.

Every effort and due care has been taken to ensure the information contained in this book is correct at the time of going to press. Bringing out such a text has been a learning as well as a gratifying experience, and I hope it lives up to the expectations of the readers. It is possible that errors are unavoidable and there is a request to the readers to point out these so that it can be rectified in the future.

Publisher's Note

Our heart pumps blood to all parts of our body without ceasing for a moment. This blood carries oxygen that our cells need. But when this dynamic relation between the heart and the veins and the vessels become disbalanced, we confront heart problems. A heart disease is any problem or disorder that affects our heart.

Ailments related to heart are on the rise. Yet it is only a few who know how best these ailments can be prevented. This is where **Dr P. R. Sinha's** *Managing Heart Problems* comes in. Through his book, he makes us understand the various heart problems that can happen to us. He explains in a simple manner, the workings of our heart, how best we can take care of it and most importantly, how best we can look after our heart even if it is too late to prevent a heart disease.

We are extraordinarily happy to publish Dr P. R. Sinha's *Managing Heart Problems* as its main aim is to guide common man how best he can keep his heart healthy through care and management.

Kuldeep Jain
C.E.O., B. Jain Publishers (P) Ltd.

Contents

Foreword   v
Preface   ix
Publisher's Note   xv

Chapters

1. Introduction   1
2. Cardiovascular Disease: A Global Scenario   7
3. Cardiovascular Disease   25
4. Amazing Heart   33
5. Atherosclerosis and the Development of Coronary Heart Disease   39
6. Burden of Coronary Heart Disease in South Asia and India   43
7. Heart Disease and Risk Factors   51
8. Coronary Heart Disease   65
9. Myocardial Infarction   87
10. Women and Coronary Heart Disease   117
11. Sex and Heart Disease   127
12. Hypertension   139
13. Diabetes Mellitus   177
14. Metabolic Syndrome   209
15. Cholesterol and Fat   215
16. Smoking and Tobacco Use   241
17. Obesity   269
18. Exercise   295

19.	Stress and Behaviour	305
20.	Complementary and Alternative Therapy	315
21.	Diet in Heart Disease	331
22.	Alcohol	377
23.	Antioxidants, Heart Healthy Foods and Herbs	385
24.	Cardiovascular Diseases–Prevention and Practice	405
	Appendix and Tables	*421*
	Glossary	*429*
	References and Suggested Readings	*441*

Chapter 1
Introduction

'One of the most devastating consequences of cardiovascular disease can be sudden death or cardiac arrest.'

The news of a heart attack or paralytic attack causes shock and horror among family and friends. They are perceived as the two most predominant forms of disease and death in the adult population. Coronary heart disease (CHD) and stroke which affects the heart and brain respectively are the two most important components of cardiovascular disease (CVD) and contribute in most of the global burden of disability and death. At the beginning of the twentieth century, cardiovascular disease was responsible for less than 10 % of all deaths worldwide. However, the scene changed for the worse and at the beginning of twenty first century it increased to an alarming level of 30 %. It is projected that CVD would be the leading cause of deaths worldwide in the subsequent years. In the middle of the twentieth century, CVD was the problem of the west only but by the end of the century the disease burden intensified in the developing countries also and emerged as one of the foremost cause of disability and death. As a result of population explosion and compounding growth of the disease burden, developing countries account for twice as many deaths due to CVD as compared to developed countries.

The onset of this century has witnessed a global spread of CVD epidemic which is not only evolving rapidly but is also shifting from developed countries (USA, European Union, Canada, Australia, New Zealand and Japan) to developing regions like Russia, China, Brazil, Mexico, India, Pakistan, Middle East, North Africa, Latin America and Caribbean with the exception to sub-Sahara Africa due to affluence and adoption of western lifestyles. Currently, almost 85 % of the world's population lives in low and middle income countries, and it is estimated that in the near future CVD will be the leading cause of death in these countries. In developing countries, CVD burden occurs amongst adults of working age or at mid-life years, the most productive years of an individual's life. Therefore, CVD not only affects the prosperity of the individual, but has an impact on families and nations too. Thus, one can imagine its adverse effect on the economic growth of the developing countries where the infectious diseases are still rampant. In five major developing countries of the world (Brazil, India, China, South Africa, and Mexico), which represent approximately 44 % of the world's population, it is estimated that at least 21 million years of future productive life are lost because of CVD each year.

If all this is true, then handling such a large number of patients in developing countries will be a mammoth task in the coming years. The treatment options for control of established heart diseases like any other chronic disease must aim to control the risk factors, reduction of complaints and suffering, stabilization or halting the disease process, prevention of future adverse events, improvement of well-being and quality of life. Tremendous advancements have taken place in the field of medical science in the recent past and today a vast variety of effective treatment options are available. However, the whole treatment process costs a fortune and it poses an immense financial burden on the individual and the nation. In my twenty years of practice in one of the developing countries, I have realized that only a few lucky ones can afford this expensive treatment and the majority will have to live with medicines only. So even though medical science has progressed a lot, it has benefitted only a handful individuals.

Cardiac disease is not only a financial burden but is also associated with a massive loss of work force. Even after decades of scientific progress, medical facility to tackle this disease is limited and is still beyond the reach of common individuals in developing countries. Medical facilities are not only limited, but are unevenly distributed. As a result of this uneven distribution, a majority of the individuals living in semi-urban or rural areas in developing countries have no access to proper medical facilities. Paucity of trained medical personnel and sophisticated costly equipment further worsen the situation. Illiteracy, ignorance and meagre income further complicate the issue. A majority of the patients cannot afford the medicines, leave aside expensive treatment modalities like angioplasty (PTCA), coronary artery bypass grafting (CABG) or pacemakers. Establishing any number of centres will not suffice for such a large number of CHD patients and will always remain inadequate and insufficient. Therefore, the only option to counter the rapid upsurge of CHD in developing countries is the adoption of cost effective preventive measures and strategies, which have proved beneficial in reducing the CHD burden in Europe and America which were facing the same upsurge of disease at the time of economic transformation 50 years ago. People of the developed world have overcome this challenge to a major extent by way of appropriate and timely modification in their health habits. It is now our turn to wake up as a developing world to our health's needs.

To combat the deteriorating heart health of the individuals, it is our duty to join hands and actively participate in the implementation of preventive measures since it is no longer the job of the government only. Prevention of heart disease involves an exceptionally wide range of researchers, clinicians, dieticians and other specialists. It has become an area of major focus for various conferences, seminars and public deliberations all across the globe. It has been the highlight of many national and international conferences. However, all efforts are futile without the active involvement of the masses who are the real beneficiaries of these measures. An individual must first understand the nature of the problem, learn what causes heart disease and what can be done to prevent before the disease manifests itself.

Today a majority of us live in the false belief that we are free from disease. We have created our own definition regarding health and believe that being healthy means the mere absence of disease or infirmity. However, contrary to this, the World Health Organization (WHO) defines health as a state of complete physical, mental and social well-being. It is true that many people might not be having the obvious disease but they may be at a risk of developing various illnesses in the future. Obesity, tobacco consumption and lack of physical activity are a few factors, which are not categorized as disease but still make the person prone to various ailments and have caused havoc in the developing countries. For a healthy life, one should have a positive approach and for a positive approach one should have a healthy lifestyle. Going for routine health check-ups is not a priority and we are also not aware or bothered about the lifestyle and dietary requisites needed to maintain a healthy lifestyle and prevent heart disease, especially heart attacks and angina. We, however, need to take note of the fact that each one of us is genetically prone to heart diseases and environmental factors trigger it. In developing countries, the environment is changing fast because of economic transformation with an enormous impact on health. The booming economy has led to changes in the lifestyle such as increased intake of unhealthy fat, calorie rich foods, and sedentary habits. Consumption of alcohol and tobacco is on the rise too. The upsurge of coronary heart disease (CHD) in the developing world correlates directly with the changes in lifestyle and eating habits rather than the changes in the genetic pool.

Education and involvement of people in the disease process before it manifests itself is the best strategy for controlling or treating a disease. Preventive strategies aim to reduce the burden of disease by making people aware of and educating them about the disease. This is a better and affordable option. It has proved beneficial and can be practiced with little effort and a positive attitude by the individual. The aim of this book is to make an individual understand heart disease, especially coronary heart disease (CHD) and properly practice the preventive measures which can reduce the burden of disease on the individual and the nation as a whole. I hope the message of *Managing Heart Problems* goes miles in making inroads into the life and health of our fellow citizens so that they enjoy a disease-free life. Protecting lives through knowledge and understanding should be a duty of all individuals. It is needless to emphasize that FAULTY LIFESTYLE HABITS have caused the disease and HEALTHY LIFESTYLE HABITS will cure it.

Chapter 2

Cardiovascular Disease: A Global Scenario

The world today is experiencing an epidemic of cardiovascular disease (CVD) that shall have a devastating effect on the human society if not combated in time. It is predicted that by the year 2020, coronary heart disease (CHD) or heart disease, which is the major manifestation of CVD, will be the main cause of disability worldwide. It is also stipulated that this trend will continue and affect the developing countries more than the developed countries and is predicted to be among the leading causes of death in the times to come. The mention of the term 'cardiovascular disease' strikes in the minds as reference to a deadly disease which catches people unawares and silently, either as a heart attack or a stroke.

Cardiovascular disease is vastly influenced by the economic status of the populace and gets promoted and supported by the prevalent lifestyle of hurry (stress), worry (strain) and curry (saturated fat) in the affluent societies. With the advances in communication technology, the world has shrunk with easy accessibility to knowledge and resources of information. Even then, majority of the people continue to be unaware of the devastating effects of the cardiovascular disease. The disease strikes more the urban population than the rural despite a high rate of literacy among urban dwellers.

The major hurdle today in curbing the disease is the laid back approach adopted by most of us in the developing countries towards health promotional measures. We continue to pay no heed to preventive measures put forth through constant advocacy and awareness campaigns.

Extent of the Problem

Heart disease knows no geographic, gender or socio-economic boundaries. The major CVDs include coronary heart disease, cerebrovascular disease (stroke), hypertension, heart failure and rheumatic heart disease. As per the reports of World Health Organization (WHO), in 2005, a total of 58 million people died in the world. Among these, an estimated 60 % of all deaths were attributed to chronic diseases or non-communicable diseases, and a majority of these deaths were due to cardiovascular disease (CVD). It has been predicted that CHD, one of the leading manifestation of CVD, would be the foremost cause of worldwide deaths by the year 2030. CVD is no longer a problem of the west only where it continues to be the leading cause of death for the past few decades but now it is also knocking on the doors of the rest of the world. Also because of the high population burden, 80 % of the deaths due to CVD and 86 % of the global burden of CVD presently is in the developing countries. Moreover, at least 20 million people survive heart attacks and strokes every year requiring lifelong, continuous, costly medical care.

A Word about CHD

Coronary heart disease (CHD) is the most important cause of CVD and therefore CVD is synonymous with heart disease. CHD is the single largest cause of death in developed countries and is one of the main contributors to the disease burden and death in developing countries. The two most common manifestations of CHD are angina and acute myocardial infarction or 'heart attack'. It is the result of hardening and blockage of arteries which supply blood to the heart. Of the two, heart attack or myocardial infarction is the most notorious and can kill the person unaware. Patients with chronic stable angina which mainly manifests as chest pain after some form of physical activity have a fairly good outcome if treated on time. Angina has an average annual mortality or death rate of 2 % or less. However, if left untreated angina may progress to unstable angina or acute myocardial infarction (AMI). Heart attack is the outcome of total occlusion of a major coronary artery with a complete lack of oxygen and nutrients leading to death of heart muscles and impairment of its function. The death associated with heart attack or AMI is very high as half of the individuals die before they reach the hospital. Even those who are admitted in the hospital, about 10 % and 30 % of them die within seven and thirty days of the event respectively. These figures are from the hospitals which have the best among heart care facilities and the scenario is worst in hospitals without such facilities where almost one third of the patients die during the hospital stay. Of those who survive from the event, a majority require costly treatment to fix up the blocked artery or lifelong medical therapy.

Impact of the Disease

The social and economic impact of cardiovascular diseases, in developing economies is enormous with a burden on the common man where access to healthcare still constitutes mostly out-of-pocket expenditure. In case of CVD, the impact is still greater because the high proportion of those affected are the working-age adults increasing the burden on the family. In South Africa, for example, costs for the direct treatment of CVD were equivalent to 2-3 % of Gross Domestic Product, or roughly 25 % of all health care expenditures. The current expenditures in developed countries are indicators of possible future expenditure in developing countries. It is estimated that the direct and indirect costs of CVD in the United States would be more than many hundred billion dollars. It is also estimated that a quarter of health care budget is spent on CVD. Thus, chronic conditions such as CVD not only kill people at economically and socially productive ages but adversely affect the growth and prosperity of the families and nations.

What is the Global Scenario?

CVD rates are changing rapidly in both developed and developing countries. Developed countries such as the United States, Canada, Australia, New Zealand and most of the Western Europe have all witnessed the epidemic of CVD spanning the latter part of the twentieth century and presently are going through the decline phase of disease prevalence. This has occurred due to better understanding and control of risk factors responsible for CVD. The majority of the CVD burden today is in the eastern part of Europe, Central Asia, South Asian countries, East Asia and the Pacific, North Africa and the Latin and South American countries like Brazil (Table 2.1). Sub-Saharan Africa is the only exception which still remains trapped in the web of infectious diseases. Not only the disease burden but the cardiovascular death rates in middle aged individuals are higher in developing countries such as Russia (680), Nigeria (410), India (405), Pakistan (400), Brazil (320) and China (280) as compared to developed countries which is less than 200 per hundred thousand population.

Table: 2.1 Cardiovascular disease deaths in the world in 2001 with special reference to the six regions of the low and middle income countries as divided by the World Bank

World Regions	Major Countries	CVD Deaths in Respect to % of Total Deaths	Number of Individuals in Million	CHD vs Stroke
High Income	USA, Canada, Australia, Japan, New Zealand,, central, north, west Europe	38.5%	29	CHD > Stroke
Eastern Europe and Central Asia	Russia, Croatia, Kazakhstan, Romania, Ukraine, Czech Republic, Hungary, Poland, Slovenia	50.1%	472	CHD > Stroke
Middle East and North Africa	Gulf countries, Egypt, Libya, Morocco, Somalia, Sudan	35%	310	CHD > Stroke
East Asia and Pacific	China, Japan, South and North Korea, Singapore, Malaysia, Indonesia, Cambodia, Vietnam	30.6%	1849	CHD < Stroke
Latin America and Caribbean	Brazil, Mexico Argentina, Chile, Cuba, Mexico, Uruguay, Venezuela, Puerto Rico, Colombia	27.8%	526	CHD < Stroke
South Asia	India, Pakistan, Bangladesh, Bhutan, Nepal, Sri Lanka, Maldives	25.2%	1388	CHD > Stroke

| Sub-Sahara and Africa | Angola, Central African Republic, Congo, Chad, Liberia, Nigeria, South Africa | 9.7% | 668 | CHD < Stroke |

Regional Burden

Europe

People in Europe can be divided into Western Europe (England, Ireland, Belgium, Holland and France), Northern Europe that is Nordic countries (Finland, Sweden, Iceland), Southern Europe (Spain, Italy, Greece, Portugal), Central Europe (Austria, Switzerland, Poland, Germany, Hungary, the Czech Republic) and Eastern Europe comprising of Ukraine, Belarus and Russia. Europe has a stable economy and is a constituent of the developed world. However, as far as the prevalence of heart disease is concerned, the eastern part suffers more as compared to the rest of Europe. Russia, Croatia, Kazakhstan, Romania and Ukraine present the worst scenario and have seen significant increases in CHD related disease and deaths which is six times higher as compared to the United States. In the Russian Federation, life expectancy for men has dropped precipitously since 1986 from 71.6 years to about 59 years in 2004, majorly because of CVD. In the Czech Republic, Hungary, Poland and Slovenia, CVD rates are three to four times higher than the rest of Europe but the positive aspect is that it is on the decline. This is in contrast to the rest of the European countries where both the disease and deaths due to CHD have declined in the last three decades. The CVD among European population is mainly attributed to the conventional risk factors responsible for increased occurrence of CHD. These risk factors include consumption of diets high in saturated fats, elevated cholesterol levels in blood, high blood pressure, smoking and diabetes mellitus. France, Greece and Italy in particular have low incidence of CHD in spite of excess smoking and high consumption of saturated fat and this is often termed as 'French paradox'. Numerous hypotheses have been put forward to explain this low prevalence. High consumption of olive oil and monounsaturated fats, antioxidants and consumption of wine may be responsible for the low rate of CHD in France.

Japan

The rise in economic prosperity in Japan, however, has not been accompanied by the rise in CVD and thus this nation has the highest life expectancy. The incidence of CVD is low as compared to many western countries. Japan has low CHD rates but high stroke rate with high blood pressure being the foremost risk factor for the disease. Average level of cholesterol is low which further explains the low level of CHD among Japanese and this may be due to the excess use of fish in diet which is high in mono-unsaturated fats. Nowadays because of the increased adoption of western lifestyles, combined with an increase in smoking, diabetes and obesity, Japan may witness a spurt in CHD in the coming years and it may surpass the stroke events which are the leading cause of death and disability due to cardiovascular diseases.

China

China is currently witnessing an increase in CHD in its population due to rapid urbanization and industrialization. If this trend continues, CHD may emerge as the leading cause of illness and premature loss of lives. The CHD prevalence rate is higher in Northern China, that is, Beijing than in Southern

China that is, Shanghai, and also it is higher in urban areas as compared to rural areas. In urban China, the death rate from CHD rose by 53 % from 1988 to 1996. Conventional risk factors such as high blood pressure, diabetes, obesity, smoking and high cholesterol levels are all important and contribute to the increased prevalence of disease. Cigarette smoking is very common amongst Chinese and may contribute to the increasing prevalence of CHD in coming years. China may face a rapid rise in the number of persons developing and presenting with CHD which may soon replace the stroke events as the number one cause of disease and death.

South Asians

'South Asians' refers to the people who originate from India, Pakistan, Bangladesh, Nepal, Sri Lanka, Maldives and Bhutan. Almost one quarter of the global population lives in South Asia. Countries of South Asia are often referred to as the developing nations have half their population living below the poverty line with limited access to healthcare. It has a significant segment of population in the higher income group including a few billionaires from India. Inequality in access to medical care is tremendous with some of the South Asian institutions offering state-of-the-art care to patients with CVD, promoting 'medical tourism'. With the current rate of economic development and increase in life expectancy, non-communicable diseases are rising. As compared to their western counterparts, South Asians do not have a high rate of conventional risk factors such as smoking, high blood pressure or high cholesterol level, yet they have higher rates of CHD. High prevalence of diabetes, impaired glucose tolerance, metabolic syndrome, central obesity, physical inactivity, high triglycerides instead of high LDL (low density lipoprotein) cholesterol, low levels of protective HDL (high density lipoprotein) cholesterol alone or in combination, make South Asians more susceptible to CHD. Few of the emerging risk factors such as elevated levels of lipoprotein Lp(a), the levels of which are genetically determined, is associated with increased atherosclerosis (hardening of blood vessels) and manifestation of disease events. The high levels of homocysteine encountered in this population can accelerate the process of blood clotting in the blood vessels, further predisposes the South Asians to CVD. It is predicted that despite the high death rates due to the communicable diseases, CVD would be the leading cause of death in the South Asian countries and India will lead with maximum number of CVD patients by 2025.

Latin Americans and the Caribbean

Non-communicable diseases are the main cause of premature death and morbidity in Latin America and in the Caribbean. It is estimated that there will be a tripling of the incidence of coronary heart disease and strokes and it is predicted that during the first decade of the twenty first century, cardiovascular diseases are expected to claim 20.7 million lives in Latin America and the Caribbean. The World Health Organization (WHO) estimates that by 2020, there will be 64 million people suffering from diabetes in Latin America and the Caribbean. The recent surge of CVD may have been partially caused by 'social transition' accompanied by 'nutritional transition' similar to that observed in South Asian countries and upper class people. Today, CVD is the leading cause of death among Latin Americans in the Caribbean and a majority suffer a high prevalence of conventional risk factors such as high cholesterol, diabetes, smoking, and high blood pressure. They also have low levels of protective HDL cholesterol, low physical activity and a higher rate of obesity. Mexico has lower rates of CHD than stroke. However, diabetes is on the rise in this country. Cuba and Puerto Rico have high CHD than the stroke events in their population and have low levels of diabetes as compared to Mexico.

Middle East and North Africa

Increasing economic wealth in the Middle East and North Africa has been characteristically accompanied by urbanization. The rate of CVD has been increasing rapidly and is now the leading cause of death, accounting for 25-45 % of total deaths. Both men and women are at high risk and the cardiovascular disease imposes the highest morbidity burden for this region. The daily per capita fat consumption is increasing and is more than 30-40 % higher than the recommended amount. Even the intake of trans-fatty acids is far higher from the recommended amount (15-30 gm per day vs < 5 gm per day). Fat along with carbohydrate consumption is highest in Saudi Arabia and lowest in Sudan. Overweight and obesity have increased two-fold or more since 1980 and childhood obesity is now a major concern. Changes in food processing, production and type of food (fast food) have affected the health in a majority of countries in the region. The population's sedentary lifestyle has also become a public health problem, with 70-80 % population being physically inactive. Conventional risk factors such as high blood pressure, diabetes and high cholesterol levels are on the rise. Approximately 75 % of cardiovascular diseases can be attributed to conventional risk factors. Hypertension affects almost 26 % of the adult population in the region. Diabetes is a major concern resulting due to obesity, and Egypt tops the list with almost 4.4 million diabetic patients (2007) in this region. CHD is the predominant cause of CVD, with about three CHD deaths for every stroke death. Non-communicable diseases and their related morbidity and mortality are becoming a significant serious public health problem in this region of the world.

Africa

Africa is a big and complex continent. It is the richest continent in terms of some natural resources, minerals and oil. Yet 34 of the world's 41 indebted poor countries are in Africa constituting one sixth of the world's population. Cardiovascular disease is the leading worldwide cause of death in all developing regions with the exception of sub-Saharan Africa. Because of their traditional dietary habits and poverty, the people of sub-Saharan Africa are still battling infectious diseases. The commonest form of heart disease in sub-Saharan Africa is chronic rheumatic heart disease which results in damage and malfunctioning of the heart valves. It is followed by dilated cardiomyopathy, pericarditis or infective endocarditis which are mainly due to poverty, nutritional and viral factors. Coronary heart disease in sub-Saharan Africa affects a small group of westernized population. The highest rates of heart disease in South Africa are found in the Indian community, followed by the white and the affluent black community. Blacks in Africa exhibit very low CVD rates. However, it may be pertinent to mention here that the same population of blacks in the US have a very high prevalence of CVD which is comparable or even higher than those among the whites in the US, underscoring the importance of environmental and social factors on the disease patterns prevalent in a population. Despite the high rate of deaths in South Africa due to AIDS, projections predict that chronic disease including heart disease is also set to increase and may account for half of the premature deaths occurring before the age of 65 years.

Currently, CHD appears to be a less important cause of illness and death than the many infectious diseases and HIV/ AIDS (human immunodeficiency virus/ acquired immune deficiency syndrome) but it is likely to escalate in the next generation. The risk factor profile (hypertension, diabetes, smoking, a diet high in saturated fats, obesity, and lack of physical exercise) for CHD is the same in sub-Saharan Africa countries as in western countries, but the haemoglobin S or C trait may be an additional risk factor for CHD unique to sub-Saharan Africa. The conventional risk factors for CHD are low in the African population with the exception of hypertension. Hypertension has emerged as a major public health concern, and hypertensive disease accounts for the dominance of stroke. Hypertension is eminently treatable and to some extent preventable. Besides hypertension, due to the changing environment in Africa, diabetes mellitus is emerging as a prominent risk factor for CVD in black Africans. Hence, with rapid westernization of lifestyle it is expected that these risk factors will increase and so will the new cases of heart disease.

Brazil

Cardiovascular diseases are the leading cause of death in most regions of Brazil, Argentina, Uruguay and other countries in South America. In Brazil, cardiovascular disease is responsible for almost one third of the total deaths. The leading cause of cardiovascular death is cerebrovascular disease or stroke closely followed by coronary heart and other heart diseases such as hypertension. Ischaemic Heart disease prevalence is estimated to range from 5-8 % in adults over 40 years of age. Major cardiovascular risk factors are similar to those prevalent worldwide such as smoking, diabetes mellitus, hypertension, abdominal obesity, high cholesterol in blood and a sedentary lifestyle. Today from among 96 million of the Brazilians above 20 years of age, 41 % are overweight and this is also increasing the number of diabetes patients which is 8 million today and projected to be almost 18 million by 2025, fourth in the world, just lagging behind India, China and USA.

Why is there a Spurt of CVD in Developing Countries?

The dramatic population, social and economic shift has witnessed a new disease pattern in the world. This has resulted in the emergence of chronic diseases especially CVD replacing infectious diseases which were prevalent a few decades earlier. The process responsible for the global shift in CVD mortality is known as 'epidemiological transition'. This transition is fuelled by rapid industrialization, urbanization and socio-economic development, and triggered by the following key factors:

Declining infant and child mortality has led to rapid demographic changes resulting in a large increase in the number of individuals surviving until middle and older age. Further, falling death rates from communicable diseases due to socio-economic development, improved medical care, vaccination, sanitation and other primary health care services has resulted in longer life expectancy which has increased the rates of chronic diseases including CVD.

Population explosion and urban development resulted in the reduction of green spaces, new housing architecture, deteriorating civic facilities, encroachment of pedestrian paths and increased road accidents which has reduced the opportunities for physical activity. Shift of large rural population in search of better jobs, insufficient health budget, inadequate and inequalities in medical treatment coupled with poverty, illiteracy and ignorance has resulted in premature and untimely deaths in large parts of the developing world.

The rise in CVD reflects a significant change in diet habits, physical activity levels and tobacco consumption worldwide which in turn is a result of rapid industrialization, urbanization and economic development. Almost all developing countries are facing a phase of 'nutrition transition' as a result of globalization of food market which is a drift from traditional diet habits to low consumption of fruits, vegetables, whole grains, cereals and legumes. One can call it unhealthy food globalization. The middle and upper class of the urban population have enough money and sufficient food, but because of poor dietary choices, they tend to select unhealthy foods which are high in salt, sugar and saturated fats. This shift in dietary pattern is a key factor leading to a rise in the prevalence of obesity worldwide. According to the World Health Organization, more than 1.6 billion adults are overweight and obese. Childhood obesity is a growing global concern and is no longer only a problem of the west. It is increasing at a fast pace in some of the developing countries like India, China, Mexico, Russia, Hungary, Brazil, Philippines, Jordan, Egypt and in a few Gulf countries. Obesity per se is not a disease but it can increase the prevalence of diabetes mellitus, hypertension and lipid abnormality in an individual which are the major preventable risk factors for CVD. Calorie rich foods when consumed over a period time, coupled with sedentary habits and excessive smoking increases the urban preponderance of CVD in developing countries.

What Can be Done?

From the pattern seen in the developed countries where the disease has declined in the last few decades we know that up to 80% of heart disease and stroke cases could be prevented by setting up healthy habits for life with a prudent diet, regular exercise and avoidance of tobacco. Fortunately, CVD shares several conventional risk factors cutting the borders of nations, baring a few regional and genetic determinants. An INTERHEART study from 52 nations revealed that 90 % of CVD burden can be explained by nine modifiable risk factors that are – smoking, history of hypertension or diabetes, waist/hip ratio, dietary patterns, physical activity, consumption of alcohol, blood apolipoproteins, and psycho-social factors. Thus a common intervention may be appropriate for the whole world.

Prevention of CHD is possible. However, it is frequently neglected, especially in the developing countries. The methods of prevention of CHD can either be based on individual or on population approach. Since more than half of the deaths due to CVD occur before the arrival of effective medical treatment, the most appropriate methods will be reducing the risk among the entire population. The population approach not only benefits a larger group of individuals but it is also very cost effective. It should be the main preventive strategy and should be the first to be considered and promoted. The second approach may be individual approach and is practiced in a few countries only. A lot of focus is being placed on one-on-one interventions among people at risk for CVD. However, it can benefit only a few and therefore has a limited role. The population based approach is the best option and all efforts should be directed towards understanding and reducing the risk factors through multiple economic and educational plans and programs. The preventive benefits may not be evident in a short span of time but it will definitely help in promoting personal health and wealth. It will save billions in the form of direct and indirect medical expenditures and thereby help in improving the quality of life and economic prosperity of the nation.

There is ample evidence which indicates that the following preventive strategies will change the CVD disease pattern, both in the developed and developing countries. It will not only effectively prevent and reduce the disease burden but will also help in managing the disease pattern and its prevalence.

Individual Preventive Measures

1. Reduce salt and sodium content.
2. Reduce total fats, especially saturated fats, trans-fatty acids and cholesterol.
3. Increase consumption of omega-3 fatty acids from fish oil or plant sources.
4. Consume a diet high in fruits, vegetables, nuts, bran, grains and whole grains.
5. Consume food in its most natural form.
6. Avoid excessively salty or sugary foods.
7. At least 30-45 minutes of daily physical activity is required. The most cost effective exercises are brisk walking, cycling and swimming.
8. Avoid tobacco use in any form and limit alcohol intake.
9. Maintain ideal body weight and avoid obesity.
10. Take care of blood pressure and blood sugar levels.

Population Based Preventive Measures

1. There should be a government-led effort to switch the main source of cooking oil from saturated fat to unsaturated fat with emphasis on traditional dietary habits and methods of cooking.
2. General community awareness levels need to be raised regarding common risk factors such as diabetes,

hypertension, cholesterol levels, obesity and its role in the development of CVD for its early detection, prevention and treatment.
3. Introduction of laws requiring labelling of packaged foods displaying calories, level of salt and trans- saturated fat contents of processed foods.
4. Effective implementation of laws banning smoking in public places and selling of tobacco products to minors.
5. Encouraging regular annual medical check-ups, mainly in urban citizens above the age of 30 years.
6. Mass awareness campaigns for prevention of childhood obesity which is emerging as a major concern for high and medium income countries.
7. Government should ensure enough green and clean open spaces to promote the culture of walking and other outdoor physical and recreational activities.

Global Burden at a Glance

A global CVD epidemic is rapidly evolving, with the burden of disease shifting to developing countries.

Twice as many deaths due to CVD now occur in developing countries as compared to the developed countries.

A vast majority of CVD can be attributed to conventional risk factors.

Even in sub-Saharan Africa, high blood pressure, high cholesterol, tobacco and alcohol use, and low vegetable and fruit consumption are already among the top risk factors for the disease.

Because of the lag time associated with CVD risk factors, especially in children, the full effect of exposure to these factors will only be seen in the future.

Information from more than a hundred countries shows that 13 to 15 year olds smoke more than ever before.

Studies show that obesity levels in children are increasing markedly in countries as diverse as Brazil, China, India and almost all island states.

This trend should alert the individuals, health authorities, medical and scientific community to take active measures in order to prevent, diagnose and adequately treat these life threatening disorders.

Chapter 3
Cardiovascular Disease

Cardiovascular system (CVS) is a broad term which includes heart (cardio) and vessels (vascular) of the body. Blood vessels include arteries and veins which are connected through very fine tubes known as capillaries. The heart works as a pump and the blood vessels work as conduit pipes which supply necessary oxygen to all parts of the body. Oxygen rich blood is supplied via arteries from the heart and oxygen is diffused or extracted by various cells of the body through capillaries and the blood, now poor in oxygen (deoxygenated) is brought back to the heart with the help of veins. The heart in turn pumps the blood into the lungs for oxygenation and the whole process continues.

Cardiovascular disease (CVD) denotes the dysfunctional conditions of the heart, arteries and veins, separately or collectively. If the oxygen and nutrients do not reach the cells of various organs of the body in sufficient quantity then the normal function will be lost and organs may die ultimately. The two most common and vital organs affected by the lack of oxygen are the heart and the brain. The brain, like a computer controls all the functions of the body and the heart, like a pump is responsible for supplying proper fuel to the body. Therefore, any affliction of the heart and brain by disease leads to catastrophic events such as a heart attack or a brain stroke respectively.

'Heart disease' is a term often used to describe a range of diseases that affect the heart, and sometimes the blood vessels. The various disorders that fall under the umbrella of heart disease are diseases of blood vessels which supply blood and essential nutrients to the heart that is, coronary heart disease, weakness of heart muscle (cardiomyopathy), failure of proper functioning of the heart (heart failure), disturbances in the heart rhythm (arrhythmias) and diseases related to valves of the heart; the commonest being rheumatic heart disease. The heart may also have certain developmental defects which are present since birth; they are clubbed together as congenital heart diseases. The diseases affecting the covering of the heart are known as pericardial diseases.

Out of all the heart diseases, coronary heart disease (CHD) is the most common and is a major killer worldwide. Thus the term 'coronary heart disease' is often used interchangeably with 'cardiovascular disease' — a term that generally refers to conditions that involve a narrowed or blocked blood vessels that can lead to a heart attack, chest pain (angina), heart failure or sudden death. Simultaneously, involvement of blood vessels of the brain (cerebral arteries) and the brain itself is equally important as they can cause paralytic attack of various severities which is also an important component of cardiovascular disease. The involvement of the brain is commonly referred to as 'stroke' or 'cerebrovascular accidents' (CVA). The narrowing of limb vessels is called peripheral arterial disease and is the commonest cause of disability, such as arm or leg pain or numbness and development of gangrene also fall in the category of CVD.

Why should I Know about CVD?

Cardiovascular disease is the world's leading killer, accounting for 17.5 million or 30 % of the total global deaths in 2005. Of these, 7.6 million were due to coronary heart disease and 5.7 million were due to stroke. As the leading cause of death and disability in adults, cardiovascular diseases are of utmost importance. Heart disease is the number one killer of men and women in developed countries and is a cause of concern across the developing countries. Today, 80 % of cardiovascular deaths are contributed by developing countries. Indians are not spared and have by far the worst problems when it comes to heart disease. Nearly 50 % of CVD related deaths in India occur below the age of retirement compared with just 22 % in the west. India is facing a double headed monster that is, both infectious diseases and cardiovascular diseases. Today in India, cardiovascular diseases lag behind the infectious diseases but the disease is assuming epidemic proportions and if the same trend continues it will soon become the cause of an infinitely large number of deaths.

It is known today that many forms of heart disease can be prevented or treated by opting for a healthy lifestyle. Also, knowledge regarding CVD helps in preventing the disease besides reducing a huge amount of financial burden, thereby saving many precious lives.

Who should Bother about CVD?

If you have any of the risk factors listed below, you may be at the risk of developing cardiovascular disease:
1. A man over 30 years or a woman over 40 years of age.
2. If overweight in relation to an individual's height.

3. Habituated to a sedentary lifestyle.
4. A smoker or someone who consumed tobacco regularly, or works with people who smoke regularly.
5. Suffering from high blood pressure or diabetes mellitus.
6. Has high cholesterol levels in the blood.
7. Who has a history of heart disease like angina, heart attack or stroke.
8. Whose parents had a heart attack before the age of 55 years.
9. Who leads a stressful life.

Causes of Cardiovascular Disease

The blood vessels, mainly arteries which supply oxygen and nutrient to the heart are affected in the process of cardiovascular disease. During childhood, the arteries are healthy that is they are clean from inside, flexible and strong. However, as the age advances, arteries are obstructed and they become hard by a process called atherosclerosis or hardening of arteries. The damage caused to arteries by the process of atherosclerosis is slow and takes many years. Over time, the thick and stiff arteries get blocked, resulting in reduced blood supply and oxygen to various organs of the body including the heart and brain. Atherosclerosis, which is the most common cause of cardiovascular disease is a normal aging process in the body. However, the process can be enhanced by an unhealthy eating pattern, obesity, a sedentary lifestyle, high blood pressure, diabetes mellitus and/or the use of tobacco. All of these are the major risk factors leading to the development of atherosclerosis and, in turn, cardiovascular disease.

How to Recognize CVD?

Cardiovascular disease is caused by narrowed, blocked or stiffened blood vessels that supply blood to the heart, brain or other parts of the body. When these organs are affected, they cause a problem in the body and are felt as complaints or symptoms. If the heart is involved in the disease process, it can cause chest pain in the form of uncomfortable pressure, fullness, aching, squeezing, burning sensation or tightness in the centre of the chest that lasts for a few minutes or longer. The chest pain that increases in intensity after doing some work or after eating may be a warning signal of heart disease. Other complaints related with the heart may include unexplained sweating, dizziness or fainting, nausea, vomiting or a feeling of severe indigestion, shortness of breath, unexplained weakness or fatigue, and a rapid or an irregular heartbeat.

When the brain gets involved, it may manifest as transient loss of memory, giddiness, difficulty in speech, blurred or double vision, vomiting, fits, loss of function of a part of the body or even coma. When blood vessels of limbs are affected it can cause pain in leg muscles during walking (claudication) or sometimes numbness, weakness or coldness in the legs or arms. As the disease advances it can lead to death of a part of a limb due to total loss of blood supply – a condition referred to as gangrene.

Atherosclerosis and narrowing of blood vessels is a slow process and thus, CVD might not be diagnosed early or may come without warning signals until the condition worsens to the point that it manifests into a heart attack, chest pain (angina), stroke, heart failure or sudden cardiac death. It is important to watch out for cardiovascular symptoms and discuss with your family physician. It is wise to suspect cardiovascular disease early and manage it in time.

Six Rules for CVS Health

Forgetting is painful. Avoiding it is more painful. Not knowing what to do is the worst kind of suffering. One should follow the rules listed below to combat and fight against cardiovascular diseases:

1. Be aware.
2. Recognize yourself.
3. Take charge of your health.
4. Act now as miracles happen rarely.
5. Prepare yourself for the priceless joys of life.
6. Think of the future generation.

Be Aware

In the west, there is awareness about heart disease, its symptoms and treatment. This is not so in the rest of the world including India and this results in late diagnosis of the disease making recovery difficult in many cases. It is important to know the warning signs of heart disease so that one can seek medical help in case of an emergency. It is always wise to recognize and prevent the disease before it manifests itself as prevention is always better than cure. One should not wait to diagnose pregnancy by labour pain and heart attack by chest pain.

Recognize Yourself

Recognize the importance of being you as it is primarily only you who is interested in your health. Health is a personal matter and only your efforts can make the change. The manner in which you eat, exercise, inculcate good habits or take medicines is entirely up to you. No one will do that for you and you cannot get a surrogate partner in the matter of health. Just listen to your body and heart. Remember it is only your active interest and involvement that will keep you one step ahead in the battle against heart and other health problems. It is possible that you may be the only person in this world but for someone you are the world, so take care of your health.

Take Charge of Your Health

Death is an irreversible immortal truth and no one can deny it, but you can certainly have a healthier, even longer life. Devote half-an-hour, out of your hectic schedule towards your health and well- being. One can influence the health for better or for worse by choices one opts for in day-to-day life. You should know the factors that can increase the risk of development of heart disease and if you have any, take charge of it to correct it or treat it with the help of your physician to safeguard the health of your heart. You should not only know the causes of heart disease but you should be aware of the complaints or warning signals or symptoms related to heart disease so that it can be diagnosed early. You scold your children to finish their homework and prepare their bags for next day stating that it is better to finish it today. Unfortunately, the same is not applied to yourself when it comes to the matter of health and a majority of us postpone it for later dates unless it affects our daily life. Getting regular medical check-ups appears to be a waste of time and money, or maybe you are afraid that if something is found wrong, it will require treatment. It is never too late to take charge of your health; act in time and do not put off for tomorrow what you can do today.

Act Now as Miracles Rarely Happen

As a result of the many advances in the medical field, expectations from medicine are very high today. Once the patient is admitted into the hospital, it is hard for the family members to accept the death of their patient. No one blames themselves for not caring for them or controlling their high blood pressure, or having poor control of diabetes mellitus or for their obesity or bad habits such as smoking and tobacco chewing. Act now as medical science can only help to fight against the disease and survival depends mainly upon the health, will power and age of the body. Remember, till date no medicine or system (pathy) has the ability which can replace a damaged or dead part of the body.

Prepare Yourself for the Priceless Gift of Life

Prepare yourself for certain unbridled joys, gladness, delight and gifts. It is the desire and dream of every individual to complete their responsibilities – owning a house, having a decent marriage and settling their children well. By the time they fulfil their responsibilities they are too old or it is too late. In my opinion, one should think beyond this and have a desire to see their grandchildren eager to cut at least their eighteenth birthday cake. These moments will be precious in life. The bond between these two extremes of age is pure and innocent, and saving and protecting a person from heart or any disease till this age will be the 'priceless' gift of life.

Think of the Future Generation

My mother and father both had high blood pressure, and my father passed away due to a heart attack when he was only 50. I have to make sure to keep my blood pressure normal and to stay healthy for my kids. It is my duty to keep my health normal so that not only me but my future generations are also risk free. Someone has rightly said – 'the past is history, future is a mystery and the present is a gift that's why it is called a present.' You cannot change your past history but you can definitely change the mystery of health through your habits. So, take care and enjoy every moment of your present health and well-being because it is the key to your future health.

Chapter 4

Amazing Heart

The heart is one of the most important and sensitive organs of the body. The main function of the heart is to push the required amount of blood throughout the body. It is a muscular organ and works like a pump. It is located in the central portion of the chest, slightly towards the left side called the mediastinum and is well protected by a bony rib cage. It is a hollow muscular structure, which receives oxygen depleted blood from the various parts of the body, and it propels oxygen rich blood into the arteries to be distributed to all parts of the body for the smooth functioning of the body. The size of the heart varies with our body build and activity, but normally it is the size of a clenched fist and weighs about 300 gm.

Functions of a Healthy Heart

There are four pumping chambers or compartments in the heart and each one is composed of a different amount of heart muscle or myocardium. The two upper chambers are called the right and left atrium and the lower chambers are called the right and left ventricles. Ventricles are the main pumping chambers of the heart and are therefore more muscular and robust than the atria. The left ventricle is the strongest of all as it has to pump blood to all parts of the body except the lungs, which receives blood from the right ventricle and therefore, the left ventricle is the major chamber of the heart. The heart also has four major valves, functioning like one way doors keeping the blood flow in one direction. Blood collected from the various parts of the body enters the right ventricle from the right atrium through the right atrioventricular (tricuspid) valve and leaves for the lungs through the pulmonary valve for the oxygenation. Blood rich in oxygen enters the left ventricle from the left atrium through the left atrioventricular (mitral) valve and reaches the aorta through the aortic valve for circulation to all body organs and structures. Each valve prevents the backflow of blood and maintains the forward direction of blood flow. The right and left heart chambers are separated by a septum to avoid mixing of blood.

The heart contracts when its muscle is excited by electrical impulses carried through its conduction system (electrical circuit) which is distributed all over the heart. The electrical impulses help in controlling the heart rate and rhythm, and may affect the strength of its contraction. On an average, a heart beats 60 to 100 times per minute in adults. However, it beats faster in children. The heart rate depends upon the level of activity; the more active the person is, the faster is his heart rate. The origin of electrical impulses is from a natural pacemaker or sino-atrial node located in the wall of the right atrium.

Functions of the Heart

In fact, the heart performs two separate pumping functions. First, the right atrium and the right ventricle are responsible for collecting blood returning from the organs and tissues of the body and pumping this oxygen depleted blood (deoxygenated blood) into the lungs where it is oxygenated by the oxygen it (lungs) receives from the inhaled atmospheric air. And the second function is where, the left atrium and left ventricle are responsible for receiving oxygenated blood from the lungs and pumping it via the aorta (the body's main artery) and the arterial system to the capillaries, the finest blood vessels of the body, to all the cells of the body. As blood flows through the capillaries, oxygen and nutrients are exchanged for carbon dioxide and wastes in the organs and tissues of the body which require oxygenated blood to perform their normal functions. The capillaries drain into the veins and the oxygen depleted blood flows from the network of veins back in to the right atrium of the heart.

Each pumping cycle of the heart consists of an ejection phase 'systole' and a filling phase 'diastole'. During diastole, the two receiving chambers (atria) receive blood from the lungs (left atrium) and other parts of the body (right atrium) while during systole, the muscles comprising of the right and left ventricle (two ejecting chambers) contract forcefully and cause the blood to be ejected into the lungs and aorta respectively. The amount of blood pumped through the heart each minute is called the cardiac output. In a normal healthy adult heart, the cardiac output varies from 4-6 litres /minute depending on the functional status of one's body. Cardiac output can be increased five times depending upon the need of the body. The heart is connected to the remainder of our circulatory system by large veins and arteries, which carry blood to and from the heart. Within the chest cavity, a thin covering or sac called the pericardium surrounds the heart. It contains a small amount of fluid called pericardial fluid which not only protects the heart but also acts as a cushion and lubricant.

Since the heart is a forever working muscular pump, it requires a continuous supply of oxygen and nutrients for its smooth and proper functioning. The energy requirements of the heart are provided by blood that circulates through a network of blood vessels, within the heart known as coronary arteries. The coronary circulation is responsible for the distribution of oxygenated blood and other nutrients to the working heart muscles.

More about Coronary Circulation

Coronary arteries are the blood vessels (like conduit pipe) that wrap around the surface of the heart and supply blood to the heart. The two primary coronary arteries are called the left main coronary artery and the right coronary artery. These originate near the root of aorta. Within the heart, the left main coronary artery runs for a centimetre and immediately splits into two different arteries which are the left anterior descending (LAD) and the left circumflex (LCx) coronary arteries. The left anterior descending and its diagonal (D) branches supply blood to the front (anterior) wall of the left ventricle (main chamber). The left circumflex and its obtuse marginal (OM) branches supply blood to the back (posterior) wall of the left ventricle. The right coronary artery and its marginal (RM) and posterior descending (PD) branches supply blood to the right ventricle and the underside of the left ventricle respectively. For the most part, these major coronary artery branches lie on or near the surface of the heart while smaller downstream branches tend to penetrate deeper into the myocardium. The size and distribution of blood by coronary arteries vary from person to person and in a majority, the left coronary artery supplies blood to major portions of the heart and is referred to as the dominant artery.

In simple words, the heart is the powerhouse of your body and maintains the lifeline. When you feel your heart beating, it is gently pumping blood throughout the body. This blood supplies oxygen and nutrients to your body and also removes wastes from the body. The blood then returns to the heart and the whole process starts all over again. The heart starts its function in the foetus and carries on unabated till the last breath. This powerhouse works daily with great efficiency and dependability, and demands no maintenance other than a sensible lifestyle.

It is important that this powerhouse of your body be properly maintained. The heart is often neglected and falls into bad shape due to your hectic, stressful lifestyles and ageing. This leads to the development of various diseases of the heart and in turn greatly affects the quality of life and may be life threatening in a few cases. Some common problems experienced by a person with a heart disease are chest pain, shortness of breath, tiredness or easy fatigability, swelling of ankles and feet, weight gain, and/or coughing. Out of these, chest pain on exertion or doing some physical activity is a strong indicator of an existing heart disease.

Heart at a Glance

1. *The heart is a hollow muscular organ with four chambers and valves.*
2. *It is situated in the middle of the chest and slightly towards the left.*
3. *It constantly supplies oxygen and nutrient rich blood to all organs for smooth functioning of the body.*
4. *Coronary arteries supply blood to the working heart.*
5. *The heart is a powerhouse of our body.*
6. *Heart beats about 70 times in a minute, about 100000 times in a day and 3.5 billion times in an average lifetime.*

7. The heart pumps 7000 litres of blood throughout your body every day and 250 million litres in a lifetime.
8. The heart beats slowly at the time of rest and faster depending on the level of activity.
9. For smooth functioning, the heart requires a simple and sensible lifestyle.

Chapter 5

Atherosclerosis and the Development of Coronary Heart Disease

'Heart disease begins when cholesterol, fatty materials and calcium build up in the arteries – a process known as atherosclerosis.'

The process of development of cardiovascular disease is complex and requires an interaction of a number of processes. The basic defect is in the vascular system of the body, precisely the arterial system. The disease in blood vessels can be in the walls or in the lumen of the vessels. The defect involving the wall and lining of blood vessels is the key process in the development of atherosclerosis (a Latin word meaning, athero – is gruel and sclerosis – is hardening) meaning the hardening of blood vessels. The second process is the interplay of various blood components resulting in the complex process of the formation of a thrombus or clot inside the lumen of the blood vessels clogging the lumen partially or totally. These two important processes are interlinked and complement each other. In a simpler way, blood vessels in the body are like roads, lanes and by-lanes of a city and various vehicles on the road can be compared to components of blood. As is common in India as well as in many developing countries, encroachment from either side, overcrowding of roads by the vehicles can mimic the process of atherosclerosis resulting in roads getting jammed so much that it can block and choke the lifeline of the city.

Process of Atherosclerosis

The blood vessels are lined on the inside by a thin layer of cells, which is termed as endothelium. This protective inner lining of vessels, endothelium, works not only as a barrier but also secretes certain substances that keep the vessels intact and maintains the smooth flow of blood. This lining of the artery can be damaged by many factors like smoking, high blood pressure, diabetes mellitus, high cholesterol levels in blood triggering and initiating the process of atherosclerosis. Therefore, the key step in the development of atherosclerosis is injury and damage to the endothelium. Once this protective lining is breached, cells present in the blood known as macrophages engulf the cholesterol circulating in the blood and get it deposited underneath the endothelium. Cells loaded with cholesterol die subsequently leaving lipids in the wall of blood vessels. Over time and as age advances, lipid continues to accumulate and forms a pool rich of fat or lipid and cell debris. This pool of cell debris and fat or lipid is known as the fatty streak or lipid core, and is the first step in the development of atherosclerosis. The second step is the accumulation of smooth muscle cells present in the wall of blood vessels along with collagen and small blood clots known as thrombi. The resultant structure is no more a lipid core; rather it is a complex structure called atheromatous plaque. When there is further addition of fibrin and calcium, it becomes hard. As the deposition continues, it grows in size, bulges in the lumen of the blood vessel and hinders the smooth blood flow, thereby hampering the supply of necessary oxygen and nutrients to the cells and body organs.

When the atheromatous plaque is damaged, which is a sudden event, then a crack can appear exposing materials to circulating blood and triggering the process of clot formation. The process of clot formation is complex and involves various chemicals and cells especially platelets, which are present in the blood all the time. When the platelets come in contact with the ruptured or damaged atheromatous plaque, they become sticky and along with circulating red blood cells and other cells form a clot, a key process of abrupt closure of vessels from inside. This clot is supposed to help heal and seal the crack or split in the blood vessel wall at the site of atheroma. When small in size and not causing too much problem in the flow of blood it is passed unnoticed. However, sometimes this clot continues to grow and blocks the artery completely. This can obstruct the flow of blood supply totally making a portion of the body organ devoid of blood supply. If it continues for a longer period it will make the body organ cry for essential oxygen and nutrients ultimately resulting in the death of the cells. When it occurs to the heart and brain it can lead to a heart attack and brain stroke respectively. Both the events are sudden, serious and can cause severe disability or even death.

Heart and Atherosclerosis

The heart is a muscular pump and like any other organ in the body it also requires oxygen and nutrients for its proper functioning. A healthy artery is that which has unruffled inner surface and is free of any blockage. This is true for the coronary arteries which supply blood to the heart, which have no blockade in the early years but as the age advances, the process of deposition of fatty substances (cholesterol), cellular debris (waste products), calcium and other substances in the inner layer of arteries by the process of atherosclerosis make it hard. This process continues unabated and progresses slowly with age. Since it is a slow process and dormant for many years, it manifests in the later years of life. In due course of time, this may result in partial or total closure of an artery resulting in diminished or no supply of oxygen and nutrients to the heart muscle. This may eventually make a portion of the heart being deprived of its blood supply. Impaired or total loss of oxygenated blood to the heart causes death of a portion of the heart muscles and prevents the heart from discharging its function properly. Therefore, in the heart this process of atherosclerosis can result in various degrees of coronary blocks and coronary heart disease (CHD).

Chapter 6

Burden of Coronary Heart Disease in South Asia and India

South Asians are individuals who live in a large geographic area that includes India, Pakistan, Sri Lanka, Nepal, Bhutan, Maldives, and Bangladesh. India is the most populous country in South Asia with more than one billion people. Pakistan, Sri Lanka, Nepal and Bangladesh are also facing a similar population trend besides sharing geographic boundaries. These countries are also economically and culturally similar to a certain extent. South Asians are experiencing an alarming increase in heart disease as well as diabetes and hypertension, two of the major risk factors for heart disease. It is fast emerging as an epicentre of chronic diseases. In the coming years, the world will be dominated by a number of patients with heart disease from South Asia, especially India. The number of productive years lost as a result of CVD is predicted to increase between 2000 to 2030 in all the leading developing countries. It is being predicted that it will be maximum with India followed by Brazil, China, South Africa and Russia. It is projected that a cumulative loss of 17 billion dollars (Rs 8500 crore) in GDP from 2005 to 2020 will be incurred due to the CVD burden in India alone.

We all will agree that South Asians, like any other low and middle income countries are still fighting poverty, malnutrition, infectious diseases as well as trying to provide hygienic conditions and safe drinking water. But little is being done and thought about chronic diseases which may take an epidemic form in the coming years. Due to an increase in the average income and change in lifestyle, non-communicable and chronic diseases are rapidly replacing infectious diseases and malnutrition, especially in the urban set up. Among all South Asian countries India is the largest and most populous. The disease trend and pattern in India may be assumed to represent the other South Asian countries. In India, the improving public health measures have led to a decline in both infectious disease and the death rate, leading to an increase in life expectancy. Further positive economic transitions in recent years have led to an increase in the average survival and longevity. However, as age advances it makes a person more prone to chronic diseases. Deaths due to communicable diseases are decreasing while that from non-communicable diseases are rising at a rapid pace. It is a shocking fact that non-communicable diseases contribute 53 % of the premature deaths in the most productive age groups in India. Cardiovascular diseases (include heart attack, high blood pressure and stroke), cancer and diabetes mellitus are becoming a serious concern and account for 28 %, 2 % and 8 % deaths respectively in 2005 as compared to 36 % deaths due to the combined effects of communicable diseases, maternal, perinatal and nutritional disorders.

Today, South Asians are facing the double burden, both of communicable and non-communicable diseases. Considering the growing population in this region of the world, we will not be able to bear the enormous cost associated with the management of chronic diseases leave alone providing adequate medical facilities. Lack of knowledge, illiteracy, ignorance and the high cost of treatment further complicates the matter.

India is an example of unity in diversity. There are different languages, economic zones, food habits but unfortunately one thing is common amongst us, that we are in the middle of a cardiovascular disease epidemic and are going to face the consequences of this epidemic in the coming years. Cardiovascular disease, more so coronary heart disease has extended its tentacles to every corner of India. The disease burden is rising in both the urban and rural population of India. The disease prevalence has increased in urban areas from 2 % in 1960 to 11 % in 2000. A similar trend has been reported for the rural population, it was 2 % in 1970, now it is 4.5 % in 2000. In 2008, there were almost 30 million patients of coronary heart disease in India and it is estimated by projections based on the Global Burden of Disease Study that by the year 2020, the burden of CVD in India will surpass that in any other region of the world. We have to ask ourselves – are we making this country the disease capital of the world? It is often felt that heart related deaths are common in the higher income group and it is the disease of the affluent society. However, worldwide majority of deaths due to CVD were reported in the low and middle income groups and also in a few developed countries. The Global Burden of Disease Study reported that in 2005 that there were 17 million total deaths from CVD worldwide and 80 % deaths were in the low and middle income groups that is, in developing countries. In 2000, approximately 1.6 million deaths were due to CHD in India. It is projected that there will be 2.6 million deaths due to CHD by 2020 out of which 1.46 will be men and 1.12 million women. The death rate compared with 1985, due to CVD in India is expected to rise by 103 % in men and 93 % in women by the year 2015. So heart attack and its related problems are becoming top killers in India.

The prevalence of CHD amongst Indians living in India is not the only cause of concern, but Indians living in different parts of the world also have a higher prevalence of this disease. It has been observed that despite low body weights and a vegetarian diet, as compared to the west, coronary atherosclerosis is widely present in migrant Indians. These groups of migrant Indians are highly educated and have access to the best medical facilities. In the United States, South Asians, also known as Asian Indians, have the highest prevalence of CHD as compared to Native Americans. Compared with the general US population, the prevalence of CHD in Asian Indians is approximately four times higher. It has been further noticed that the risk for CHD was highest amongst Indians. It was six times higher than the Chinese and four times higher than other Asian Americans. In addition, although death due to CHD has declined in many western countries in the last three decades, it has increased in immigrant Asian Indians. CHD in Indians is characterized by extreme prematurity and severity, and this population has more adverse cardiovascular events for any given degree of atherosclerosis than other ethnic groups. Studies have suggested that this increased CHD risk can be attributed to genetic disposition, which is exacerbated by a westernized lifestyle, more sedentary and dietary habits that include simple sugar and foods rich in saturated fats. The high rates of CHD in Asian Indians are accompanied by low rates of conventional risk factors except diabetes and this has been referred as 'Asian Indian paradox' by Enas A Enas.

Industrialization and urbanization has led to various changes in our lifestyle. This has led to certain environmental changes which include an unhealthy lifestyle such as stress, physical inactivity, tobacco and alcohol consumption, intakes of fats and calorie rich foods, obesity, increased incidence of diabetes and high blood pressure. Lack of awareness and ignorance coupled with environmental changes has further worsened the scenario. Vegetables and fruits are consumed less and fried foods are consumed more. Frequent consumption of junk food has caused havoc, especially in the lifestyle of kids. Let us ask ourselves – why are we playing with our kids lives by providing them junk food so often? We have to accept and understand that the burden of heart disease is rising and we have to act fast to curb it as early as possible, not only for ourselves but for our future generation also. In view of the existing burden of heart disease and to save millions of people, we have to take the initiative to prevent the disease before it manifests itself.

Today, South Asians have the highest CHD mortality compared with individuals of Chinese, Japanese and European descent. In addition, South Asians are prone to develop CHD at a younger age, often before the age of 40 years in men. South Asians represent one fifth of the global population and a majority are still residing in rural or semi-urban areas. There is also a large immigrant population from these countries settled all over the world, both in developed (US, Canada, UK, Australia) and developing (Caribbean, Africa, East Asia, Gulf) countries. Considering the disease burden and the pattern of risk factors, concentrated efforts are urgently needed to prevent the epidemic of cardiovascular disease in South Asia, and it is possible that preventive strategies applied to this part of the world may be applicable to the remaining developing countries.

CHD is the number one killer in the world today. While death rates of CHD have been declining in developed countries, it has been increasing in South Asian countries, especially India. In South Asians, acceleration of the disease process (atherosclerosis) seems to have some genetic predisposition but is largely influenced by the changing lifestyle. Protective factors such as moderate to heavy exercise, moderate alcohol consumption, daily intake of fruits and vegetables are lower in South Asians than in other countries. Since we cannot change the health care facilities overnight, we can definitely try and change the health of our heart by adopting a healthy lifestyle and food habits which have been the novel method with proven results in the developed countries, where the disease is on the decline since the last three decades.

Alarming Facts

1. South Asians appear to be the most affected by the rising trend for CHD, diabetes and hypertension.
2. It is projected that India will be the world capital of CHD by 2025.
3. It is expected that India would lead the world in CHD related deaths within the next 15 years.
4. Of the projected 62 million CHD patients in India by 2015, 23 million will be younger than 40 years of age.
5. CHD in India is going to affect the younger and productive population.
6. Today, almost 30 million people have CHD in India. Actual number may be more if silent heart attack and asymptomatic CHD are included.
7. Almost 50 % CHD deaths are reported under the age of retirement.
8. A large number of people die suddenly without getting medical aid or without being hospitalized.
9. Tobacco sale and consumption is increasing, especially in the younger generation.

10. *Rise in obesity is a major cause of concern and almost 50 % of the urban adults are unhappy with their shape.*
11. *Physical inactivity is a common habit amongst South Asians.*
12. *Cardiovascular diseases are increasing at a fast pace in developing countries in general, and particularly in South Asians.*
13. *It is taking epidemic proportions as a result of rapid urbanization, industrialization and changing lifestyles.*
14. *Urbanization and industrialization of South Asians is still ongoing and the disease has still not shown its final impact.*

Chapter 7

Heart Disease and Risk Factors

'We are still living in a world where almost one third of the patients die before we are aware that these people were ill or that their lives were in jeopardy.'
—F. Manson Sones, Father of Coronary Angiography

It is important to know whether you are at a risk for developing heart disease or not. Till date there is no single known cause of coronary heart disease (CHD). Various studies have identified certain danger signs which are called 'risk factors' that increase the chances of CHD. The progression of heart disease is a long process and the risk factors tend to speed up the development of heart disease. By reducing the risk factors, one can stop the progression of the disease and decrease the chances of having a CHD. The more risk factors you have, the greater is your chance of developing CHD.

Types of Risk Factors

Risk factors for heart disease can be classified under two headings. The risk factors which are not under our control and cannot be modified are classified as non-modifiable and those risk factors which can be changed or modified with the help of lifestyle or drugs are termed as modifiable risk factors.

Non-modifiable Risk Factors

These include:
- Age
- Family history of heart disease
- Gender
- Ethnicity

1. **Age**

   The risk of heart disease increases with age that is, age is directly proportional to risk of heart disease. The precise relationship between heart disease and aging is difficult to define but atherosclerosis or hardening of blood vessels is universally present. This increases in severity as the age advances. Therefore, age in itself is a powerful risk factor. Studies have shown that the risk rises sharply for men after the age of 45 years and for women after the age of 55 years. In developing countries, heart attack occurs 10 years earlier than western countries and a majority of the people suffer and die of heart attack complications in adulthood. Lack of exercise, poor nutrition, associated diseases, financial constraints, neglect in family, depression and loss of better half are a few causes which increase the risk further as the age advances.

2. **A family History of Heart Disease**

   If one of your family members such as, father, mother, grandparents, brother or sister have had a heart attack before the age of 55 years, it is possible that you are also at a higher risk of getting a heart attack. This is because of some genetic conditions, which are poorly understood, make you prone to heart disease. Certain other risk factors of heart disease run in families such as high cholesterol level in blood (familial hypercholesterolemia), high blood pressure, diabetes mellitus and/or obesity. A family's lifestyle and eating habits also contributes to heart disease. It has been observed that most of the people who have a strong family history of heart disease have one or more other risk factors also. Since, family history cannot be controlled, it is even more important to control other risk factors, if present.

3. **Gender**

   In the initial years of life, it is a male dominant disease and men suffer more from heart disease as compared to women till 50 years of age. Female gender is protected till menopause by the hormone oestrogen but after menopause they have a similar risk as their male counterparts.

4. **Ethnicity**

   In a study conducted in seven countries, the CHD mortality varied more than fivefold among populations with the Japanese having the lowest and the natives of Finland having the highest mortality. Coronary heart disease risk is 50 % higher in North Europeans as compared to South Europeans. In Asia, Japanese and Chinese have a lower rate of CHD as compared to South Asians. This may be due to increased physical activity, use of fish in their diet making their cholesterol favourable with high protective good cholesterol and low levels of bad cholesterols, despite rapid urbanization and heavy smoking in these countries. South Asians are becoming more prone to CHD due to a low level of overall physical activity, a recent surge in tobacco use, obesity which can partially explain the alarming increase in incidence of diabetes mellitus, unfavourable cholesterol milieu such as high level of bad cholesterol and low level of good cholesterol. Increased use of vegetable or vanaspati oil rich in trans-fats and saturated fats, overcooking of vegetables, less use of fruits in the daily diet and use of refined cereals with whole milk further contribute to heart disease. Simple sugars and sweets are commonly consumed which are loaded with excess of calories and fats. More use of red and organ meat products instead of fish also contribute to the high incidence of CHD in South Asians.

Modifiable Risk Factors

Certain risk factors that can be controlled or can modify the disease process and outcome are classified as modifiable risk factors and are as follows:

1. **Hypertension**

   Hypertension is the term used for high blood pressure (BP) and this condition increases the burden on the heart and makes it work harder and stronger. High blood pressure can damage blood vessels and lead to serious health problems. Studies reveal that a 7 mmHg rise in blood pressure over the baseline reading increases the risk of CHD by 27 %. Blood pressure tends to increase with age as the blood vessels become stiff and more susceptible to injury, further enhancing the process of atherosclerosis. High blood pressure not only affects the heart but also the brain, eyes, kidneys and other important organs of the body. Unfortunately, high blood pressure results in no or little complaints and causes no early warning signals. It may manifest as a heart attack, paralytic attack, blindness or kidney failure. Therefore, if it is ignored it can kill you silently.

2. **High Cholesterol or Fat in the Blood**

   It is normal to have cholesterol in the blood but when its levels become high in the blood, it becomes an important risk factor for CHD. There is a linear relation between the risk of heart disease and the level of cholesterol in blood. The risk of heart disease increases as the cholesterol level in the blood rises that is 'higher the level, higher the risk'. The chances of developing heart disease increases even more when the high level of cholesterol is associated with other risk factors. Since high cholesterol is a number, it cannot cause any complaints and people are usually unaware of their high cholesterol level unless it is measured in the blood (serum to be more specific). Not all cholesterol numbers are bad. High density lipoprotein (HDL) cholesterol is good cholesterol and its level should be kept high. Low density lipoprotein (LDL), total cholesterol and triglycerides (TG) are bad cholesterol and should have lower levels to prevent heart disease. In India, it is triglyceride (TG) cholesterol which is bad as compared to LDL cholesterol which is higher in Americans and Europeans. Unfortunately, good HDL cholesterol is also low in Indians. After 30 years of age, it is important to know your various components of cholesterol in the blood. Every Indian should get it measured and your physician may prescribe it as your lipid profile. If your cholesterol level is found to be high or you are suffering from diabetes mellitus or you smoke, it is wise to get it checked frequently and regularly.

3. **Diabetes mellitus**

Glucose (sugar) in our diet is an important source of energy. The hormone insulin, which is produced in the pancreas, is responsible for shifting the glucose out of the blood and into the cells for our bodily function. When insulin is insufficient or the body is unable to use (insulin resistance) it properly, the sugar level rises in the blood, and this condition is termed as diabetes mellitus. To diagnose diabetes mellitus, the overnight twelve hour fasting sugar estimation in blood should be more than

126 mg/dl on two different occasions. The cause of concern is that the prevalence of diabetes mellitus is increasing at a rapid rate in Indians. There were 41 million diabetics in the year 2008 and it is projected that it will reach up to 79 million by the year 2030.

Diabetes mellitus affects all cells of the body and all organs. The heart is not spared and diabetes is associated with an increased risk of heart disease and heart attack. A majority of deaths in diabetic patients are due to heart disease and related problems. Diabetics are also prone to develop lipid abnormalities and high blood pressure which are also major risk factors for heart disease and explain such a high incidence of heart related deaths in diabetics. Diabetes is more risky in women than in men. It increases the risk of heart disease by two to four folds in men and three to seven folds in women.

4. Metabolic Syndrome

This syndrome consists of high blood pressure, apple or central obesity, insulin resistance, abnormal lipid levels (high TG and low HDL) and glucose intolerance. Metabolic syndrome is a precursor of diabetes and has a five-fold risk of developing diabetes mellitus in the next five years. Metabolic syndrome is closely associated and is a risk factor for the development of heart attack and related problems. People suffering from metabolic syndrome have a two-fold risk of developing premature heart attack. All or few components of metabolic syndrome are common in Indians.

5. Physical Inactivity

It is true that stagnant water decays fast and so too the inactive body. Various studies have proved beyond doubt that an inactive lifestyle, in itself, is a strong risk factor for coronary heart disease. Reduced or no physical activity is also associated with obesity, diabetes mellitus, high blood pressure and abnormal lipid levels, especially low levels of protective good HDL cholesterol. All these risk factors further increase the chances of developing heart disease. Regular exercise plays an important role in our overall well-being. It tones up your heart and also maintains the elasticity of blood vessels. Thus, regular exercise not only helps in preventing heart and blood vessel diseases but also prevents the development of other risk factors. Studies have shown that risk of heart disease can be reduced by as much as 50 % by performing regular aerobic exercises.

6. Obesity and Being Overweight

Obesity or excess weight is an independent risk factor for coronary atherosclerosis. Obesity is also associated with an increased risk of high blood pressure, diabetes, high cholesterol and physical inactivity. Framingham Heart Study suggested that obesity in young subjects could account for as much as 23 % cases of CHD in men and 15 % in women.

The distribution of fat in the body plays an important role in the development of heart disease as compared to total body fat. The distribution of fat around the waist is called central or apple obesity, while fat distribution around the hip is termed pear or gynoid obesity. Studies have shown that central obesity is associated with more adverse metabolic consequences and with an increased risk for heart disease than pear obesity. Central obesity is not only common among Indians but also more dangerous as far as heart disease is concerned. Obese people or those with excess body fat are at a higher risk of heart disease even in the absence of other risk factors. Thus, obesity can be considered as an independent risk factor for CHD.

7. Tobacco use

All forms of tobacco use are unsafe and hazardous for health. It is the biggest risk factor of heart attack and related diseases. Fortunately, it is the most preventable cause of death. Lung cancer is the most well-known disease associated with smoking but smoking makes you 2 to 4 times more at a risk for a heart attack. In INTERHEART study, smoking amounted for 36 % of attributable risks of the first heart attack.

If you smoke and have had a heart attack, you are more likely to die early and suddenly than a non-smoker. The carbon monoxide present in smoke reduces the amount of oxygen in blood. Nicotine present in tobacco is a known poison and is a powerful toxin which can kill a person in high doses. Nicotine damages the inner lining of blood vessels and triggers the formation of blood clots. Both these processes clog the blood vessels. Smoking also decreases the good HDL cholesterol in blood. Smoking stimulates certain hormones in the body which may disturb the rhythm of the heart and may lead to sudden death due to cardiac or heart arrest. In a nut shell, smoking even one cigarette or bidi has harmful effects. It raises your blood pressure, makes your heart work harder, increases your risk of blood clots and causes spasms of coronary arteries. In India, it is emerging as the single most risk factor strongly associated with CHD in young and rural Indians.

8. Stress

Depression, hostility, anger and anxiety are associated with CHD. Stress has not yet been established as a proven independent risk factor for heart disease. However, more and more evidence suggests a relationship between the risk of cardiovascular disease and environmental and psychosocial factors. In response to stress, certain substances such as adrenaline hormone are released in the body, which in turn increases the heart rate and blood pressure. These hormones are termed as 'stress hormones'.

Acute and chronic stress may affect other risk factors and behaviours, such as high blood pressure and cholesterol levels, smoking, physical inactivity and overeating. Anger is associated with a two to three fold increase in the risk development of angina, heart attack or sudden cardiac death. Certain day to day stress factors such as money/bills, traffic jams, job related stress, work load, overcrowding, lack of support, financial crunch, health related issues, scarcity of free time, tense relationships, divorce, marriage of children, long legal battles, family and friends can all contribute or precipitate CHD.

9. Lipoprotein (a): A Genetic Risk Factor

Lp(a) is a strong independent risk factor for CHD in many populations in Asia including India. Lipoprotein (a) is a variant of 'bad' LDL attached to an extra protein particle. Its effect in the body is ten-fold higher than LDL (bad cholesterol) and that is why it is classified as a deadly cholesterol. Its level is genetically influenced and it is slightly influenced by environmental factors. Trans-fat consumption may influence and increase its level. Its level during childhood is a marker and predictor of future CHD in young adults and partially explains premature CHD in Indians, especially under the age of 40 years. High level of Lp(a) and triglyceride coupled with a low level of good cholesterol that is, HDL in Indians forms a lethal combination and is the most common abnormality.

10. Homocysteine Level

Recently, a high level of homocysteine has been identified as a marker of heart disease. It was initially a marker for the risk of stroke. This has prompted a lot of studies over several years. Initial observational evidence suggested that a 25 % lower homocysteine level was associated with huge differences—about a 60 % lower risk of coronary events and strokes. Homocysteine is the end product of metabolism of methionine and its normal level ranges between 5-15 micromol/L. Deficiencies in vitamins B6, B12 and folic acid are known to be associated with high levels of homocysteine in blood. Homocysteine levels are higher in Indians as compared to whites as overcooking of food, especially vegetables is a common practice in India. This overcooking food destroys most nutrients and vitamins, especially folate. This probably accounts for high levels of homocysteine found in Indians. Folic acid and vitamin B which is present in fruits in abundance can reduce the levels of homocysteine in blood. Thus, food fortification with folic acid is practiced in many developed countries to reduce CHD risk and burden.

11. C-reactive Protein

It is thought that inflammation and infection can cause cardiovascular disease. In the last decade, research has shown that bioactive molecules and cytokines which are characteristic of inflammation are involved in every step of atherosclerosis and cardiovascular disease is a result of this inflammatory process. Today, it is regarded as an emerging risk factor. However, the problem is how to use markers of inflammation in clinical or day to day practice. Of the current inflammatory markers, hs-

CRP (high sensitivity C reactive protein) estimation has been recommended by various scientific bodies to be used in clinical practice. Today its levels are used as an independent risk factor. It may also be used to guide the treatment besides motivating the patients to improve their lifestyle behaviours. It is derived from the liver and may be raised under a few other conditions such as chronic infection, high blood pressure, diabetes, cigarette smoking and obesity. Studies show that lowering hs-CRP with medicines may be protective for future coronary events even if your cholesterol levels are normal. A healthy diet and exercise also reduces cholesterol and CRP levels with no side effects. This approach could be more beneficial as diet and exercise also take care of other risk factors.

12. Alcohol

Is whisky too risky? Excess and irregular alcohol intake is associated with high blood pressure, heart failure and an increase in triglyceride and cholesterol levels. All are established risk factors for heart disease. Drinking a moderate amount of alcohol on a regular basis has been found to protect one from a heart attack by raising good HDL cholesterol and reducing clot formation in blood. The pattern of alcohol intake is entirely different in the Indian culture. Here, moderation and regular alcohol intake is not practiced. In fact, in India, rather large quantities are consumed at irregular intervals. Binge drinking is common and studies have revealed that it is associated with an increase in heart related deaths. Fried foods and snacks are commonly consumed along with alcohol, which are full of saturated fats and hidden calories. Alcohol consumption is also associated with liver disease and various social problems. Therefore, in India, alcohol may not have a protective role and may even be considered as a risk factor. Various studies have found that alcohol consumption per se is not a considerable risk factor for heart disease in South Asians.

Impact of Risk Factors

The precise aetiology and mechanisms leading to the development of CHD remains incompletely understood although a number of risk factors have been identified over the past several decades. One can argue that my neighbour who was a strict vegetarian, teetotaller and fitness fanatic died suddenly of a heart attack or my grandfather lived 80 years and he ate everything. These can be exceptions but not rules to generalize disease pattern and they remind us of the fact that this disease occurs in one third of the patients without warning and with no risks attached.

The total individual risk assessment is of paramount importance and it can help in the management of heart disease. In a majority of individuals, the chances of development of heart disease in the future depend upon the particular risk factor profile, age and sex. An elderly man is more at risk than a young woman. An individual with multiple mild risk factors may be more prone to develop the disease than someone with just one major risk factor. The individual risk profile of the person helps in deciding the intensity of preventive interventions such as dietary restrictions, intensity of physical activity, pharmacological therapy and when and what drug is to be prescribed to control the risk factors. No risk factors should be judged in isolation as it is a multi-factorial disease and needs a comprehensive approach.

We should not get confused with this knowledge. In fact, we need to understand the impact of various risk factors.

Heart disease is influenced by multiple factors and the most important is the way we live. In the race for advancement, we have forgotten to follow a healthy lifestyle and how to nurture our body as nature nurtures it. We gorge on high fat and calorie rich foods more frequently which not only increases the level of bad cholesterol in our body but makes us prone for other important risk factors such as obesity, diabetes and hypertension. Tobacco is consumed with no known benefits. You will be surprised to know that birds or animal do not consume this plant product except us, the most intelligent race. A decrease in physical activity is common and it has caused havoc in the modern life. A bicycle is a pleasure of childhood which is replaced by a motorbike even before the law permits its use. Majority of schools do not have proper playgrounds and parks are a rarity in residential colonies these days. With no option left, children are forced to watch television. Many patients enquire why my parents had this disease in the sixties while I had it in the forties. They just fail to realize and accept that physical activity was routine for their parents and the new generation has left physical activity when they left their school, 20 years earlier. Stress levels were also low in yester years as compared to today. Earlier people were more satisfied even with less money. We should realize that a faulty lifestyle has triggered this epidemic and only a healthy lifestyle can overcome it. The only problem is that we have created the time frame for our convenience and today we have become the slaves to time and find it difficult to manage time. A common lame excuse – I do not get enough time for myself – can no longer be accepted. Try to understand, heart health is non-negotiable, it is either there ……or not. A broken heart may find a companion but a damaged heart has no replacement. You have to sit, think, listen to your heart and act fast as your heart needs your attention urgently.

Chapter 8

Coronary Heart Disease

A heart attack is a sudden and dramatic event in anyone's life and often comes as a complete shock with unpredictable and disastrous results. The irony is that it affects the person in their most productive age. Thus, the loss is many folds and it puts enormous financial burden with loss of work hours and sometimes precious lives. Studies clearly show that lifestyle modification is a novel way of preventing and protecting one from heart disease. Though it is unlikely to substitute the conventional treatment modalities in established heart disease cases but it could have an essential and positive impact in ameliorating the disease in the person.

What is Coronary Heart Disease?

For the smooth functioning of the heart, the heart muscles need blood and oxygen just like any other organ of the body. The blood vessels feeding the heart muscle are called the coronary arteries. When the normal blood supply to the heart is jeopardized because of coronary artery disease, it results in coronary heart disease. The commonest cause is the narrowing or blockage of the coronary artery or arteries by deposition of fatty build up. This fatty build up, starts early during childhood and continues throughout life. The fatty build up grows in size and blocks the passage of blood inside the coronary artery, either partially or completely. The process starves the heart muscles of necessary oxygen and nutrients. When the supply of blood is insufficient to a critical level such that it can no longer meet the normal demands of a working heart, it can result in various problems. A complete block and total cessation of blood supply can permanently damage the heart muscles. This can result in the manifestation of coronary heart disease in the form of chest pain or heart attack, deterioration in heart function, heart failure or sudden death.

Cause of Concern for Indians

Indians have small and narrow coronary arteries. Coronary heart disease and related problems occur a decade earlier in Indians as compared to people from the west. Not only does it affect the younger population in India but the disability and death rate associated with this disease is very high. Indians settled abroad have a higher occurrence of heart disease and other chronic diseases when compared to the native Indians suggesting that environmental factors do have a vast influence on an individual's health.

What will happen if the Coronary Artery is Blocked Incompletely?

Partially blocked coronary artery (50 – 70 %) gives sufficient oxygen and nutrients to the working heart at rest, when the heart is not strained. Under certain situations where the body demands more oxygen and energy such as, during exercise, emotions or anger, the heart has to work extra hard. The heart is now unable to increase the blood supply to its vigorously contracting muscles through this partially blocked artery. Since there is no increase in blood supply due to the blockage in the flow, heart muscles receive insufficient amount of blood and are deprived of a proper supply of oxygen and nutrients causing injury to the heart muscles. This is manifested as chest discomfort or pain. Once the person takes rest, the blood supply required to meet the extra burden on the heart is removed and the person gets relieved of chest pain. This is known as angina pectoris, meaning choking or squeezing sensation in the chest. It is a warning signal for the presence of significant coronary heart disease. Patients with angina are always at a high risk of developing a heart attack (myocardial infarction) or related complications.

What is Unstable Angina?

If the angina is ignored or not treated in time then the block in the artery will increase and so will the problem of chest pain. This pain will get aggravated and may occur after routine household activities or on least effort, at rest or sometimes even at night. If the episodes of angina pain increase in duration (lasting longer), severity (more intense) and frequency (happening more often), then it suggests that the disease process is worsening and coronary artery is significantly narrowed or blocked. This is called unstable angina. Not only worsening of stable angina is termed as unstable angina but even a single episode of angina of less than six weeks duration occurring at minimal exertion or at rest is also classified as unstable angina. Chest pain after a heart attack and after bypass surgery is not a normal feature and if present, it can also fall in the category of unstable angina. As the name suggests, its fate is unstable and can lead to a heart attack or even sudden death. This is an indication that progression of the disease process has reached a critical level and is a warning sign that a heart attack may occur soon. It is like sitting on a health bomb which can explode any time and may result in painful and tragic events such as heart attack and death if no immediate action is taken. Thus, unstable angina is a serious medical condition that should not be ignored. It demands urgent attention and action.

Postprandial Angina

Some people complain of chest pain or angina while having their meal or walking within 30 minutes of ingesting a meal. Such people who complain thus feel no pain while walking on an empty stomach or during a morning walk. Postprandial angina is a marker of severe disease and is associated with unstable angina. It sometimes occurs after a heart attack or in patients suffering from diabetes as it is often passed and ignored as a gastric problem by majority because it is linked with meals.

What Will Happen if the Coronary Artery is Blocked Completely?

If the coronary arteries are completely blocked it means no blood flow to a portion of the heart supplied by the said coronary artery. As the heart does not get sufficient nutrients and oxygen, it results in INJURY or ISCHAEMIA of heart muscles. Injury to the heart muscle causes chest pain and pressure. If blood flow is not restored within 20 to 40 minutes, irreversible damage of that particular portion of the heart muscle will begin. If the supply is not restored within 6-8 hours, the heart muscle will die or may be damaged permanently. In due course of time, the dead heart muscle is replaced by scar tissue. This results in the improper functioning of the heart. Permanent damage to a portion of the heart because of complete cessation of blood supply results in a heart attack. The pain of a heart attack lasts for more than 30 minutes, is often severe and not relieved by rest or any manoeuvre. Heart attack in itself is a very serious condition and may cause death instantaneously. About 50 %

patients do not get sufficient time to reach the hospital, or even those who reach the hospital 50 % may die within 48 hours.

Can I Get Angina With No Block in the Coronary Artery?

It is sometimes possible to have typical angina pain among few patients. However in these patients coronary angiography reveals no block in the coronary arteries and the flow of blood is normal. Such patients are often elderly women and are referred as suffering from Syndrome X. These individuals are difficult to manage and require thorough investigation to rule out other causes of chest pain including psychological disorders. However, all such patients should not be referred to a psychiatrist. This is supposed to arise because of endothelial dysfunction with no significant block in the major arteries or the disease is in the small coronary arteries which are not visualized in the angiography. In contrast to other types of angina, syndrome X patients have an excellent outcome despite repeated episodes of chest pain. All patients should be assured that it is a difficult problem to cure/solve but not a life threatening disease. No specific hospital therapy can be offered, rather reassurance, conventional anti-angina drugs and control of associated risk factors remains the only treatment and often patients improve in due course of time.

Who Will Get the Angina or Heart Attack?

Any adult can have a heart disease after the age of 30 years. Coronary heart disease in the second and third decade of life is rare but not unknown. It is difficult to predict who will get a heart disease. However, people who suffer from diabetes mellitus, high blood pressure, have a family history of CHD, smoke or use tobacco in any form, have high cholesterol, lead a stressful life, sedentary style or are obese, are at a higher risk of develop a heart problem. Almost one third of the people develop heart disease despite having no known risk factors. Therefore, it is very clear that no single factor can be attributed to the disease.

What Does Angina Feel Like?

Angina pain often feels like a pressing, crushing, burning or squeezing pain. It is not a piercing or stabbing pain. It could feel like heartburn. In some cases it may cause sweating, tiredness, shortness of breath or occasionally nausea. Some people, especially diabetic patients sometimes have no pain at all. The chest pain is mainly located in the middle of the chest or slightly towards the left side, but it may also occur on the right side, neck, jaw, or may radiate into the back or left shoulder. It is often felt going down the left arm or both arms. Any pain which is above the jaw and below the umbilicus is not due to angina. Similarly, chest pain lasting for a few seconds or hours is less likely to be angina. However, angina pain may feel different for different individuals.

What Precipitates Angina?

The pain of angina is usually precipitated by anxiety, exercise (such as walking, climbing stairs, jogging), emotions or mental stress, post sexual intercourse, walking in cold weather or after heavy meals. Recently angina or sudden death has been noticed after watching exciting programmes on television, the so-called 'match of the day angina'. It is relieved after rest or after taking medicines such as nitroglycerine or glyceryl trinitrate or GTN. If pain is not relieved after taking a few tablets of GTN then it reflects unstable angina or a heart attack.

A classical description on part of the patient is, *'Doctor, I am fine when I am at rest. However, I feel discomfort in the form of heaviness, burning or pain in the chest while I walk or climb stairs or when I am in a hurry and get relieved once I stop the activity or there is belching or release of gas from the abdomen. The whole process repeats if I do the same again.'*

Angina at a Glance

1. *Angina is a condition in which chest discomfort occurs when the oxygen supply to an area of the heart muscle does not meet the demand.*
2. *It is not an emergency.*
3. *It is not sudden in onset.*
4. *Heaviness, pain or tightness in chest is common.*
5. *It is usually aggravated by exercise and relieved after rest.*
6. *It disappears immediately once the precipitating factor is removed.*
7. *Pain usually radiates towards the left hand, jaw, shoulder or back.*
8. *It is unaffected by swallowing, pressing or breathing.*
9. *Routine resting ECG may be normal in a majority of cares.*

Historical descriptions of CHD

The Roman philosopher Lucius Annacus Seneca (4 BC – 65 AD) described his own symptoms, *'The attack is like a storm. To have any other malady is to be sick, to have this is to be dying.'*

Charak, an Indian physician described the symptoms as *'a disorder of the chest which was fatal and when the pulse falls from the root of the thumb and becomes imperceptible and there is a burning sensation in the heart, life only continues as long as the burning sensation lasts and ends when the burning sensation ends.'*

In the modern era, the first and best description was by William Heberden in the late eighteen century. *'There is a disorder of the breast, marked with strong peculiar symptoms. Those who are afflicted with it, are seized while they are walking and most particularly when they walk soon after eating, with a painful and most disagreeable sensation in the breast, which seems as if it would take their life away, if it were to increase or to continue, the moment they stand still, all this uneasiness vanishes. After it has continued some months, it will come on, not only when persons are walking, but when they are lying down and oblige them to rise up out of their beds every night for many months. Most of them are men who are obese and are above 50 years of age. In a few cases it has been brought by the motion of horse or carriage, and even swallowing, coughing, going to school, speaking or disturbance of mind. The natural tendency of this illness be to kill the patient suddenly.'*

What to Do if Angina is Suspected?

One should consult one's family physician first. Angina, if suspected can be diagnosed by taking a detailed history from the patient, as the diagnosis of stable angina in the majority is based on a history of effort-related chest discomfort. The presence of risk factors attributed with heart disease makes the diagnosis more likely. As the person is symptom free at rest, a majority of tests done in the resting state are usually normal. If all tests are normal and there is a high degree of suspicion, then the person should be subjected to more specific tests which help in clinching the diagnosis of angina.

Initial Investigations for Angina

The investigations include tests which are mandatory not only for diagnosis of angina but also to know about the associated risk factors and to decide the treatment plan. Initial investigations of angina include resting and stress electrocardiogram (ECG) coupled with echocardiography. Certain blood tests such as haemoglobin and total blood count, fasting and post meal sugar estimation, urea and creatinine for kidney, and a total lipid profile estimation are all helpful. Ordering X-ray of the chest is necessary to rule out other causes of chest pain and to assess the size of the heart. Out of all these tests, stress ECG or treadmill test, a form of exercise test, reproduces the complaints of angina and is considered the most reliable and diagnostic test for angina.

What is the Need for Screening Tests in CHD?

It is a common complaint and argument on the part of people who suffer from CHD where they argue, that how can they have a heart disease when they did not have any complaints earlier. The heart attack and sudden death may be the first manifestation of coronary heart disease in many patients and it is often not preceded by any chest pain or warning signs. For this reason, people are advised to undergo screening tests so that the heart disease is detected before any serious medical problem occurs.

Who Should Get the Screening Test?

It is advisable to undergo screening tests if you are above 30 years of age. Screening tests are of immense importance for a person who has any of the risk factors for CHD. Coronary heart disease results in damage of the heart to a varying intensity, and a damaged heart cannot be repaired to normalcy by any mode of treatment. If the disease is detected before it manifests itself, then the treatment offered gives the best results, saves a lot of money, embarrassments and precious lives.

What are the Common Screening Tests?

Commonly employed tests for diagnosis of coronary heart disease are resting electrocardiography (ECG), stress or exercise ECG commonly known as treadmill test (TMT), and resting and stress echocardiography.

What is Electrocardiogram (ECG)?

It is the most readily available, cheap and bed side investigation for heart disease. It records the electrical activity of the heart with the help of surface electrodes and a recording machine. Unfortunately, an ECG done during the resting phase may be normal in a majority of angina patients. Sometimes it is possible that a resting ECG taken during pain may show certain changes suggestive of angina or heart pain. ECG can be recorded both during rest or exercise. In cases of heart attack, diagnosis in a majority of cases can be reliably obtained with the help of this simple test, as the ECG is abnormal in the majority of heart attack patients.

What are the Types of Stress Tests?

There are two methods of stressing the heart. Stressing the heart means increasing the heart rate and increasing the demand for oxygen, nutrients and measuring the various parameters necessary for the smooth functioning of the heart. The heart can be stressed either by exercise or through medicines. The commonly used stress test is, where a person is asked to exercise on a treadmill (widely used) or bicycle. Out of the two stress modalities, treadmill is more popular than the bicycle. The less commonly performed stress test is done with drugs, such as adenosine or dobutamine, and then it is called as pharmacological stress test. TMT is the most common screening test and is synonym of 'stress test'.

What is the Basis of TMT?

As mentioned, angina is caused by incomplete or partial blockage of the coronary artery. Thus, during rest the partially open artery provides sufficient blood, oxygen and nutrients for the heart to function. However, when exercise is done, more blood and oxygen are required by the exercising muscles and the duty of the heart is to meet this extra demand by increasing the blood supply to itself and to the exercising muscles by increasing its own function. In a normal healthy heart this is met without any difficulty but in case of partially blocked arteries, sufficient blood is not supplied to the heart and it is not able to meet this increased demand. Thus, the heart cries for help or it gives a signal that the heart is at strain and the exercising must stop. These changes in the heart are recorded both during exercise and after exercise. Thus, considering the physiology of angina, an ECG taken during exercise or stress will be more informative in diagnosing angina than a resting ECG.

What is TMT?

The most common stress test for the diagnosis of coronary heart disease is TMT (treadmill test). In this test, the person is asked to exercise over a treadmill and a computer generated ECG is taken throughout the test to check the changes in the heart while one is exercising. Heart rate and blood pressure are monitored simultaneously. A positive test is associated with a significant shift in the ST segment of ECG (depression is more common than elevation) which may or may not be associated with chest pain. The severity of disease depends upon how early and how marked the ECG shift is and how long it takes to disappear after exercise or during the recovery period. It is one of the most frequent and reliable non-invasive test used to assess a patient with chest pain.

How is the TMT Performed?

The person is asked to come in a state of fasting and with all the previous medical records. He or she is asked to exercise on a motor driven treadmill according to a standardized protocol with a progressive increase in the elevation and speed of the treadmill. There are various protocols for TMT but the majority of stress labs follow Bruce protocol. In this protocol, speed and inclination of the treadmill machine changes every three minutes and is known as a stage, and there are in total seven stages in this protocol. During this the person's ECG and heart rate are displayed on a computer screen and monitored along with the blood pressure. This monitoring is carried on throughout the exercise and also after an average of six minutes of exercise known as recovery period. Care is to be taken that the TMT be performed under the supervision of a qualified doctor.

How Sensitive is this Test?

The accuracy of TMT depends upon the degree of exercise performed and the severity of the underlying disease. If one performs good exercise (average of 9 minutes on Bruce protocol) and achieves at least 85 % of the target heart rate (target heart rate = 220 – age of the person) then it is unlikely that he has a heart disease. However, if exercise performed is poor (less than 6 minutes on Bruce protocol) and there is a strong suspicion of disease and ECG changes are not there then other tests may be performed. If there is involvement of two or three coronary arteries or severe disease then accuracy of this test is very high as compared to a mildly blocked, single blood vessel. Individual interpretation is done by the doctor and his or her advice must be followed. If one performs a good exercise, achieves the predicted heart rate and there is no risk factor for heart disease, TMT is sufficient as a screening test. If one performs the stress test between 6 – 9 minutes with no chest pain and with no ECG changes then the likelihood of a disease is very low. However, such a person should be followed up closely and should be advised a healthy lifestyle.

How Safe is TMT?

TMT is a very safe test. However it should not be performed during a heart attack, unstable angina or angina with rest pain, uncontrolled high blood pressure or severe narrowing of the heart valves. The risk is more if it is performed soon after an acute heart pain or ischaemic event. It should not be performed against the will of the person and therefore a written consent is mandatory and should be obtained.

Treadmill test or stress test still remains the most useful test because of its wide availability, reasonable cost, proper safety and easy interpretation.

What is Echocardiography?

Echocardiography is an ultrasound based test. It can be performed at outdoor clinics and is affordable. With the help of echocardiography, structures of the heart, valve functions, blood flow across the various valves and contraction of the heart muscle are estimated. Since echocardiography is a resting test it may be normal in a majority of angina patients. However, it may be helpful in ruling out the angina caused by narrowing of heart valves such as aortic stenosis. Echocardiography is of immense use in diagnosis of various complications of coronary heart disease.

Who Requires the Additional Tests?

It is possible that in some people, the results of TMT do not accurately reflect the disease and there is a high degree of suspicion regarding a heart disease. In such a situation, it is better to undergo additional tests for diagnosis. People who cannot exercise because of joint problems, breathing problems, morbid obesity or any other related problems also require additional tests.

What are the Additional or Special tests Done for Angina?

There are other available tests which may be of immense use, if TMT alone is not helpful. The following special or additional tests may be undertaken on such people to ascertain the cause of chest pain:

1. Stress echocardiography
2. Dobutamine stress test

3. Stress thallium
4. CT or MR angiography
5. Coronary angiography

What is Stress Echocardiography?

When the resting echocardiography is coupled with exercise then it is called stress echocardiography. If the heart muscles are not supplied with the proper amount of blood then its contraction and function is affected and this abnormality of contraction (wall thickness) or motion of heart muscles can be detected reliably by echocardiography. This is interpreted as wall motion abnormality and presence of such abnormality is diagnostic of coronary heart disease. It is also useful to detect changes in heart function during rest and after exercise. If the heart function improves during the test then it suggests good blood circulation and heart function. Stress can be induced with the help of a bicycle or treadmill while taking the echo simultaneously or taking echo pictures during the resting phase and immediately after exercise, and comparing the various images to derive a conclusion.

What is Stress Thallium?

Various radioactive substances, when injected in the body are taken by the healthy heart muscles and their distribution in the heart muscles in health and in disease is of immense value; in not only detecting the disease but also to know the possible benefit to the heart muscle after treatment. The most commonly performed imaging procedure is single photon emission computed tomography (SPECT) which is imaging of heart muscle perfusion. In this procedure, images are obtained after injecting a radiotracer in the blood. The isotope is taken up by the heart muscles from the blood. The healthy heart muscles, called viable myocardium take up and retain the isotope for some period. A gamma camera is used to capture the gamma ray photon and convert the information into digital data giving an idea of the area and amount of uptake.

The most commonly used tracer agents are thallium 201 and technetium. Thallium is a potassium analogue, and is taken up by the healthy heart muscle cells in proportion to the blood flow. The test is performed after overnight fasting and after stopping certain drugs used by patients with heart disease (for example, beta-blockers) so that the result is not influenced by these drugs. Thallium is injected at the peak of exercise and its uptake and redistribution in the heart muscle is detected by the gamma camera. The result is a hypo-perfused (getting less than normal blood) area of the heart, detected as less uptake or 'cold spot' of isotope than normally perfused healthy heart muscle (getting normal blood supply). The hypo-perfused or ischaemic area of the heart will show less or no uptake and in the next few hours, if this hypo-perfused area shows concentration of the isotope equal to the normal healthy heart muscle then it suggests that this muscle is viable and this defect is called reversible defect and restoration of blood supply to this area will benefit the person. Areas of infarction, dead heart muscle or scar will have no or reduced uptake and it will not change in the next few hours and suggest irreversible change in the heart muscle or death of that particular portion of heart. Restoration of blood supply to this dead tissue is of no use and passes no benefit whatsoever to the patient.

What is Pharmacological Stress Test?

Most cardiac stress labs and nuclear medicine departments use exercise stress tests as a reliable diagnostic tool as it is most close to the normal body physiology. This test is commonly employed on people who cannot perform exercise due to certain reasons. Thus, certain chemical agents are injected into their body which induce a stress-like physiology. The commonly used agents are dobutamine and adenosine. The test is performed initially at rest and then subsequent studies are performed after injecting these drugs. The dose of the drug is increased to achieve an increasing level of pharmacological stress and heart rate. A normal and healthy heart muscle will contract more vigorously with increasing stimulation and this effect is minimal or lost depending upon the degree of ischaemia. If a person has lung problems such as asthma or allergic bronchitis, adenosine should not be used.

What are the Newer Imaging Techniques for CHD?

Advances in magnetic resonance imaging (MRI) and computed tomography (CT) have markedly improved the speed and resolution of imaging, making these modalities useful in the clinical evaluation of CHD and improving their safety and convenience. Contrast material is injected in the body through a superficial vein. The contrast labelled blood reaches inside the heart and blood vessels and is not only helpful in defining the structures of the heart but is also useful in identifying areas of impaired blood supply.

What is MR Angiography?

Magnetic resonance (MR) applied to the cardiovascular system has been termed as cardiovascular magnetic resonance or CMR. MRI has shown to be capable of imaging the coronary arteries and demonstrating stenosis without catheterization. In addition, MRI is useful in identifying the location and thickness of myocardial scars.

What is 64 Slice CT Coronary Angiography?

A new tool for the diagnosis of coronary heart disease is multi slice CT coronary angiography with 64 slice or higher technology. This is emerging as the most reliable non-invasive diagnostic test. In CT angiography (CTA), X-rays are used to visualize blood flow in the coronaries. After injecting a contrast material through the intra venous route, beams of X-rays are passed from a rotating device through the heart from several different angles to create cross-sectional images, which are then, stored and reconstructed with the help of a computer to form three dimensional pictures of the heart and to detect plaque within the coronary arteries which are responsible for the blockage of one or more coronary arteries.

Emerging Role of Coronary CT Angiography

This diagnostic tool takes super- fast pictures of a moving heart using X-rays and displays it in a 3-dimensional (3D) format on a computer monitor. As it provides many more details regarding the heart's function and structures, the 64 slice CT scan helps experts detect the earliest stages of heart disease so that they can treat it and prevent it from progressing further. A cardiac CT (64 slice or more) scan can provide an image of the heart and its arteries in such fine details that the presence of plaque, narrowing or stenosis of the arteries, calcium scoring and abnormal heart vessels can be determined with a comparable degree of detail and accuracy, previously only available through an invasive procedure such as cardiac catheterization or angiography. The 64 slice CT angiography is useful for patients who are asymptomatic but are at high risk of having coronary heart disease that is, a person with chest pain or shortness of breath where heart disease is to be ruled out. The test is of immense value in people who are chronic smokers, suffering from diabetes mellitus, high blood pressure or having a strong family history with premature deaths.

Today, neither MRI nor CT has replaced conventional X-ray angiography for the diagnosis of narrowing of coronary blood vessels. It is possible that in the near future these tests may be very useful in certain cases of heart disease.

What is Coronary Angiography?

X-ray angiography is the gold standard for identifying the coronary artery distribution and narrowing. It is not only helpful in determining the extent of the disease but also has an advantage that a blocked artery can be opened during the procedure. The process is invasive, that is, after giving local anaesthesia the site of entry is punctured with a wide bore needle and the catheters (hollow plastic tubes) are advanced under the guidance of X-ray. The tip of the catheter is placed and hooked at the opening of coronary arteries one by one and a non-ionic contrast (dye) is injected into the arteries and the images are recorded. This gives excellent pictures and information regarding the location, degree and severity of narrowing of arteries. This information is transferred and stored in the computer. The report is expressed in percentage of luminal narrowing of the coronary artery. This procedure is done under local anaesthesia while the patient is awake, alert and conversing with the performing doctor.

How Safe is Coronary Angiography?

With advancement of technology and use of non-ionic contrast material, it is a very safe procedure in the hands of trained cardiologists. It requires hospitalization for one or even less than one day. If it is done from the groin (femoral) approach then the hospital stay is for 24 hours and if it is done from the arm (radial artery) approach then the stay is only for 12 hours.

It should be performed by a trained cardiologist and at a fully equipped centre.

Is the Contrast Use Safe?

Nowadays, non-ionic contrasts are used which are very safe. The hydration status is important as the person should not be dehydrated at the time of the procedure. Since the majority of the dye is excreted through the kidney and patients are in the fasting stage, the procedure should be done early in patients with diabetes and kidney disease so as to avoid precipitation of any kidney impairment due to dehydration caused by long standing fasting and delay in procedure.

What Are the Tests Best Suited for the Majority?

I would recommend resting and stress ECG (TMT) as the basic screening tests to detect significant blockage or narrowing in coronary heart disease coupled with echocardiography because this is widely available, cheap, non-invasive and the majority can afford it.

Nuclear scanning, dobutamine stress test and CT angiography are available at select centres and expensive as far as the common Indian is concerned. Recently, 64 or more slice multidetector-row CT angiography (CTA) has shown promise as an alternative to X-ray angiography for the identification of coronary blockages. All these tests are of immense importance if there is a strong suspicion regarding CHD. Since 64 slice CT scan is available in major cities of India it may be the choice of investigation in asymptomatic people with a high degree of suspicion for CHD. If there is evidence of CHD, then X-ray conventional coronary angiography should be performed as it can tell the extent of lesion, and if required, the problem can be fixed by angioplasty at the same sitting. The test best suited for the person can be decided on an individual basis and I would recommend letting your doctor decide about the test which will yield maximum information in the given circumstances.

Chapter 9
Myocardial Infarction

Myocardial infarction is the medical term used for heart attack and results from complete cessation of blood flow to one of the major coronary arteries. Lack of oxygen and other nutrients, which is the result of the abrupt closure of the artery that supplies blood to that particular area of heart muscle, causes injury and death of the heart muscle. It will lead to deterioration of heart function and finally heart failure. A heart attack is the commonest cause of sudden death in adults and elderly people. Advancements in medical science have led to the opening of the culprit or blocked artery to restore blood supply and to minimize the death of the heart muscle. But whatever may be the advancement in treatment, a dead tissue cannot be revived or repaired. Damage once established will remain so and will be replaced by scars which are made up of dead tissues. Scars formed will adversely affect the smooth and proper functioning of the heart and in due course of time, the heart will enlarge and fail. Therefore, even if one has access to the best medical facilities and finances, a heart once damaged cannot be repaired or returned to normalcy. To live a healthy and trouble free life, it is wise to prevent heart attacks or to minimize the effects by adopting preventive measures in time.

'When I was studying, one of my neighbours, who was a Professor in the Institute of Technology, had a heart attack. It was my first close encounter with the disease. He was young, dynamic and a learned scholar. The only drawback was that he was a chain smoker though he used his cycle frequently. One day he had severe chest pain in his class and was rushed to the University hospital. There he was thrombolysed immediately for his heart pain. Things looked okay till evening and he asked for coffee which his wife went home to prepare. A phone call an hour later changed the life of this happy family when they learnt that the professor was no more. This was the untimely, unexpected, severest blow for the family with three children of less than 12 years age. The lady had to go back without pension to Hyderabad, the native place to which she belonged. After 12 years the younger son came to study in the same Institute in which his father was once a professor and he narrated the courage of his mother who joined as a school teacher and with her determination she made her sons, engineers and daughter, a medical graduate. Now during my practice, whenever I come across this disease, the only thing which I am afraid of is that this family should not be shattered by the claws of heart disease.'

Is There Any Time for Heart Attack?

A heart attack can occur at any time of the day, but it is more frequent in the winter season and at early morning hours. The majority of adverse changes which can enhance the chances of a heart attack occur in the body during the morning hours. The most important is the presence of a hormone known as adrenaline (stress hormone) which is released in excess from the adrenal glands. Increased level of adrenaline in the blood at this hour may contribute towards the rupture of cholesterol plaques and cause narrowing of coronary arteries. It has also been observed that, a blood component-platelet, which helps in clotting, becomes sticky and aggregates or clusters more in the morning hours resulting in the formation of blood clots which can choke the artery abruptly. Human beings are warm blooded. It means their body temperature does not vary according to the temperature outside. During winters, when it is cold, the heart has to work more vigorously to maintain the temperature of the body by increasing the blood circulation. Therefore, demand for blood is increased in this season which poses as an extra burden on the heart and can precipitate a heart attack.

What are the Complaints at the Time of Heart Attack?

Chest pain is the foremost complaint during a heart attack and is usually felt as severe pain, pressure, heaviness, tightness or burning sensation in the middle or left part of the chest. It often radiates to the left arm, back, jaw, even both arms, or shoulders. Rarely, chest pain may be restricted to the right side of chest or right arm or jaws only. The pain of a heart attack lasts for more than 30 minutes and is excruciating. It may be associated with nausea, vomiting, sweating, syncope, and /or difficulty in breathing. It is often associated with an impending sense of death. The chest pain is unbearable and is not relieved by any change of posture or intake of oral medicines, and often the patients are in great distress.

What is a Silent Heart Attack or Silent Ischemia?

It has been observed that people may be suffering from coronary heart disease without being aware of it because many of them may not have typical complaints like chest pain. These are the cases which can go undetected for many years and this is common in the older age group or patients who have diabetes. These people may have a sole presentation of profuse sweating, severe difficulty in breathing, gaseous discomfort or syncope, while the main complaint of chest pain is missing. A heart attack without chest pain is termed as a silent heart attack and may lead to sudden death. Patients with diabetes have twice the chance of getting silent heart attacks or sudden death. It is advisable for elderly and diabetic patients, not to ignore chest discomfort of any severity or atypical complaints. They should consult their doctor promptly.

Heart Attack at a Glance

1. *Heart attack is a condition in which chest discomfort occurs when the blood and subsequent oxygen supply to an area of the heart muscle is totally blocked.*
2. *It is sudden and may not give warning signals.*
3. *Chest pain is a major complaint and is often very severe. It does not disappear immediately.*
4. *It is associated with a high death rate.*
5. *Blockade is not temporary and complete.*

Thus it is an Emergency

Common complaints of a heart attack are:
- Tightness or severe chest discomfort
- Pain may radiate towards the left or both arms, left shoulder, neck or back
- Vomiting and/or nausea
- Sweating
- Fainting
- Shortness of breath
- Diabetics may not have chest pain

Why are there No Warning Signals in Heart Attack?

Atherosclerosis is responsible for a heart attack which is a slow process in itself. Partial blockage of arteries sets in over several years and has no or little symptoms of any kind. However, complete blockage of an artery at the site of a partial block develops in a short time and is sudden. Therefore, it comes without warning signals and is unpredictable in a majority of cases. Due to our modern lifestyle, we are not fond of physical activity unless it is the need of the day. Therefore, a majority of us do not have complaints unless the disease has progressed to a critical severity.

What are the Types of Heart Attacks?

Depending upon the blood supply by the respective coronary artery and the area of damage in the heart, various types of heart attack have been categorized. As mentioned earlier, the left coronary artery supplies blood to a major portion of the heart while the right coronary artery supplies blood to the under surface and back of the heart. However, the pattern of blood supply may vary from person to person. Heart attacks are termed as anterior, inferior, extensive anterior, lateral, posterior and right ventricular depending upon the area of heart involvement. It has been found that anterior, extensive anterior and inferior heart attacks involve large portions of the heart and major coronary arteries. Also, it may be associated with more complications as compared to lateral or posterior heart attacks. It is a misconception amongst people that a person will die only after he has had the third heart attack. It must be stressed that a patient may die in his first attack itself, if a large portion of the heart muscle has been affected.

What should be Done if a Person has Severe Chest Pain Accompanied with Sweating?

Most likely, any person with the above complaints is suffering from a heart attack. Thus, immediate action must be taken. A doctor must be called in or an ambulance must be summoned urgently. The patient should be advised rest. Meanwhile, a tablet of ASPIRIN, a common pain killer, dissolved in a cup of water should be administered. Another tablet known as CLOPIDOGREL, in a dose of 300 mg should also be administered along with aspirin. If possible, a pain killer injection may be given and the patient should be transferred to the nearest hospital without any further delay. If the person has a known case of gastric ulcer (stomach) or is allergic to aspirin, it is better to avoid aspirin.

What is the Role of Aspirin?

Aspirin inhibits platelet accumulation, helps in thinning the blood and thus restores smooth flow of blood. Actually aspirin breaks the fresh blood clots rich in platelets and if given early during chest pain, can restore the blood supply through the blocked arteries by breaking down the clots. Various studies have proved beyond doubt that if a 325 mg of aspirin tablet is given early, it improves the survival in case of a heart attack and reduces major complications among heart patients such as recurrent chest pain, heart failure and death.

What should be the Dose of Aspirin?

There is enough scientific data to suggest that a dose of 75-150 mg per day of aspirin after meals is sufficient for the primary and secondary prevention of coronary heart diseases.

Since aspirin may result in gastric upset and rarely causes gastric ulcer, enteric coated aspirin is a better choice and it should be taken after meals. However, in case of a heart attack the first dose of aspirin should be 325 mg and the type of aspirin should be such that it dissolves in water completely to achieve immediate and maximum effect.

If Aspirin is Beneficial should I Take it to Prevent Heart Attack?

Answer is NO. Various studies have shown that long term use of a tablet of aspirin after 40 years of age per day without any risk factor and heart disease is not beneficial. However, a subset of patients such as diabetics with a history of smoking or hypertension may benefit. Therefore, an aspirin should always be taken after consulting your doctor. Remember, self-medication is always harmful and a little knowledge is a dangerous thing. Also, aspirin can take care of one part of risk while lifestyle management and other remedies can take care of all the risk factors.

What is Thrombolytic Therapy for Heart Attack?

It is known that myocardial infarction or heart attack occurs due to sudden and total blockage of one of the coronary arteries and this block is due to the formation of a thrombus (platelet and fibrin-rich blood substances) that clog the artery and cause sudden cessation of blood flow to a portion of the heart muscle. If the total blockage of blood flow to the heart is continued for more than 6 hours then that particular part of heart muscle becomes dead. There are certain drugs (streptokinase, urokinase or tissue plasminogen activator) which have the property of dissolving that thrombus, and if given within 6 hours of onset of chest pain in a heart attack, it may open the blocked artery, reduce the damage and save the heart muscle, and someone's life. This thrombus dissolving therapy is called thrombolytic therapy and should be given by a trained person with close cardiac monitoring and preferably in an intensive coronary care unit (ICCU) set up. It should be offered to all patients suffering from heart attack unless there is a contraindication for it. Whether it should be given after 6 hours and before 24 hours, will be decided by your physician according to the condition of the patient. This therapy usually has no benefits if given after 24 hours except in on-going or persistent chest pain. This therapy may be administered in an ambulance, while transferring the patient to a hospital by a trained personal.

Why 6 Hours for Thrombolytic Therapy?

A heart attack results in the death of heart muscle from the sudden blockage of a coronary artery by a blood clot. Blockage of a coronary artery deprives the heart muscle of blood and oxygen, causing injury to the heart muscle. Injury to the heart muscle causes chest pain and pressure. If the blood flow is not restored within 20 to 40 minutes, irreversible death of the heart muscle will begin to occur. Muscle continues to die for six to eight hours by which time the heart attack is usually 'complete'. The dead heart muscle is replaced by scar tissue. Therefore, if treatment is given within 6 hours it can save the dying heart muscle and can improve the survival. Today it is stressed that 'time is muscle' in heart attack, the earlier the treatment administered, less is the damage to heart muscle or in simple terms, 'saving time means saving heart muscle'.

Should Every Patient of Heart Attack be Hospitalized?

Yes, because it has shown that the majority of deaths due to heart attack occur in the first 48 hours. Treatment in the hospital, where a patient is kept in an intensive coronary care unit (ICCU) under close medical supervision saves more lives than any other form of therapy. An isolated set up in a hospital gives physical and mental rest to the patient and poses reduced burden to the fragile heart which is crying out for proper blood supply. A fractured bone can be rested in a plaster case, but a beating heart cannot be stopped. Therefore, the function of the heart should be minimized. It can be achieved only by giving proper and necessary rest to the ailing heart in a calm and quiet set up like an ICCU. This helps in restoring the health to the ailing heart. Moreover, a majority of the complications which can cause death can only be recognized under close supervision and can be tackled in the hospital, promptly and properly.

How Long shall I be Hospitalized?

In an uncomplicated heart attack it is usually for a week or so, because by that time a majority of the complications are averted and the blood supply to the damaged heart muscle is partially restored. However, people with complications may require a longer hospital stay.

Is my Heart Permanently Damaged?

To a certain extent, may be yes. After an attack, not all, but a varying degree of heart is damaged permanently and the remaining heart takes over the functioning. In a heart attack, the blocked artery is unable to supply blood and the damaged heart muscle dies in due course. The extent of heart muscle damage depends upon the time between injury (onset of chest pain) and treatment, the site involved and type of coronary artery involvement. Proximal involvement or involvement close to the origin of right coronary artery and left coronary artery causes more damage as compared to mid or distant lesions. This damaged heart tissue heals in 4-6 weeks and is replaced by dead tissue, that is, the scar tissue. Even though the scar is a dead tissue, the remaining healthy heart muscles keep working. This causes weakening of the heart. A weak heart cannot pump blood properly. The damage to the heart can be minimized or prevented by administering treatment in time and by a healthy lifestyle.

Will I Recover from my Heart Attack?

The answer is most likely yes. The damaged heart muscle which has been replaced by scar tissue does not help in proper contractions and pumping functions of the heart. This means, the pumping action of the heart is reduced. The degree of loss of heart function depends upon the location and size of scar. Thus, recovery in survivors of heart attack depends upon the extent of damage and the treatment received. Every year, millions of persons survive heart attacks, go back to work and enjoy a normal life. You have every reason to be confident about a full recovery. If you are taking proper care, your heart is healing and with each passing day you'll become stronger and more active. It is advisable to make necessary lifestyle changes along with the treatment to enjoy a full and productive life, and to prevent future heart attacks.

Is Chest Pain Normal After a Heart Attack?

Recovering from a heart attack means a pain-free life. However, some patients may experience chest pain after suffering a heart attack, and this is not normal. If you're experiencing chest pain, that is occurring after exercise or after eating heavy meal and is bothering you in your day to day activities, then you should immediately consult your doctor. Angina immediately after a heart attack should not be ignored. It is an indication that probably your disease is worsening despite medical therapy and you need urgent coronary angiography and further treatment in the form of angioplasty or bypass surgery.

How Long Will I Not be Fit for my Normal Work?

It all depends upon the type and severity of heart attack, and the modality of treatment which you have received. The treating doctor is the best judge. However, if there is no complication, you can walk around by the end of the first week and about 10–30 minutes by the end of the second week. Within 4 weeks you can join your duties with some precautions. If you have received angioplasty for your heart attack, you can resume your duties in 2 weeks time.

Your doctor will determine when you can go back and how much activity is suitable for you. Mind, hurry in one's mind, worry in one's nature and curry in one's food should be avoided at all costs by all.

When Can I Drive my Car?

Driving does not consume a lot of energy and in an uncomplicated heart attack one can drive safely after 4-6 weeks. The person should enjoy driving and should not be nervous or tense in different road situations which are beyond their control, as sometimes it may increase the heart rate and blood pressure which may be detrimental to health. The individual should learn the skill to combat unhealthy situations such as traffic jams, noise and air pollution. Reckless and rash drivers should be ignored. Long distance or professional drivers should avoid lengthy hours of driving. Drivers who earn their wages should be advised to choose small distance or city driving for their livelihood.

Can I Board a Flight?

Today, flights are quit safe in modern, pressurized airplanes. Flying for 1-3 hours does not pose any special discomfort or danger. Even taking a flight for a longer duration in a stable heart patient is quiet safe. However, precautions have to be taken to move the legs and body regularly so that the blood vessels are not blocked in the lower limbs due to stasis or sluggish blood flow.

Can I Use my Mobile Phone?

There are only a few scientific reports regarding the effect of mobile phones on people exposed to the radiations. Few studies claim that microwave radiations from mobile phones can damage the DNA sequence and may cause brain tumours, especially Glioma. It can increase the risk of disturbed brain functions, hearing problems and decreased spermotozoal counts in a few if used for more than ten years. Long term mobile use has not been reported to cause heart disease or serious health problems. However, patients having pacemaker implants and automatic implantable defibrillator devices (AICD), should be cautious and know the effect of mobile phone or cordless phones. Mobile phones emit radio signals and electromagnetic energy. There is possibility that it may interfere with the functioning of the implanted device when the phone is held directly over or is held very close to the device that is, within 6 inches. Mobile phones may cause interference only if it is in use or in standby mode, not when it is switched off. Few mobile phones have a magnet and can activate the magnet mode of the device. The program of the device may change and the pacemaker will start operating at a fixed rate. However, it will not stop working in this mode and will revert to normal operation when the magnet is removed. It is important to note that any effect resulting from the interaction between a mobile phone and an implanted device is temporary and a rare one in 100000. Simply moving the phone away from the implanted device will return it to its proper state of operation. The potential for a mobile phone to interfere with a pacemaker or implantable defibrillator can be minimized by maintaining a separation of at least 6 inches between the mobile phone and implanted device. This can be achieved by keeping the phone in a pocket away from the site or the belt position and use of ear connections when operating the phone or use the phone against the ear that is farther away from the pacemaker.

Should I Undergo TMT After a Heart Attack?

Yes, in 4-6 weeks time you can undergo TMT and it helps in deciding further treatment for you and also boost up your confidence. Stress tests may be done in a few patients just before discharging them from the hospital, especially in those where a heart attack recovery is uncomplicated. It is better to defer TMT in patients with recurrent chest pain, heart rate disturbances and who feel difficulty in breathing (features of heart failure). TMT after a heart attack should be done under supervision and the choice of protocol for exercise (bicycle or treadmill) which is suitable for the individual patient will be decided by your physician.

Why is the Heart Attack Diagnosis Delayed or Missed in the Indian Subcontinent?

Lack of knowledge, ignorance, poverty, associated with limited medical facilities are major reasons for delay in diagnosis and treatment of a heart attack. It may occur anywhere but is more common in rural or semi-urban areas. Few important reasons are:

1. In a majority of individuals, symptoms occur during the night or early in the morning when medical facilities are not available or are attended by local doctors who are not qualified enough. They inject pain killers which relieve the initial complaint of pain but miss the real diagnosis.

2. In some individuals, the predominant symptoms are belching, vomiting and heaviness of lower chest and upper abdomen which mimic abdominal complaints, especially when the lower surface (inferior) of the heart is involved which lies over the stomach. In such a case, it is generally passed off as a gastric problem. A majority of patients try to convince themselves and their doctor that it is a gaseous problem and has nothing to do with the heart.

3. If the complaints are few and atypical, people do not accept that they are having such a serious problem (they find it hard to believe that they are having a heart attack) and argue why they should get prompt medical attention and hospital admission which requires money, especially from elderly and diabetic patients.
4. In remote places or in rural areas, the facility for an ECG is not available or is infrequent and then it is delayed.
5. Limited or lack of transport facilities for patients to higher centres is another reason for delay in diagnosis and treatment.
6. The life-saving thrombolytic therapy is delayed or not administered as the patients are diagnosed late or reach late at a medical centre or cannot afford the treatment.

How to Treat Coronary Heart Disease?

The goal of treatment for CHD is to make people not only feel better but also live longer. The initial treatment modality is medical management which includes the use of medicines and modification of risk factors. The patient and family members should understand the nature of problem. They should know what should be done to prevent worsening of their symptoms. Drug therapy is only half the treatment. The rest of the treatment includes correcting lifestyle that has contributed to their problem which is as important as taking medicines. Ideally each and every patient should undergo coronary angiography after a heart attack. However, this is not possible in our country as it is expensive and available only at select centres. Opening of a blocked artery by coronary angioplasty and where it is not possible, operation and putting grafts (coronary artery bypass graft) to restore blood supply may be required in a few. These treatment modalities are costly and who needs it, will be decided by the treating doctor.

Apart from all this, lifestyle modifications which include regular physical activity, modifying and controlling various risk factors are of paramount importance. Lifestyle modifications especially exercise, diet and cessation of tobacco use is more easily said than done. Therefore, it is you who will be responsible for its practice as taking drugs alone is not a guarantee that you are not susceptible to a second heart attack. A majority of people live in the false belief that since they are not having complaints, they are fit merely by taking the drugs; then why should they undergo costly tests and follow lifestyle modifications. It is better to get check-ups at regular intervals as complications of CHD, especially heart failure is a slow process and its diagnosis, if done at an early stage can save life and money as success of various treatment modalities depend mainly on the strength of the heart. A poorly functioning heart has the worst outcome as compared to preserved heart function. You have to understand that your heart is under your control, you have to take charge of it.

What is Revascularization Therapy?

The blood flow to the diseased heart muscle can be restored either by opening the blocked artery by a procedure known as angioplasty or putting another blood vessel from your own body and attaching it before and after the blocked artery. The latter procedure is surgical and is known as bypass surgery. It is similar to what each one of us in India experience and follow once a road is blocked or jammed by taking the help of a bypass road. Revascularization therapy is a treatment of choice for all patients of CHD who have no or little relief with medicines.

What is Angioplasty?

Coronary balloon angioplasty was first performed by Andreas Gruentzig in 1977. This novel method of treatment has gained tremendous acceptance and has expanded dramatically over the last three decades. Today, it is an effective and accepted mode of treatment and the number of procedures has surpassed bypass surgery. It is commonly referred to as PCI (percutaneous coronary intervention) or PTCA (percutaneous coronary angioplasty) or simply angioplasty. Angioplasty is a procedure in which a balloon is inflated and deflated to open a narrow or blocked blood vessel of the heart (coronary artery). It is not a surgical procedure. The procedure is performed in a catheterization lab and by trained cardiologists. It is done under local anaesthesia and the person is awake. A guide wire is inserted into one of the coronary arteries through the groin (femoral artery) or wrist (radial artery) under local anaesthesia. The balloon catheter is positioned at the blocked area and once positioned, is inflated and deflated a few times. This procedure compresses the blocking material and debris along the inner portion of the arterial wall. The result is of restoring patency or opening of the blocked artery and improvement of blood flow beyond the blocked area. If required, medicines can also be delivered through the catheter to dissolve a blood clot in an artery. The major advantage of this procedure is the relief of complaints and reduction in future complications.

What is Primary Angioplasty?

Recently, studies have shown that if the blocked artery can be opened up within 90 minutes of onset of chest pain with the help of balloon angioplasty, the survival is best as compared to any other modality of treatment. This process is called primary angioplasty. However, it is a dream treatment for developing countries because of lack of awareness, unavailability of equipped centres, round the clock accessibility of trained personnel and of course, the cost.

What is a Stent?

A stent is a small metal coil or mesh tube that is placed in a narrowed artery through a catheter which holds the artery wide open, compress plaque and helps blood flow through the coronary artery. It helps in preventing restenosis of the opened coronary artery by balloon angioplasty.

What are Drug Coated Stents?

The process of balloon angioplasty alone is associated with 30 % incidence of restenosis or re-blockade and to prevent it initially bare metal stents were used. Nowadays, the stents are coated with certain drugs or chemicals and are known as drug coated or drug eluting stents (DES). Today, the use of drug eluting stents in patients with acute myocardial infarction is safe and improves clinical outcome by reducing the risk of restenosis and need for future interventions compared to bare metal stents.

Complications and Success Rate after PTCA

The success rate of this procedure is as high as 98 %. It all depends upon the patient's subset, skill and competence of the operator. Restenosis rate which was 33 % with bare metal stents has come down to 5 % after the advent and use of drug eluting or coated stents. Restenosis usually occurs within 6 months of the procedure and it is rare after 6 months of procedure. Death rate associated with the procedure is less than 1 %. Death rate is high in patients with poor heart function, low blood pressure and in patients with long standing, poorly controlled diabetes. A heart attack or myocardial infarction can occur in 1-2 % after angioplasty. Stent thrombosis or fresh clot formation over the stent is less than 1 % after the use of antiplatelet (aspirin and clopidogrel/prasugrel) and antithrombotic medicines (heparin and Gp IIb/IIIa inhibitors), and may occur within 24 hours of the procedure. All patients should undergo a TMT test after 4-6 weeks of the procedure to know the patency and complications related with angioplasty. Considering the risks after a heart attack and the subsequent cardiac complications such as recurrent pain and heart failure balloon angioplasty of coronary artery is definitely a safe and effective treatment in the hands of trained persons.

How Long should one Stay in the Hospital?

Majority of the angioplasty and stent deployment procedures are done at the time of angiography and usually one has to stay for one or two days in the hospital following angioplasty.

What is the Cost of the Procedure in India?

In India, one angioplasty with a drug eluting stent costs approximately 1 lakh (US $2000) rupees in government run and 1.5 to 2.5 lakh rupees (US $3000-5000) in a private hospital depending upon the set up and the type of stent used during the procedure. Though bare metal stents are comparatively cheap but because of the high rate of stent restenosis, it is not preferred. One of my patients underwent three stent deployment 10 years earlier and his reaction was heart touching, *doctor sahib* it was equivalent to marrying a daughter.

What is Bypass Surgery?

Coronary artery bypass graft surgery is popularly known as bypass surgery or CABG and is a common operative procedure for restoring blood flow to the heart tissue that has been deprived of blood because of coronary artery disease. It creates an extra route for blood flow. The principle of the procedure is that the blocked artery is bypassed with a vessel taken from another part of the body. This allows the blood to flow to your heart again. A blood vessel from your leg, arm or chest is taken and attached to the blocked coronary artery. The commonly used blood vessels are saphenous vein from the leg, radial artery from the arm and internal mammary artery from the chest. The CABG should be undertaken by trained surgeons and hospitals equipped with ICU facilities as you have to spend the initial few days in ICU after surgery and then you may be discharged from the hospital in a week's time depending upon your condition. After surgery you may feel weakness and pain at the site of surgery for a few weeks but always keep in touch with your doctor, physiotherapist and dietician. Even after the surgery, regular exercise and control of risk factors are important to prevent further blocking of the grafted arteries. Leg veins (venous grafts) block early as compared to arterial grafts (arm and chest arteries). It takes an average of 10 years to block these grafted vessels but this can occur earlier or later depending upon the lifestyle changes you have adopted and control of the co-existing medical illnesses such as diabetes and hypertension after surgery. CABG has an excellent outcome and 5 years survival after CABG is 94 % and 10 years survival is 84 %. 10 years of survival may be reduced to 69 % for those continue to smoke or have uncontrolled lipid or sugar levels.

What Are the Risks of CABG?

Today, coronary artery bypass surgery is safe and with the advent of beating heart surgery, risks have been reduced to 1-2 %. Death after CABG is less than 1 % and depends upon the patient subset. Complication rate following CABG depends upon the age, sex, weight and other diseases present in the patients at the time of surgery. The most important determinant is the functional capacity of the heart; better heart functions are associated with better results. Concomitant presence of diabetes mellitus, hypertension and obesity influences the surgical outcome and poses excess risk. Hospital complications include heart attack, infection, bleeding from the wound, stroke or paralytic attack. However, for many patients, discomfort and healing of the wound, both at the site of chest and legs or arms from where the graft has been taken are major problems and even a slight discomfort or chest pain not only causes unnecessary worry but also limits the activity and recovery.

How Long does one has to Stay in the Hospital?

Normally one has to stay for 7-10 days in the hospital following an uncomplicated CABG procedure.

When can one Resume his Normal Activity After CABG?

In 4-6 weeks time, one can resume his normal activity and can perform moderate exercise by 8-12 weeks.

What is the Cost of CABG?

On an average an uncomplicated bypass surgery costs 1-2.5 lakhs rupees (US $2000-5000) depending upon the centre. It is less expensive in government hospitals as compared to private hospitals. The cost may increase when it is coupled with valve replacement, resection of thin and dilated portion of heart or associated post-operative complications such as infection.

PCI vs Medical Therapy

Considering the cost associated with percutaneous intervention (PCI), majority of the patients in India are forced to continue medical therapy. PCI is not superior to medical therapy in a case of stable angina if the person is asymptomatic and can perform fairly good exercise with no chest pain. PCI should be advocated to all if the symptoms persist even after optimum medical therapy. PCI gives better results in the initial years as it provides better quality of life by relieving the chest pain. However, after 5 years, the symptoms may reappear in a few cases. Stent restenosis is still not solved and remains a problem even after the advent of drug eluting stents (DES). Patients on medical therapy and those who are symptom free on routine work but have a positive exercise test can be benefited more by PCI. Similarly, angina after CABG may require PCI for the blocked grafted vessels.

PCI vs CABG ?

Today, because of the advancement in techniques and availability of suitable hardware the number of angioplasty procedures are more than the number of bypass surgeries. The most important reason is that not only the hospital stay is reduced but there is no surgery involved and the procedure is less traumatic. Moreover, it is the patient's mentality to avoid surgery which has further increased the acceptance of PCI. An ideal candidate for PCI is one who has single or two vessel involvement with preserved heart function and the block is closer to the origin involving short segment of the arteries. Long lesions, diffuse diseases, narrowing at the bifurcation of the artery, opening of the left main artery and all the three arteries require not only skill but huge finances. However these lesions are fixed successfully nowadays, reducing the burden of bypass surgery. PCI is an excellent mode of treatment. However, it should be kept in mind that it may require more interventions due to restenosis in the future and does not improve or worsen the prognosis in multi-vessel disease. It definitely improves the quality of life and the number of angina episodes. Complications such as death and heart attack are similar following PCI and CABG in stable patients. Patients with multiple, long, diffuse lesions or with involvement of all three arteries are the best candidates for bypass. Initially left main disease or narrowing at the origin of left coronary artery was only amenable to bypass surgery, but today in some patients, angioplasty may also be the procedure of choice and is effective.

Who are the High Risk Patients?

Heart disease should not be taken lightly and one should not live in the false belief that once he is taking medicines and following a healthy lifestyle, he will be fine or the disease will be cured in the future. With the advancement in medical field and the effective treatment, majority of patients are comfortable with optimum drug therapy and enjoy a fully productive life. However, some of the patients may develop problems in the future. If any of the following problems are noticed, the patients should immediately consult their physicians:

1. Chest pain occurring at rest or during usual household activities.
2. Chest pain after heart attack.
3. Heart attack in diabetics.
4. Experiencing chest pain even after optimum medication.
5. Angina with poor heart function.
6. Angina episodes associated with low blood pressure.
7. Elderly patients > 65 years.

Elderly with Heart Disease, are they Different?

Elderly patients with heart diseases have the same complaints as the young or adult patients. However, they are often ready to accept the disease and continue on medical therapy rather than consider angioplasty or bypass surgery. The reasons are the high cost of therapy, financial strains, and last but not the least, they are very concerned about being a burden on others. Other co-existing medical problems such as high blood pressure, cataract, diabetes, arthritis, etc.

not only increase their worry but also limit their mobility. Elderly patients often have a more diffuse disease, affecting multiple coronary arteries and may have low heart function. Elderly patients with heart disease should be offered the same treatment protocol as younger patients. The complication rate may be slightly high in elderly patients after bypass surgery because of the co-morbid medical conditions, advanced age, less physical activity and often due to fear of total recovery and future dependency. Their physical physiology is also different from that of young patients and the drug bioavailability changes with age which should always be considered while prescribing medicines. One should start with lower doses of drugs and build it up slowly to achieve an optimum response. Often patients receive medicines for other diseases, hence the number of tablets being ingested is again a cause of concern and utmost care should be taken to prescribe fewer tablets. Combination therapy and of course, cost of the drug must be kept in mind while prescribing medicines.

Why should I Take All Chest Pains Seriously After 35 Years of Age?

Even though symptoms of a heart attack at times can be vague and mild, it is important to remember that heart attacks producing no symptoms or only mild symptoms can be just as serious and life-threatening as heart attacks that cause severe chest pain. A majority of people, due to ignorance and lack of knowledge try to pass heart attack symptoms as indigestion, gaseous distension, fatigue, or as common cold and consequently delay seeking prompt medical attention. Involvement of the lower surface of the heart (inferior heart attack) is often associated with belching, vomiting as the inferior surface of the heart rests upon the stomach. For many of these cases, heart attack may be the first sign of coronary heart disease and a majority of such patients never reach the hospital. Therefore, it is important to seek prompt medical attention in the presence of symptoms that suggest a heart attack. Early diagnosis and treatment saves precious lives, and delay in seeking medical assistance can be fatal. Out of many causes of chest pain probably this is the only chest pain which if ignored can cost you your life.

Are All Chest Pains, a Heart Attack?

Chest pain is a common complaint in angina and heart attack and it requires urgent medical attention. However, there are other causes of chest pain which should be kept in mind while evaluating a person. If one fails to establish heart disease as a cause of chest pain even after repeated tests and medical examinations, it is wise to look for other common causes of chest pain. Some of the common causes of chest pain apart from angina and heart attack are:

1. Pain in chest wall muscles. This is called myalgia. It increases by movement or during the act of breathing, or on directly pressing the area. It may come and go or persist for hours.
2. Costochondritis or Tietze's syndrome can mimic angina or sometime heart attack. It is inflammation at the site of rib joining the bone and cartilage.
3. Pain due to infection of lungs (pneumonia) or in the membrane covering the lungs (pleurisy). It increases on deep breathing or coughing and may be associated with fever. Prescribing a chest X-ray may be sufficient for diagnosis.

4. Upper abdominal discomfort that is, gastritis or hyperacidity is often referred to as heartburn and is associated with belching, feeling of fullness, nausea and a burning sensation. Upper abdominal endoscopy is the investigation of choice.

5. Presence of gall bladder stone (cholelithiasis) is accompanied with severe pain in the right upper abdomen; may be felt in the back region. A simple ultrasound of the upper abdomen will clinch the diagnosis in a majority of cases.

6. Pancreatitis or inflammation of pancreas causes upper abdominal pain, which is severe. It may radiate to the back and is associated with nausea and vomiting. It is associated with a rise in serum amylase and lipase. A CT scan of the abdomen will further help in establishing the diagnosis.

7. Pericarditis or infection of the covering of the heart may be another cause. It is often associated with fever and pain persists for a longer period. The intensity of pain is mild to moderate. It has no relation with the act of breathing. On examination, one can detect a scratching sound over the left side of chest which varies with posture. Echocardiography will show excess fluid between the heart and its covering- the pericardium.

8. Compression of nerve roots, pain from spine, either because of tuberculosis of spine (common in India) or cervical spondylitis or pain at the nape of the neck often radiates to the left or right arm with chest pain and may be associated with a tingling or numb sensation. X-ray of the spine coupled with a MRI, if necessary in different views will help in the diagnosis. Pain in nerves can also be due to an infection from a virus known as herpes zoster. This infection (herpes) is associated with blisters along the course of the nerve on the chest wall.

9. Anxiety and panic attacks can also mimic heart attacks. It is common in young individual especially the female gender. It is often associated with a racing heart, lack of sleep, uneasiness and vague pain of varying degree and duration. It should be diagnosed once all common causes of chest pain are ruled out.
10. Two serious conditions can also imitate a heart attack. Firstly, pulmonary embolism (blockage of blood flow to the lungs), that is, blockage of one of the pulmonary vessels causes pain and is common following delivery, surgeries involving the lower limb, immobilization or after prolonged bed rest. In this condition, blood clot from a lower limb vein breaks and travels up to the lungs and blocks one of the major pulmonary vessels. The second condition is tearing of aorta (a main blood vessel connected with the heart which carries blood from the heart to the rest of the body). It is called dissection of the aorta. It causes severe chest pain, often radiating to the back or only manifests as back pain. Both the conditions are rare, life threatening and require high degree of suspicion.

CHD at a Glance

1. *Coronary heart disease occurs because of atherosclerosis and subsequent blockage of the coronary arteries which supply blood to the heart muscles.*
2. *Development of CHD and its outcome is determined by a number of risk factors.*
3. *The important risk factors are family history of premature CHD, use of tobacco, diabetes mellitus, high blood pressure, obesity, high cholesterol and physical inactivity.*
4. *Excessive use of tobacco, increased prevalence of diabetes and physical inactivity are most important and these have led to the recent epidemic of CHD in India.*

5. CHD can cause many complaints. The common ones are chest pain, breathlessness, tiredness and a racing heart. Effort induced chest pain is most suggestive of CHD and should not be ignored.
6. The commonest screening test is resting and stress ECG or TMT.
7. Effort angina, especially after meals is a precursor of severe underlying disease.
8. Heart attack or myocardial infarction is an acute presentation of CHD and requires urgent treatment. If ignored, it can kill the patient.
9. Diabetics and the elderly have a greater chance of suffering from a silent heart attack, mild complaints and sudden death.
10. Risk of CHD in a society can be reduced by adopting a healthy lifestyle and regular exercise apart from the daily routine.
11. A majority of patients are benefitted by lifestyle changes and the use of medicines.
12. Some patients may require balloon angioplasty (PTCA) or bypass surgery (CABG).
13. A combined strategy of medical therapy, lifestyle modifications and selective intervention in the form of PCI or CABG will be the most rational approach.
14. Once the damage has occurred, the heart muscles cannot be repaired. Hence, prevention may be the only cure.

Chapter 10
Women and Coronary Heart Disease

Heart disease in women has received less attention than men. If one asks for the leading cause of death in women, many will respond 'breast cancer' or 'cancer of the cervix'. On the contrary, heart attacks and related heart diseases are problems affecting not only men but are a leading cause of death in women in many countries of the world. Thus, heart disease in women is of equal concern across the world and results in millions of deaths every year. It is largely preventable.

Developing countries including India are no different. Heart diseases are rising amongst women. However, the actual statistical data regarding its prevalence is not yet available. The data available on the prevalence of heart disease is male dominated. Some of the available studies from India reveal an increasing prevalence of heart disease in women. It is more prevalent in urban India as compared to rural areas. The reduced prevalence of the disease in rural areas may be attributed to a healthier and more active lifestyle such as low incidence of obesity, less use of alcohol, better dietary habits, reduced stress and increased physical activity. Now the scene is changing in India and there is a surge of heart disease and related complications in women because of the increased prevalence of diabetes mellitus, hypertension, obesity, stress and physical inactivity in urban Indians and the excessive use of tobacco, lower rate of literacy, and health care inequities in rural women.

The occurrence of heart disease and its related complications are very low in women of reproductive age, but it rises to a significant level after menopause. In women, the disease manifests 10-15 years later than in men. The fact is that, between 25-34 years, heart disease is twice as common in men then in women. By 45-54 the two sexes have equal prevalence but after 55 it is the female gender which takes over as leaders in heart related ailments. One of the possible explanations of this difference is the protective effect of oestrogen hormone (secreted up to menopause) which is reduced in women as the age advances. The complaints related with heart disease are slightly different in women as compared to men. Also because of lack of knowledge and awareness, the complaints are ignored in general. Social taboos prevalent in a major part of India, especially rural India prevent them from getting better medical treatment and therefore they manifest the disease once it is full blown such as heart attack, stroke or heart failure. In rural India where tobacco consumption (smoking or tobacco chewing) is common, the situation is worse as the diagnosis is overlooked or delayed due to a lack of education in the family and women getting less attention as compared to men. The medical facilities in rural India are either far away or beyond the reach of many and the disease remains undiagnosed or the treatment is delayed. Today, the impact of heart disease in women in India is equally enormous and as important as in other parts of the globe.

A shocking but humble submission

'She had rest angina and was having little relief with medicines. I insisted several times for her to undergo coronary angiography and

to fix the blocked arteries with either angioplasty or bypass surgery. The advice was not complied with and then I explained the prognosis of the disease to her son who always accompanied her. I told him to come with his father so that the whole process can be explained to him also and the financial implications associated with the treatment process can be discussed. Before the boy could answer she interjected, 'Doctor sahib, please write the prescription only. They have enough money only to purchase agricultural lands but not for my treatment. The medicine which I get is procured by the boy out of his hostel fee.'

Presentation

Presentation of heart disease in females is slightly different as compared to males. Women tend to present with more of atypical symptoms like back pain, arm pain, upper mid abdominal pain, jaw pain, shortness of breath, nausea, indigestion, silent heart attack or even sudden death. Not only is the presentation different, the complications associated with heart disease are higher in women. Unfortunately because of narrow coronary arteries women tend to have a high death rate, more frequent recurrence of disease and related complications like heart failure. The death rate is almost double that of men due to heart related problems. Women are also more likely to present with chest pain that is not related with heart disease. This leads to missed diagnosis or delay in diagnosis resulting in detection of the disease once it is full blown or complicated, and the situation further worsens as treatment is not rendered in time.

Investigations

In women, frequent atypical presentation, social taboos and lack of awareness along with limitation of the diagnostic tools make the situation worse. A high degree of suspicion is necessary, especially in post-menopausal women as diagnostic tools such as electrocardiography (ECG) and treadmill test (TMT), which are commonly employed for diagnosis, are often misleading. Non-specific resting ECG changes are more common in females as compared to males. The second most common test employed for diagnosis of heart disease is exercise ECG or TMT. TMT is less specific when compared to males as false positive test is more common in females, posing a greater challenge in diagnosis. The other common limitation of the exercise test (TMT) in Indian women is that, a majority of them are unable to perform the desired level of exercise on the machine making the interpretation of result and diagnosis difficult. Coronary catheterization and stress echocardiography are costly and only available at select cities in India. All this not only makes the diagnosis difficult and delayed, but also prevents women from getting appropriate treatment in time. Recently, multi-slice computed tomography coronary angiography, a non-invasive test may be more helpful where there is a strong suspicion of disease and the ECG and TMT are inconclusive.

Treatment

Early recognition of symptoms and accurate diagnosis of coronary heart disease are of great importance if proper treatment strategies are to be implemented. This will reduce the number of women dying from heart attacks and related diseases. As far as the treatment is concerned, it is similar to men. Each woman should be approached separately, their associated risk factors if any, should be assessed and measures should be taken at the earliest to treat or correct them. All this requires an individual approach, assessing the associated risk factors and correcting them in time. It is also important to give special emphasis to opening up the blocked blood vessels of the heart. However, these procedures are costly and only a few can afford it. The requirement of angioplasty and coronary artery bypass grafting (CABG) are the same as men, but complications related with these treatment modalities are higher in women as compared to men.

Heart Disease Risks After Natural Menopause

Menopause is associated with an adverse effect on lipids including increase in total cholesterol, low density lipoprotein (LDL) and triglycerides, and a reduction in good cholesterol such as high density lipoprotein (HDL) in blood. Reduced levels of oestrogen hormone after menopause can result in high blood pressure, obesity, increased incidence of blood clotting, impaired glucose metabolism and may lead to diabetes. All these changes occurring after menopause place women in the high risk group for heart disease.

Heart Disease Risks After Hysterectomy

There is a significant increase in the risk for heart disease in women who have undergone bilateral oophorectomy (removal of ovaries) and hysterectomy (removal of womb or uterus) and who have not taken exogenous oestrogen. Whether or not hysterectomy alone increases heart disease risk is controversial but, hysterectomy may lead to subsequent ovarian failure and makes the female devoid of protecting benefits of the oestrogen hormone.

Heart Disease in Young Women

Heart disease in young women is a rarity. The protective reasons are not only hormones but it is further enhanced by low levels of blood pressure, low levels of LDL and TG and high levels of HDL cholesterol compared to men. Heart disease, if it occurs in young women is often associated with one or two risk factors such as hypertension, diabetes mellitus, a family history of heart attack, obesity and / or smoking. These diseases are becoming more prevalent in young women, especially in urban areas, thereby, increasing the chances of heart disease. Use of oral contraceptives at a young age rarely increase the risk of heart attack unless one of the known risk factors for heart disease is also present. In a few, an increased incidence of heart attack might be caused by early menopause, development of diabetes or high blood pressure.

The environment in which we are living today is changing at a rapid speed, increasing the number of younger women getting heart disease. Therefore, it is important to recognize vulnerable young women and adopt the preventive measures early. These days, young women of both developed and developing countries are dynamic and health conscious. Thus, all efforts should focus on reducing the risk of heart disease among young women in the same way as in others. Young women should receive counselling about lifestyle modifications which are applicable to all. Regular exercises, cessation of tobacco use, consumption of vegetables and fruits regularly, maintenance of ideal body weight, yoga and meditation to combat stress and drugs to control diabetes, high blood pressure and lipid abnormality must be strongly advocated.

Hormone Replacement Therapy (HRT)

One area of women's health which has perhaps generated the maximum amount of controversy and confusion is hormone replacement therapy. Until recently it was thought that this therapy, consisting of oestrogen and progestin in varying combinations was protective for the heart. However, results from recent studies have contradicted these findings. The current scientific recommendations for hormone replacement are:

1. HRT should not be advocated in all post-menopausal women as routine preventable measure to control heart disease.
2. If post-menopausal women, who are already on hormone replacement therapy (HRT) develop heart attack or angina, they should discontinue hormone therapy.
3. If post-menopausal women who are not suffering with pre-existing heart disease require HRT therapy for non-heart indications, HRT should be given.
4. There is a small excess risk of venous thromboembolic for (clogging of blood vessels, especially of lower limbs) events in women who are on HRT.
5. HRT should not be continued while patients are confined to bed rest.
6. The only reason for taking hormone replacement therapy, should be relief from the symptoms related to menopause. It should be started only after consulting the doctor.

Prevention of Heart Disease

Heart disease in women is of special concern in today's modern society and they should be made aware that heart diseases are as important as breast or cervix cancer. Unfortunately heart disease in women in developing countries, including the Indian subcontinent is under diagnosed, under treated and under researched. All preventive strategies known today must be practiced to gain maximum benefit. Efforts should focus on reducing the risk of heart disease among women in the same way as in men. They should be encouraged to say NO to smoking and/ or use of tobacco consumption, to increase physical activity, to watch their weight and waist, to consume fresh fruits and vegetables. If they are suffering from high blood pressure and diabetes mellitus then it should be controlled. Guidelines specific for women are:

Waist circumference	: < 80 cm
Weight	: Maintain close to ideal
Blood Pressure	: Maintain at 120/80 mmHg
Blood sugar	: Fasting sugar < 110 mg/dl
HDL cholesterol	: > 50 mg/dl
LDL cholesterol	: < 100 mg/dl
Triglycerides (TG)	: < 150 mg/dl
Physical activity	: 45 minutes of daily exercise/ brisk walking

Women and the Heart Disease, at a Glance

1. *Women live under the false belief that they are less likely to have heart disease. Also, very few physicians are aware that more women die each year from heart attacks after 55 years than men.*
2. *Women have similar or even more risk for heart disease as men do, but are protected by their hormones till they reach menopause.*
3. *Women, who smoke or use tobacco in any form develop the disease early.*

4. Women often have atypical symptoms, more than men and the disease is diagnosed late and often with complications.
5. Diagnostic tools have their own limitations in women and coronary angiography is costly and beyond the reach of many in India.
6. Women in India are so involved in taking care of their family that they often neglect themselves.
7. Social taboos and gender disparity in the society prevent women from getting aggressive treatment than men.
8. Women have a greater risk of developing heart failure and other complications after heart attack compared to men and a greater risk of dying (higher death rate and related complications following heart attack when compared to men).
9. Women are two times more prone to die following bypass surgery (CABG) as compared to men.
10. Angioplasty related complications are more frequent with higher recurrence of symptoms and less relief as compared to men.
11. Preventing strategies such as education and screening regarding heart disease which is lacking should be employed early and aggressively to all.

Chapter 11

Sex and Heart Disease

Heart attack is a serious event in one's life, but it is not the end of it. You can recover and live a fully enjoyable life with a little change in your daily routine. You should know and understand what happened to you and how to reduce the risk of further adverse or unpleasant events. No drastic change is required, rather you have to practice a few necessary healthy lifestyle changes for your own good health. Regular physical exercise and activity after a heart attack is a part of the treatment and is good for the heart. Sex after heart attack is also another form of exercise and normal sexual activity is equivalent to mild to moderate exercise.

People are often reluctant to engage themselves in sexual activity because of the fear of precipitating another heart attack. Depression after a heart attack is quite common and is often associated with loss of libido and poor sexual performance. Associated risk factors such as smoking and diabetes along with certain medicines increase the erectile dysfunction and result in a low interest in sex. People who use tobacco or who are diabetics have two to three fold increased chances of poor sexual performance. The situation is further complicated by the fact that neither the doctor nor the patients are willing to discuss sexual history and advice is often neglected, uncommon, incomplete and neither rendered nor asked for. The question concerning sexual activity and heart remains unanswered, more so in the Indian set up where talking about sex is regarded as indecent behaviour and is a social taboo. People who have experienced a heart attack or heart surgery will be more cautious while indulging in sexual activity or a majority give up sex all together. A thorough understanding of sex after heart problems is mandatory and will help the person to improve their sexual life. In this, an individual counselling approach is the treatment of choice. In the western world and affluent countries, a majority of the patients of heart disease get full treatment that is, angioplasty or bypass surgery. In India and other developing countries, because of lack of finances and availability, only a few of the patients get the complete treatment of a heart attack and related heart disease. Thus a majority of the patients have to continue on drug therapy. It appears that the risk of development of heart related problems may be more during sexual activity in the developing world and thus appropriate recommendations regarding the safety of sexual activity should be a part of the treatment protocol for every heart patient. A thorough knowledge and counselling of both partners will help all patients to enjoy their sexual life.

It Haunts the Partner More than the Patient

'Doctor, he is shy of asking questions about sexual life after the illness. I also do not know how to talk to you as a majority of the time you are busy and his attitude prevents me from discussing it with you in front of him so, I am writing to you. The foremost fear which makes me shiver is that if something goes wrong during sex I shall be not able to handle the situation. I don't know what to do at that time and what to tell my doctor as to why this has precipitated or worsened? You also know the limited medical facility available at night. I am afraid that if this situation ever occurs I will not forgive myself and the guilt will haunt me all my life. This feeling in me compels refusal from my side, either gently or forcibly. The nervousness and tension

during this period bothers me and I cannot share this with anyone in the nuclear family. Because of this he is losing interest in sex, his depression is mounting and probably, he feels that the disease has made him impotent. His irritation and loss of interest in the surroundings and children is obvious. As a result I feel a sense of frustration, irritability in him and fear of the end of our physical relationship. When I want to discuss the situation he snubs me and ends up assuring me that he will talk to you. I know I may be wrong but I am unable to handle this situation. It's my humble request to you that having taken care of his heart attack kindly help us in this matter also and please do not reveal this to my husband.'

What Bothers Patients After a Heart Attack?

The question of sex after a heart attack bothers them so much so that most patients give up sex. Couples worry about triggering a second heart attack, or even that a patient could die in the bedroom. In fact, the chance of another heart attack during sex is so low that its not worth worrying about.

Does Sexual Activity Increase the Chances of Heart Attack?

There is little danger in having sex after a heart attack. The incidence of heart attack following sexual activity in patients with heart disease is negligble and therefore patients who are stable on therapy may safely engage in sexual activity. For healthy people, the risk is a scant two in a million. If a person has coronary heart disease, the odds rise to only twenty in a million, or 1 in 50,000. Sex usually does not increase the chances of a heart attack except in high risk heart patients.

What is the Effect of Sex on the Heart?

Sex in general is a physical and emotional experience and puts pressure on your heart equal to a brisk walk of 20 minutes. The physiological changes in the body are similar to any physical activity and as you get aroused, your breathing rate, heart rate and blood pressure increase. At the same time your skin also gets flushed and the muscle become tense. As the sexual tension builds up, heart rate and blood pressure rises even more. During orgasm you release this built up tension. The heart beat increases from resting 80 to 180 per minute and systolic blood pressure from 150 to 190. After you attain orgasm, the body relaxes and the built up tension along with heart rate, blood pressure and respiration all return to normal in 3-5 minutes. The individual response is variable and a young and fit person will have a lower heart rate, blood pressure response and energy expenditure as compared to elderly and sedentary people. The energy expenditure during sexual activity is equivalent to a mild to moderate physical exercise and various studies suggest that rarely heart attacks are precipitated by sexual activity.

What Are the Concerns on the Part of the Patients?

A heart patient's sexual activity depends upon the type and severity of heart attack, related complications and the modalities of treatment received. It is also influenced by the age and previous physical activity. People who have recovered from heart attacks will be more aware of their heart beat and the breathing pattern. The slightest chest pain makes them alert. If you are not ready to resume sexual intercourse after a heart attack, it is better that you talk about it to your treating physician. Exercise test after an attack is not only important to decide about the recovery and future treatment protocol, but is also helpful in knowing the individuals performance and this can be used to check their physical capacity. A fair exercise without discomfort is an indication that you can safely resume sex.

When should the Person Resume Sex After an Attack?

If your heart attack is uncomplicated and recovery is uneventful, you can safely resume sexual activity after a couple of weeks. If the routine household activities such as climbing stairs is not causing any discomfort then you can safely have sex after 10-14 days.

How Should One Assess to Safety?

Heart attack patients should not be debarred from sexual activity. In medical terms, the actual energy costs of sexual activity range between 2-6 metabolic equivalents (Mets). This is equivalent to mild to moderate exercise in life such as brisk walking for 20 minutes, or able to walk a couple of flights of stairs or if they can complete four to six minutes of Bruce protocol on a treadmill (TMT). If the said physical activities are performed without any chest discomfort or without any severe shortness of breath, then one can safely resume sexual activity. Patients who are stable on drugs may engage in sexual activity with no discomfort.

When to Perform Sexual Activity?

A heart patient should know and practice healthy ways of life which include a nutritious diet, enough daily exercise and use of medicines. Use of tobacco and alcohol in any form should be avoided. You and your mate must adjust with each other's emotions, feelings and timing. Choose a particular time, depending upon the situation when both of you are mentally and physically relaxed. An early morning or an afternoon session may be more suitable after a good sleep or rest. As applied to any exercise, a heavy or full meal should be avoided and may be taken at least two hours before having sex. A short acting nitrate, a drug used to control angina can be taken an hour before the performance.

Is There any Particular Posture which Helps Heart Patients?

Sexual positions after a heart attack or heart surgery must be taken into consideration. It should be comfortable for the patient and should not pose much physical strain or pressure on the chest wall. It is better to lie by the side or with him or her in front or behind. Utmost care must be practiced not to give undue pressure on the chest or obstruct the proper breathing of the mate. If you have had a bypass surgery and the wound is no longer painful, then be assured that nothing will fall apart, and the stitches will remain intact. You can have full enjoyable experience. Penetration may not be the only way of sexual satisfaction. One can attain it by lying close, caressing or hugging the person, having fore play, masturbation or oral sex. Oral sex will not hurt your heart as long as both you and your partner are comfortable with it. The most important aspect is the realization of the need of the patient. The active part must be played by the healthy partner and the patient should be passive. The role of the healthy partner is very important and he or she should not only know and recognize the symptoms of discomfort but should also realize the ability of the patient and prevent them from overdoing it. Recognizing the ability is important for stability in a sexual relation. A good relation and return to normal sexual life is a boon to the patient giving him or her the confidence that he or she can have a normal life with some precaution.

What is the Overall Impact of Resuming Sexual Activity?

After you have had a heart attack, you may leave the hospital concerned. You may be worried about having sex. You may fear that sex will cause another heart attack or even death and are thus, reluctant to resume sexual activity. Many couples mistakenly believe sex is risky and avoid it. These fears may place a strain on your life and your relationships. They are often afraid, tired, depressed and irritable. Sex is a normal and healthy part of relationships and is important to bring self-confidence, boost morals and ease tension. Thus, having sex after a heart attack often gets you closer to your partner and the reality of life.

What is the Role of the Sexual Partner?

Many patients, especially their spouses, are afraid to have sex because they think it might be very dangerous and may precipitate a second heart attack. The psychology of a heart patient affects his sexual life to a large extent and it is the healthy partner who is the best companion and guide at this hour of need. It is needless to emphasize that the partner is the physician at this select moment of life. Patients are often worried and afraid. They will feel tired and weak all the time with the diet restriction. They may have sleepless nights or they may be sleeping too much under the influence of drugs. They will be more worried about the heart beats, breathing and muscle tension. Full recovery is always in the back of their mind and this makes them more vigilant, concerned and worried while resuming sexual activity. Patients often become hypochondriac. Even a slight chest discomfort makes them alert, which may not always come from the heart. The heart patient's partner must recognize these changes. Do not get panicky or deny or overprotect them from their physical needs. The best solution is to provide moral, emotional and physical support after consulting your doctor or psychologist.

What is the Role of the Treating Doctor?

Sex is an essential aspect of one's life and its importance must be emphasized. A positive impact should be discussed in length without inhibitions. It should be a part and parcel of the treatment protocol. Even in today's modern era, patients rarely ask about this because of embarrassment. Therefore, the doctor should take the lead. The doctor should sense the complaint of their patients as they try to convey it by just saying they are having internal weakness or they get easily fatigued at night. All these are indirect indications that they want to discuss their sexual life. Sex is an individual's choice, act and enjoyment. Therefore, the doctor must talk to both, the patient and the partner. The doctor must first listen carefully to the problems and then suggest the solution which suits them best. In this matter it is not the drug but a danger in having sex after a heart attack which should be explained and will be more helpful in tackling this tricky situation. It is the duty of the doctor to bring back not only the years in their lives, but also the life in their years.

When to Consult Your Doctor?

If you have a chest pain or pressure, upper abdominal pain, a jaw pain, back pain, extreme shortness of breath or an irregular heartbeat during sex, stop the act immediately and rest. If the problem does not subside in a short period of time then do not panic, consult your doctor or hospital. You should always keep nitroglycerine tablets or spray in your bedroom. It should be taken (beneath your tongue) once you experience chest pain (angina) during or after sex.

Who Should Avoid Sex After a Heart Attack?

Certain high-risk patients do need to be more cautious. Patients who had developed complications after the heart attack such as, heart failure or heart pain or dangerous heart rhythms, as all these make them prone to heart attack, fainting or sudden death. If you are having chest discomfort during household activities then you require further investigations and additional treatment. Until these treatments are rendered, work and reduce the cardiac risk one should avoid sex. Also, you should get in touch with your doctor before resuming sexual activity.

Can Anyone Die During Sex?

One can die any time and that includes during sex. We all have heard about deaths occurring during international soccer games to well-trained players. Even after this, soccer is still played, so do not be afraid of sex. The risk is very low or negligible and is no higher than the chances of dying during normal daily activities. Death is common if you are suffering from heart failure or dangerous heart rhythms and you are symptomatic at rest or skipping medication frequently.

Any Heart Drug which Reduces the Sexual Performance?

There are certain medicines which if used for heart problems can affect the sexual desire and performance of the patient. These medicines include those for blood pressure (beta-blockers), fluid pills (diuretics), tranquilizers (for better sleep), antidepressants and some medications used for chest pain and irregular heartbeats. These medicines may cause an inability to maintain an erection in men and frigidity or orgasmic dysfunctions in women. Erectile dysfunction is also common in people addicted to tobacco, alcohol, cocaine, heroin and marijuana- all these should be avoided.

What is the Role of Sildenafil?

Sildenafil citrate or Viagra as it is popularly known is used extensively for the treatment of erectile dysfunction either by choice or by prescription. Erectile dysfunction is common in the elderly, diabetics and heart patients. Very few patients are aware that nitrates, a common drug used in heart patients to control angina, should not be used with sildenafil, 24 - 48 hours before and after, as both these drugs result in dilatation of blood vessels causing lowering of blood pressure and syncope or unconsciousness or even death occasionally. This drug should be avoided by heart patients who take nitrates or nicorandil to control angina as concomitant use of both drugs can lead to severe lowering of blood pressure or hypotension.

Sex and Your Heart at a Glance

1. *Sexual activity is another form of physical activity. Do not feel embarrassed to consult your doctor about it.*
2. *Sex in CHD patient is safe and there is negligible chance of getting chest pain if your symptoms are controlled and if you can perform moderate grade of exercises.*
3. *Anxiety, depression, concern of ability and discomfort, all may affect your sexual life.*
4. *Psychological impotence or lack of desire is common, talk to your partner and physician.*
5. *Always be positive and take medicines as prescribed; a few of the medicines may affect your desire and performance.*
6. *Do not consume tobacco or alcohol.*
7. *The healthy partner should understand and support the patient.*
8. *Having heart disease does not mean the end of an enjoyable sex life.*

Chapter 12

Hypertension

Hypertension, the medical term used for high blood pressure is the most common disease and is a major public health problem for both developed and developing countries. Almost a quarter of the world's population was hypertensive by the end of the twentieth century and it is projected that by the year 2025 almost 30 % of the world population will suffer from high blood pressure. High blood pressure is one of the major risk factors and is responsible for paralytic attacks (stroke), heart disease (heart attack and heart failure), kidney failure and/or vision problems. Out of these, stroke is the major complication due to high blood pressure accounting for millions of paralytic attacks. Various studies have shown beyond doubt that the higher the blood pressure, the greater is the risk. This relationship is consistent in different populations, in younger and older subjects and in men and women alike. Anyone can have high blood pressure and as the age advances, the chances of getting high blood pressure increases. It has been proved beyond doubt that benefits of reducing blood pressure to the normal levels significantly reduce the disability and death associated with it. Hypertension can be easily diagnosed with the help of a simple instrument called a sphygmomanometer. Although cheap and effective therapy is available for this disease, most people with high blood pressure are unaware of their status and fall victim to this dreaded disease unknowingly. Today, the diagnosis and treatment of hypertension is very simple and is within the reach of the common man. Lack of knowledge and ignorance is increasing the disease prevalence and it should be a priority for health personnel and the public to reduce the burden of high blood pressure at all levels.

The Truth of Life

He had retired from an intermediate college as a principal and was one of my jolly natured patients. He was God fearing, satisfied with life and what he had achieved from it. He was also blessed with a stamina and determination that was difficult to duplicate. He was enjoying his life after retirement at his native village and was running a school for the poor and elderly. He was a widower, had a son and a daughter, both of them happily married and settled.

On his visits to my clinic he would ask me not to worry about him as he had completed all his social responsibilities, had seen all walks of life, was fit as a fiddle, performing yoga, taking a brisk walk for an hour and would question the rationale of being on medicines. I use to tell him, you live alone, and your blood pressure is under control both because of your healthy lifestyle and medicines. I know you have no complaints but if you leave or skip the medicine it may cause some problem which may include a heart attack and brain stroke. His comment used to be, 'Doctor are you telling me the truth or are you afraid of the perils of high blood pressure.'

Conversations like this continued. Then one day he walked in after a long gap clutching onto the hand of a boy. I sensed something wrong by the look of his eyes-they were blank and the way in which he was desperately holding onto the hands of his grandson. Sitting down and with tears in his eyes he narrated how he had performed the last rites of his only son sometime back whom he had lost in a tragic roadside accident. He continued that since he was the only earning member and the whole family now depended on his pension, he needed another fifteen years of life for the sake of the family. He further went ahead and promised that he will never skip his medicines. I assured him that his treatment would be looked after by me and his life by God.

Before leaving my chamber he stressed onto the same wish, and this time I could sense a real determination in his voice and a sense of hollowness and desperation in his eyes. Now it was an embarrassing situation and the silence in the chamber was deafening. As it is a well-known fact that nobody can guarantee life in years but his faith towards medical science wanted assurance from me so that he had the moral courage to fight against the odds of life for which he was not prepared. I assured him I shall always be with him. I looked towards the child who was probably unaware of the world around him and feeling secure with his grandfather. The innocent child was holding the hand of his grandfather and waved me goodbye with a cute smile and left me wondering as to what was in his mind? I still imagine whether the old man was holding actually onto life in the form of his grandchild's hands.

Burden of Hypertension in Developing Countries Including India

Hypertension is a major public health problem both for developed and developing countries. The prevalence pattern of hypertension in developing countries is different from that in the developed countries. It is expected that developed countries with an ageing population will have a higher prevalence of hypertension than in a developing country. Hypertension, today, has also become an important health problem in almost all developing countries. As a result, blood pressure related diseases are rapidly rising in developing countries such as China, India, Brazil, Mexico, Russia, Japan, Pakistan, Indonesia, Egypt, Middle East etc. which are currently undergoing rapid epidemiological transition. In China and India, the total number of hypertensive patients is expected to increase to more than one hundred million by the year 2025. Even in some parts of sub-Saharan Africa, a huge burden of blood pressure related diseases are on the rise. The epidemiological transition has a positive impact that it has resulted in an increased life expectancy and concomitant increase in the prevalence of hypertension. This is obvious from several urban and rural studies in India. In India, community surveys have documented that between three and six decades of life, prevalence of hypertension has increased by about 30 times among urban dwellers and by about 10 times among the rural inhabitants in the last three decades.

Various factors might have contributed to this rising trend. Among others, the consequences of urbanization such as changes in lifestyle, food habits, household and work stress, meagre income, increased population and shrinking employment have been named. Lack of physical activity due to automobile revolution has also contributed further to the rise in hypertension. Obesity, both in adulthood and childhood, is on the rise and is expected to further increase the mean blood pressure level in the population of developing countries.

High prevalence of rise in only upper reading of blood pressure that is, systolic hypertension, is cause of concern and is common as the age advances. The studies revealed that almost 50-70 % population suffers from isolated hypertension after 60 years of age in India and the Parsi community has the highest prevalence.

What is Bothering Us?

Hypertension is one of the most easily detectable of diseases, and can be identified by a paramedic. However, measurement of blood pressure, an essential part of the physical examination of any adult, is often neglected in India. Blood pressure measurement is not practiced routinely in every outdoor clinic and is left for medical and cardiac clinics only. Even in large hospitals, blood pressure is not checked regularly in certain clinics. Auxiliary nurses and midwives at the community level should examine blood pressure as a part of antenatal care, as pregnancy-induced hypertension is a major contributor to maternal mortality in India, yet this is rarely done. An urban Chennai study revealed that only half of the hypertension cases were detected, of which only half received therapy, and a further half of it were adequately controlled. The situation in rural areas is worse. Only 7 % of patients in a study from Rajasthan were aware of their hypertension.

What is Blood Pressure?

When the heart pumps, it forces blood through your blood vessels. This force is exerted on the walls of the blood vessel or artery. Thus, blood pressure is the amount of force exerted by the heart against the walls of the arteries. The measurement of blood pressure is recorded in two numbers and measured in millimetres of mercury (mmHg). It is expressed as 120 over 80 (120/80 mmHg) as the blood pressure reading. The upper number is termed systolic blood pressure. It represents the force of the blood in your blood vessel when the heart pumps and the lower number is called diastolic blood pressure which denotes the force of blood in the blood vessels when the heart is at rest. The blood pressure readings vary with the age, sex and built of the person. It also varies according to the activity, mood and behaviour of the person. In a normal adult, the systolic blood pressure ranges from 100 to 140 mmHg and diastolic blood pressure 60-90 mmHg.

What is High Blood Pressure?

A person's blood pressure is considered high when the readings are higher than 140 mmHg systolic (the upper number in the blood pressure reading) or 90 mmHg diastolic (the lower number). A consistent blood pressure reading of 140/90 mmHg or higher in an adult is considered high blood pressure. To diagnose a person having high blood pressure, the readings should be more than 140/90 mm Hg at least on three different occasions and times of day. A very high single reading of blood pressure can also indicate hypertension.

Definition of Hypertension

To reduce confusion and provide more consistent advice to doctors across the globe, the definition and classification provided by JNC VII (Joint National Committee on Prevention, Detection, Evaluation and Treatment of high blood pressure) is used in clinical practice (Table - 12.1). This is followed widely in India for the diagnosis of hypertension. The following classification for diagnosis of hypertension and its treatment is applicable for person of more than 18 years:

Table -12.1: JNC VII Classification of Hypertension

Category	Systolic or higher blood pressure (mm of Hg)	Diastolic or lower blood pressure (mm of Hg)
Normal	<120	<80
Pre-hypertension	120-139	80-89
HYPERTENSION		
Stage 1	140-159	90-99
Stage 2	160-179	100-109
Stage 3	>180	>110
Isolated Systolic Hypertension	>140	<90

Why should one Worry about High Blood Pressure?

High blood pressure is a major health hazard and is responsible for adult disability and death. The disease goes undiagnosed or is detected late, as it causes no or little discomfort to the person. The problem is further aggravated due to ignorance. Effective therapy has been available for more than 50 years but most hypertensives in India do not have their blood pressure under control as they are unaware of the risks associated with high blood pressure.

What are the Health Risks Linked with High Blood Pressure?

With high blood pressure, the heart works harder and the arteries are stressed.

The maximum adverse effects of high blood pressure are observed on various important organs of the body. The chances of getting brain haemorrhage (paralytic attack), heart attack or heart failure, vision loss and kidney problems are greater with uncontrolled or poorly controlled high blood pressure as compared to normal blood pressure.

Why Hypertension is Termed as the SILENT KILLER?

In a majority of people, symptoms related to hypertension are few and vague. This is because hypertension doesn't cause problems over a short period of time. As the blood pressure rise is slow, the heart adjusts by making its muscles stronger. This compensatory mechanism along with excess reserve of heart tries to overcome the ill effects of high blood pressure till it fails. Therefore, it usually takes several years for high blood pressure to cause noticeable complaints. During this period, the patients generally have no problems. Even when it does cause a problem, the complaints are often mild and non-specific. It has been found that 10 % patients present with life threatening complications of hypertension as their first presentation such as paralytic attacks (brain, haemorrhage), heart attack, heart failure, blindness or end stage renal disease (terminal kidney problem), bleeding from nose, and they land up in the emergency room of hospitals without any prior warning signal or symptoms. That is why high blood pressure is termed as a SILENT KILLER.

What are the Symptoms of Hypertension?

High blood pressure often has no complaints or symptoms. There are very few who feel the problem related with high blood pressure, and some of the common symptoms are headache, confusion, giddiness, weakness, fatigue, shortness of breath, and/or getting irritated or tense easily. These symptoms are so vague that they are often overlooked or ignored. This is the main reason why many people don't seek medical advice, until they have more severe symptoms from organ damage that chronic hypertension can cause.

Why should I Get my Blood Pressure Checked Even if I am Healthy?

High blood pressure in the initial stages rarely gives any problem. Having a regular check up enables your doctor to detect any problem early and start the treatment in time. Timely treatment ameliorates the harmful effects related with high blood pressure. Hence, its dangers can be avoided or postponed. The only way to determine if you have high blood pressure is to be tested for it. Using a simple blood pressure instrument, your doctor or health giver can easily tell whether your blood pressure is high or not.

What are Blood Pressure Fluctuations?

The body is a dynamic structure; therefore, blood pressure fluctuates throughout the day depending upon the state and need of the body. Blood pressure normally rises early in the morning, varies during the day depending upon the activity and falls during sleep. When the body is at rest, such as during sleep, the blood pressure can be as low as 100/60 mmHg and at routine working conditions it may be 120/80 mmHg in healthy adults. When you are exercising like running, swimming, playing, it may rise upto 160/100 mmHg or even more. Blood pressure can rise during anxiety, stress, emotions or excitement. This fluctuation of blood pressure is the need of the body and is a normal phenomenon. It returns to the normal level quickly once the body is at rest or relaxed. The myth that my blood pressure should be 120/80 mmHg is not true as it is not a static number. It only represents an average reading.

What Contributes to Hypertension?

Even after so much of advancement in medical knowledge, it is difficult to pinpoint what contributes to high blood pressure in the majority of individuals. Apart from advancing age, faulty living style and habits which increase the risk or chances of high blood pressure, a few contributing factors are:

1. Age: Blood vessels may become stiffer and narrower with advancing age. Thus, age predisposes to high blood pressure.
2. High Salt Intake: Retain excess water in the body and building up pressure on the heart.

3. Sedentary or easy going lifestyle.
4. Tobacco smoking or chewing.
5. Alcohol abuse.
6. High levels of saturated fat in diet.
7. Obesity.
8. Stress.
9. Diabetes mellitus.
10. Family History of hypertension: Siblings have a greater chance of blood pressure if either or both parents are hypertensive.

What is Primary Hypertension?

Primary hypertension means that high blood pressure is present without any detectable or known disease in the body. It is also known as idiopathic hypertension and constitutes the major chunk. In 90 % of hypertensive patients, there is no obvious underlying disease responsible for high blood pressure.

What is Secondary Hypertension?

Secondary hypertension is defined as high blood pressure caused by some underlying disease in the body and it contributes to almost 10 % of all causes of hypertension. Kidney disease is the commonest secondary cause for hypertension.

What are the Common Diseases which can Cause Secondary Hypertension?

There are certain diseases which can cause secondary hypertension. Some of the common diseases are:
1. Renal disease (kidney ailment).
2. Renal artery stenosis or blockage of blood supply to the kidneys.

3. Phaechromocytoma-a disease of the adrenal glands which are situated above the kidneys.
4. Hyper-function of thyroid gland or thyrotoxicosis (a gland in the neck).
5. Coarctation of the aorta, narrowing of descending aorta in the chest, a birth defect of the aorta, the main artery emerging from the heart which supplies blood to all parts of the body.

How can you Differentiate Between Primary and Secondary Hypertension?

People with primary hypertension belong to the relatively older age group with few symptoms and require only one or two drugs to control their high blood pressure. On the contrary, people with secondary hypertension are young, presenting with more symptoms and hypertension related complications. Secondary hypertension is difficult to control even with multiple combinations of drugs.

(It is advised to consult the treating doctor before making any inference from this text.)

Is High Blood Pressure Harmful if Left Untreated?

Yes. Initially high blood pressure is tolerated by the reserves in the heart, and it usually takes several years for problems from hypertension to become noticeable. Unfortunately, if left untreated or uncontrolled, then in the coming years, serious irreversible damage may occur to the body resulting in serious complications. Once high blood pressure is controlled, then the only difference between you and other healthy subjects of your age is that your high blood pressure is controlled on drugs and in others it is naturally controlled. You enjoy the same risk-free life as your healthy counterparts.

When to Consult Your Doctor Immediately?

There are situations when a person should immediately contact the physician. The few of the reasons are as follows:

1. If your blood pressure is not controlled, despite the drugs and lifestyle measures.
2. If you develop swelling of the body or oedema.
3. If you are pregnant.
4. If you get giddy on standing.
5. If you are short of breath, either at rest or during exertion.
6. If your sexual performance has deteriorated as some drugs and high blood pressure can cause this.
7. If you are having visionary problem, chest pain or headache.

What are the Common Drugs which can Cause High Blood Pressure?

High blood pressure can be caused by certain drugs if used for long. Use of oral contraceptive pills is the commonest drug which can raise the blood pressure. Anabolic steroids used for boosting performance and increasing the muscle mass may be associated with high blood pressure. Some of the pain killers and antipsychotic drugs, if used for a longer period may be associated with high blood pressure.

How to Evaluate Hypertensive Patients?

All patients should be evaluated to know how long they have been suffering from high blood pressure. Is anyone else in the family like mother, father, brother, sister also suffering from high blood pressure or is there a family history of high blood pressure. If either of the above situation exists then what treatment needs to be undertaken? The evaluation should also include assessment of the severity of high blood pressure, its effect on various organs of the body, any underlying disease or drug which can cause or aggravate the high blood pressure and the response to the therapy. The data for evaluation are acquired through medical history, physical examination, lab testing and special diagnostic procedures in some cases.

Investigation for all Patients with Hypertension

Certain blood and urine investigations are mandatory for all patients suffering with high blood pressure. It helps in detecting the cause, effect and other commonly associated diseases with or due to hypertension. The routine tests are as follows:

1. Examination of morning urine sample.
2. Complete blood count.
3. Blood chemistry (potassium, sodium, urea and creatinine).
4. Glucose estimation after overnight fasting and after two hours of meals.
5. Fasting total cholesterol and lipid estimation.
6. Standard 12-leads ECG.
7. X-ray of chest.
8. Ultrasound study of whole abdomen.
9. Echocardiography.

Investigations for Specific Patient Subgroups

For those with diabetes or chronic kidney disease or patients of secondary hypertension, additional specific tests are required.

One should assess urinary protein excretion, since lower blood pressure targets are appropriate if protein leak is present in urine. For those suspected of having an endocrine cause for high blood pressure, specific tests such as thyroid function tests, urinary excretions of catecholamines, metanephrines and vanillylmandelic acid for phaeochromocytoma are required. Evaluation of arteries supplying to the kidneys or aorta with the help of an angiography should be done to know about the reno-vascular and coarctation of the aorta respectively as a cause for hypertension may be needed in a few cases. Other secondary forms of hypertension require specific testing which may include a CT scan of the causative organ in the body.

What is the Treatment of Hypertension?

It is important to keep your blood pressure under control. The treatment goal is to keep blood pressure below 140/90 mmHg and even lower than 130/85 mmHg for people who suffer from diabetes and kidney disease. Adopting a healthy lifestyle is an effective first step in both preventing and controlling high blood pressure. If lifestyle changes alone are not effective in keeping your pressure controlled, it may be necessary to put you on medicines. It is advised that drugs should be used under the supervision of your doctor and self-medication should be avoided and discouraged. A common practice in India is people indulge in self-medication. Once they know that they are hypertensive, they frequently use and try medicines prescribed to either their spouse or parents without consulting a doctor.

Can I Stop my Medicines Once my Blood Pressure is Controlled?

No. Your high blood pressure is controlled because of the medicines and lifestyle modifications and you have to continue it lifelong unless the treating doctor advises on the contrary. A majority of the patients stop their medicines either assuming that they are cured or require it for a limited period so they fail to turn up at the scheduled appointment. Do not stop the medication by yourself and without consulting your doctor.

Are the Medicines Harmful if I Take them for a Longer Period?

No. It is a false belief that taking medicines to control high blood pressure for years can damage your liver or kidneys. On the contrary, if high blood pressure is not controlled in the long run it will cause damage to the brain, kidneys, eyes and heart. The second common myth is if the medicines are taken for years they will lose their potency and will not be effective which is again not true. As age advances, arteries become stiff and further raise your blood pressure. Because of this the person may require a new medicine or an increase in the dose of the same medicine.

Do I have to Take the Medicine Life Long?

May be yes, since high blood pressure cannot be cured and the only remedy left is to control it properly. To enjoy the benefits linked with the control of hypertension, it is advisable to continue the medicine unless suggested by your doctor either to stop or reduce the dose. Even if the blood pressure is controlled by lifestyle modifications only, still it must be closely monitored and supervised.

What is the Role of Salt?

Excess of dietary salt can increase the chances of high blood pressure or it can create difficulty in controlling it. Excess salt increases the likelihood of the body to retain water thereby contributing to the development of high blood pressure by creating an additional pressure on the heart.

If I Stop Salt Intake Altogether, can I Control my Blood Pressure?

No, it is a myth that merely removing salt from diet can control high blood pressure. It should not be practiced as a routine because salt is essential in Indian climatic conditions for the proper functioning of the body. In tropical countries, including India because of the hot and humid weather conditions, sodium is lost through sweat and this loss is maximized during summer season. Considering this, a salt-free diet can lead to an electrolyte (sodium, potassium and chloride) imbalance in the body and can result in fatigue, muscle weakness and sometimes unconsciousness. Salt-free diets do more harm than any benefit. As it is not palatable, patients are uncomfortable, go into depression, lose weight and become weak. It cannot be practiced for long periods and should not be encouraged in India unless and until it is associated with severe heart failure.

How Much Salt should I Take?

A normal person requires 6-8 gm of common salt per day. In India 90 % of salt requirement is met by the salt which is added during cooking. Excess salt is present in pickles, papad, chutneys, chips, salted wafers, canned foods, packaged soups, butter, bread, ketchups and sauce. Salt dressing on salads is also one of the extra sources of salt in Indian food. A key to healthy eating is choosing foods lower in salt and sodium. The current recommendation is to consume less than 2.4 gm (2,400 mg) of sodium a day. That equals 5 gm (about 1 teaspoon) of table salt a day. People with high blood pressure can safely consume 3-5 gm of salt per day. Considering the Indian subcontinent climate, consuming common salt in diet such as that used for preparing vegetables and pulses may be sufficient. However, one should curtail the intake of all the extra or table salt. This saves the burden of not only preparing extra food for the person in the family who is having high blood pressure, but also makes his food tasty (just try salt-free meals a few times and you can experience the agony). If a person is suffering from heart failure with high blood pressure, then the salt intake must be reduced and for this the person can take the help of the doctor or dietician. Low sodium salt preparations are available in the market. However, these are expensive and increase unnecessary financial burden with little benefit.

What is the DASH Plan?

This dietary and lifestyle plan helps not only in preventing high blood pressure but also helps in controlling high blood pressure. The National Heart, Lung and Blood Institute (NHLBI) in the United States have released guidelines designed to help, prevent and treat high blood pressure. The guidelines recommend that Americans follow the Dietary Approaches to Stop Hypertension (DASH) plan, which involves eating a diet rich in fruits, vegetables and non-fat dairy products. The NHLBI also recommends several types of lifestyle changes. These include losing excess weight, becoming physically active, limiting alcoholic beverages and following a heart-healthy diet, including cutting back on salt and other forms of sodium.

The DASH diet with a low sodium (1500 mg) or 1.5 gm of salt led to mean systolic blood pressure that was 7.1 mmHg lower than in participants without high blood pressure and 11.5 mmHg lower in hypertensives.

Is there any Herbal Treatment for High Blood Pressure?

The answer is NO. Till date no herbal treatment gives long lasting, smooth control of high blood pressure. At best it should be avoided. Even some herbs like licorice, ma hung and yohimbine can increase blood pressure.

Measuring Blood Pressure

Whether I should Measure my Blood Pressure at Home or Not?

Having your blood pressure tested is quick and easy. People with high blood pressure should be taught how to measure blood pressure at home and they should be encouraged for the following reasons:

1. It increases the awareness and involves the person in the treatment.
2. It gives an idea of the overall control of blood pressure.
3. It increases the responsibility of the person and gives them an opportunity for healthy interaction with the treating doctor.
4. It increases the adherence with the treatment protocol because patient's non-compliance is the commonest cause of drug default.

What Precautions should I Take Before Getting my Blood Pressure Checked?

The following precautions should be taken care of before a blood pressure check, either at home or in a clinic:

1. Wear loose clothes so the arm can be fully exposed for the cuff.
2. Sit quietly for at least 5 minutes and relax yourself before getting the blood pressure tested.
3. Bowel and bladder should be empty before the measurement.
4. Do not consume coffee, alcohol or smoke before measuring your blood pressure.
5. Get two readings. If the values vary widely, talk to your physician.
6. Keep your hand steady and instrument at the level of your heart.

Which Instrument is Best for Blood Pressure Measurement?

Of course, mercury blood pressure (sphygmomanometer) instrument is the best but it requires trained personnel and help of another person during the measurement. Electronic and digital instruments are becoming popular. In these devices, blood pressure readings are displayed on a small screen and no stethoscope is required for measurement. These instruments are best suited for home or self-measurement as they are handy and require no assistance. To measure the blood pressure at home, it is advised to sit on a chair and rest your arm on a table in front of you. Place the blood pressure instrument on the table so that it is at the level of your heart and take at least two readings. Do not move your hand or body while measuring your blood pressure. The instrument should be calibrated once in 6 months and the first reading must be taken in front of your doctor who can assist or guide you with the correct method and how to tie the cuff around your arm.

Is there any Difference in Right and Left Hand Blood Pressure and in which hand should it be Measured?

The blood pressure may not be equal in left and right arm. There may be a difference of 5-10 mmHg in systolic pressure that is, upper blood pressure which is normal. It should be measured in both arms and if there is a difference then in subsequent visits it must be measured on the arm with the higher reading. If the difference is more than 10 mmHg then consult your doctor for further advice. The blood pressure of both arms in paralytic patients should be monitored routinely as blood pressure is either high or low in the paralytic arm of stroke patients as compared to the healthy arm.

How to Increase the Patient's Compliance for drug Therapy?

Even though blood pressure detection is easy and there is effective treatment with proven benefit, drug compliance is the biggest problem in proper control of blood pressure in both developed and developing countries. In India, the asymptomatic status of disease, lack of knowledge, fear of taking medicines for longer periods and the myth that allopathic drugs may damage body organs prevent people from taking drugs properly. The cost of the drug and multiple pills are also important reasons for drug non-compliance in India. All the patients should be encouraged to take drugs regularly and the following measures should be practiced:

1. They should be taught the benefit of controlling high blood pressure.
2. They should know the harm linked with leaving or skipping drugs.

3. Minimal drugs should be prescribed and frequent dose schedules should be avoided. If possible use of combination drugs may be encouraged.
4. Drug intake must be linked with the daily routine, such as taking drugs after brushing one's teeth, at the breakfast table or after dinner
5. Drug intake must be assisted by the family members for children or for elderly, patients with diabetes mellitus and people with vision problems.
6. Keep a reminder note either on the refrigerator, or the dinning table, study table, at the place of worship or *pooja ghar*, an alarm in your cell phone or computer.
7. Try to prescribe drugs which are pocket friendly to patients.
8. The name of the drug should be written in local language also.

Hypertension During Pregnancy

Pregnancy is the most beautiful phase of a woman's life and all over the world the desire to be a mother is very high in family and society. Staying healthy during pregnancy is of utmost importance and mainly depends on you. It is in the best interest of your health as well as the child to get yourself checked regularly. Throughout pregnancy, it is mandatory to check the weight, blood pressure, haemoglobin and urine samples of the mother. Low levels of haemoglobin or anaemia in women is very common in countries with low and middle income, but high blood pressure during pregnancy is equally important and can complicate the issue. It may be dangerous for the well-being of the mother as well as the foetus. High blood pressure may be present before pregnancy or in a few it may develop during pregnancy. Whatever is the time of development of high blood pressure it should be monitored and controlled throughout pregnancy and even after delivery.

What are the Normal Changes in the Heart During Pregnancy?

During pregnancy, the growing foetus gets all its nutrition from the mother through the placenta via the umbilical cord. This increased demand is met by increasing the blood volume of the mother which may rise upto 50 %. Increase in the heart rate of the mother to the tune of 10-20 % is also normal. Both the effects help the heart to pump 30 % more blood to meet the extra requirements for the healthy development of the foetus. Slight swelling of feet is also common during the later phase of pregnancy. Throughout pregnancy, the blood pressure remains normal or lower to a certain extent but having high blood pressure is not a normal feature during pregnancy.

What is Pregnancy Induced Hypertension?

Some women develop high blood pressure while they are pregnant (often called gestational hypertension or pregnancy induced hypertension). Gestational hypertension is noticed during pregnancy only and it disappears within 6 months of termination or delivery. It is usually not more than 160 mmHg and often noticed after the third month of pregnancy. Studies suggest that gestational hypertension apart from the immediate effect, may increase the risk of high blood pressure and stroke later on in life.

What are the Effects of High Blood Pressure During Pregnancy?

Many pregnant women with high blood pressure have healthy babies without serious problems. However, high blood pressure during pregnancy can be dangerous for both the mother and the foetus. Women with pre-existing, or chronic, high blood pressure are more likely to have certain complications during pregnancy than those with normal blood pressure. The effects of high blood pressure range from mild to severe. High blood pressure can harm the mother's kidneys and other organs, it can cause low birth weight and early delivery or premature abortions. In more serious cases, the mother develops pre-eclampsia or 'toxaemia of pregnancy' which can threaten the lives of both the mother and the foetus.

What Is Pre-eclampsia?

Pre-eclampsia is a complex disorder that affects 3 to 8 % of pregnant women. Pre-eclampsia, also known as toxaemia, is a severe complication during pregnancy, which causes soaring blood pressure and swelling of the hands and feet. It starts in the later part of pregnancy, usually after the twentieth week and is related to increased blood pressure and a protein leak in the mother's urine. Pre-eclampsia affects the placenta, and it can also affect the mother's kidney, liver, and brain. Pre-eclampsia can develop slowly or at a rapid pace and its effects are mild to severe. When pre-eclampsia causes fits or seizures, the condition is known as eclampsia and is a serious condition. Eclampsia is one of the leading causes of maternal death during pregnancy in a majority of developing countries including India. It can cause premature delivery, maternal and foetal illness, and even death.

There is no proven way to prevent pre-eclampsia. Most women who develop signs of pre-eclampsia, however, are closely monitored to lessen or avoid related problems. If it progresses fast or gets worse then the only way to 'cure' pre-eclampsia is to get the baby delivered.

Prevalence

In India, the incidence of pre-eclampsia in hospital delivery varies widely from 5 % to 15 %. Imperfect documentation and lack of uniformity in the diagnostic criteria are responsible for the wide variation in frequency. Women in their first pregnancy suffer more commonly as compared to those with multiple pregnancies (15 % vs 5 %). It is as high as 20-25 % in women with a history of chronic hypertension.

Who is More Likely to Develop Pre-eclampsia?

There are a subset of women who are prone to develop pre-eclampsia and they are:

1. Women with chronic hypertension (high blood pressure before becoming pregnant).
2. Women who developed high blood pressure or pre-eclampsia during a previous pregnancy, especially if these conditions occurred early during the pregnancy.
3. Women who are obese prior to pregnancy.
4. Pregnant women under the age of 20 years or over 40 years.
5. Women who are pregnant with more than one foetus.
6. Women with diabetes, kidney disease, rheumatoid arthritis (joint problems), certain skin disorders such as lupus or scleroderma.

How to Detect Pre-eclampsia?

Unfortunately, there is no single test to predict or diagnose pre-eclampsia. Key signs are increased blood pressure and presence of excess protein in the urine (proteinuria). Other symptoms that seem to occur with pre-eclampsia include persistent headaches, blurred vision or sensitivity to light, oedema of lower limbs and abdominal pain.

When to Consult Your Doctor Urgently?

There are situations when patients of pre-eclampsia should get prompt attention and urgent admission in hospital to save both mother and foetus. If a woman complains of blurred vision, headache, pain in the abdomen and difficulty in breathing, and her diastolic blood pressure is more than 110 mmHg, there is new onset of protein leak in urine or there is deterioration in kidney function such as when serum creatinine rises to more than 2 mg/dl. They should be immediately hospitalized to avoid further complications. Even growth retardation in the foetus should be taken seriously.

How can Women with High Blood Pressure Prevent Problems during Pregnancy?

If you have hypertension and want to become pregnant or you are already pregnant you should consult your doctor and take certain precautions such as:

1. Blood pressure should be controlled before and during pregnancy.
2. You should avoid alcohol or tobacco use.
3. If you are obese or overweight, try to reduce it.
4. Take the prescribed medicines regularly. Only a few blood pressure lowering drugs should be avoided during pregnancy and your doctor is the best guide.
5. Get your urine checked on every visit for protein leak or when your doctor advices.
6. Always go for hospital and supervised delivery by qualified personal. Avoid home delivery or delivery administered by midwives or untrained hands.

I have High Blood Pressure. What Precaution should I Take if I want to Become Pregnant?

One should not worry as women with high blood pressure can become pregnant safely. They should not leave the drug prescribed for high blood pressure. They should consult their doctor before planning their pregnancy as some medicines used for high blood pressure may be harmful to the foetus. A person should be advised to take only those medicines before conception and during pregnancy which are safe for the mother and have no adverse effect on the growing foetus. Utmost care must be taken in the first three months of pregnancy as this is the time when maximum foetal development occurs. Pregnancy is precious for both the mother and the child. It should be monitored closely with meticulous control of blood pressure. Delivery of pregnant women with high blood pressure is normal in a majority of cases. However, a few may require caesarean section to deliver and this procedure is safe as long as the blood pressure is under control.

Special Situations in Hypertension

What is the Role of 24 Hour Ambulatory Blood Pressure monitoring?

Ambulatory blood pressure monitoring (ABPM) takes numerous readings of your blood pressure over a 24-hour period or longer. It provides accurate and reliable information and can give you and your doctor a true picture of your blood pressure than occasional visits and readings taken at your doctor's office.

Who Benefits from Ambulatory Blood Pressure Monitoring?

ABPM is not popular in developing countries including the Indian subcontinent. However, it is now a routine procedure in Europe and the United States to evaluate hypertension and related conditions such as:

1. **'White Coat' Hypertension:** This means that you only have high blood pressure when you are in the doctor's chamber.
2. **Resistant Hypertension:** This is diagnosed when multiple drug regimen fails to control high blood pressure as measured in the doctor's clinic.
3. **Borderline Hypertension:** Sometimes people have high normal blood pressure readings.
4. **Episodic Hypertension:** ABPM can help detect periodic high blood pressure that indicates another medical problem. ABPM can also help detect high blood pressure associated with some anxiety syndromes.

What is Pre-Hypertension?

There is a situation in which patients are not hypertensive but most of the time their blood pressure is on the higher side of normal. Pre-hypertension is defined as systolic blood pressure between 120 and 139 mmHg and a diastolic blood pressure between 80 and 89 mmHg. About one-fourth of adults have pre-hypertension and some of them may develop high blood pressure in the future. The chances of getting high blood pressure is high, if they are obese, have a family history of high blood pressure, smoke, consume alcohol, lead a sedentary and stressful life. Since these people are more prone to develop high blood pressure in the future, they should be encouraged to adopt a healthy lifestyle to prevent the development of high blood pressure. They may also require a more aggressive approach than people with normal blood pressure.

What is Accelerated Hypertension?

About 1 % of the people with high blood pressure can develop a severe form known as accelerated or malignant hypertension. This is due to skipping medicines or receiving inadequate doses of medicines.

There is a severe elevation in the blood pressure, especially the lower one, that is, diastolic blood pressure (DBP) is higher than 130 mmHg. In this condition, it is not the absolute value of blood pressure but the rate in rise of blood pressure, which is more important. Rapid rise in the blood pressure can damage vital organs of the body. This may be life threatening. When hypertension becomes so severe that it can threaten the life of the person, it is compulsory to admit all such patients into a hospital. People with malignant hypertension often present with blurred or loss of vision, headache, nausea or vomiting, confusion and/or delirium or coma. In principle, all people suffering from DBP more than 130 mmHg should be treated under close supervision of a physician, irrespective of their complaints or complications.

Isolated Systolic Hypertension

Both numbers in a blood pressure reading are important. As we grow older, systolic blood pressure becomes more important because of the hardening of blood vessels. When only the upper pressure that is, systolic blood pressure is high and the lower one that is, diastolic blood pressure is normal it is called isolated systolic hypertension (ISH). Isolated systolic hypertension is equally important and it must be treated to prevent the complications linked with isolated systolic hypertension. The prevalence of isolated systolic hypertension is rapidly increasing with the increased life expectancy in India. Isolated systolic hypertension is diagnosed when only systolic blood pressure is more than 140 mmHg. It is the most common form of high blood pressure for older people across the globe. It occurs in more than two thirds of the individuals after 65 years of age. In this age group it is the cause of concern as they have the lowest rates of blood pressure control. Risk factors for isolated systolic hypertension include being older, being overweight, smoking and having diabetes. If left uncontrolled, isolated systolic hypertension can lead to all the complications of hypertension, especially brain haemorrhage or stroke which is the leading cause of death at this age.

What is Low Blood Pressure?

Low blood pressure is defined as, when blood pressure readings fall below 90/60 mmHg. In many countries, low blood pressure is regarded as a sign of excellent health, and it is certainly true that it is associated with a good outlook from the point of view of risks of strokes and heart attacks. In other countries, such as Germany and in India, it is regarded as a disease responsible for symptoms of weakness and fatigue.

Is Low Blood Pressure Harmful?

As long as low blood pressure is not associated with symptoms such as giddiness, fatigue, weakness or a feeling of being run down, it is thought of as beneficial for heart's health. Low blood pressure does not cause any pressure or burden on the functioning of the heart and blood vessels. If low blood pressure is due to certain medical conditions such as, following the excessive loss of fluid or blood or following heart attack or high fever it should be treated promptly.

What is Postural Hypotension?

Postural hypotension is defined as a drop in blood pressure (hypotension) due to a change in the body's position (posture) resulting in an inadequate supply of blood to the brain. It is also known as orthostatic hypotension. It is defined as a 10 mmHg drop in diastolic or a drop of 20 mmHg or more in systolic blood pressure occurring within three minutes of getting up. This occurs when a person moves to a more vertical position that is, from sitting to standing or from lying down to sitting or standing. Postural hypotension is more common in older people. It is also seen in a water depletion state or dehydration, after prolonged bed rest, in patients of diabetic neuropathy, and certain drugs which cause dilatation of blood vessels (vasodilators). A person suffering from postural hypotension can experience dizziness, blackouts or fainting.

What is the Treatment For Postural Hypotension?

Usually no treatment is needed for postural hypotension. If someone with postural hypotension faints, consciousness can be regained by simply sitting or lying down or raising their feet. Since there is no treatment, the person is advised to stand up slowly and in stages, take plenty of fluids, avoid self-medication and avoid a certain class of drugs such as vasodilator drugs.

Coffee or Tea and Its Relation With Blood Pressure

Caffeine in coffee as well as in other drinks, such as tea and colas are consumed daily by a majority of Indians. It raises the blood pressure slightly in normal people but more so in cases of high blood pressure. A normal person can continue to take 3-4 cups of coffee or cola per day safely without any adverse effect on blood pressure as the rise is temporary and harmless. Beyond the possible pressure effect, increased coffee consumption is also associated with an increased risk of worsening of existing coronary heart disease due to rhythm disturbances and it is better to avoid or limit it in patients with heart disease. Data suggests that you should continue to have drinks that contain caffeine, unless you are sensitive to it or have heart disease and your doctor advises against it. Heart patients should be aware of the caffeine content in their drink.

Alcohol and Blood Pressure

The consumption of more than 2 pegs (60 ml) of ethanol per day is associated with a higher prevalence of high blood pressure. Light or moderate consumption of alcohol daily may be associated with a better heart health. However, this positive effect of alcohol consumption must be weighed against other consequences of alcohol consumption. It should be avoided in all, as unrestricted increased consumption and binge alcohol drinking is common in India and may result in the rapid surge of blood pressure as well as alcohol abuse. The simultaneous intake of snacks rich in salt and fat will not only increase the blood pressure but also make control of blood pressure difficult and contribute towards weight gain.

Oral Contraceptives and Blood Pressure

Women taking oral contraceptives experience a small but detectable increase in both systolic and diastolic blood pressure. This rise in blood pressure is less with the newer formulations and most of the women who develop high blood pressure, the disease is mild; and blood pressure returns to normal once the oral contraceptives are stopped. Only a few women develop hypertension and require treatment. Talk to your doctor about a possible rise in blood pressure and if it occurs, other forms of contraception may be adopted. Women who smoke and use oral contraceptive pills are at a greater risk of heart disease, stroke and development of hypertension. The same is true with women suffering from diabetes. They should all be encouraged to quit smoking and control their diabetes.

Stress and High Blood Pressure

Stress can make blood pressure go up for a while, and it has been thought to contribute to high blood pressure. However, the long term effects of stress are as yet unclear. Stress management techniques do help in preventing high blood pressure. Such techniques may have other benefits, such as making you feel better or helping you to control overeating, so they should be adopted by all.

Can Children Suffer from High Blood Pressure?

Yes, children can also have high blood pressure. However, there is no cut off definition for children. It is defined according to their age, sex, height and weight. Secondary causes of hypertension such as kidney disease, coarctation of the aorta (a congenital narrowing or constriction of the aorta), disease of adrenal gland are more common in children.

How Helpful is the Lifestyle in the Treatment of Hypertension?

Lifestyle modifications to a certain extent help in the prevention and control of hypertension. Lifestyle changes which have a proven scientific role are losing weight if you are overweight (losing weight can reduce blood pressure by 5-20 mmHg), increasing physical activity (45 minutes per day can reduce blood pressure by 5-9 mmHg), intake of sodium or salt reduction (2-8 mmHg reduction), alcohol consumption in moderation, choosing a healthy eating pattern that includes fruits, vegetables and low fat products. If lifestyle modifications alone are not helpful in controlling your blood pressure, today different groups of safe drugs are available which can be added as per the advice of your physician.

Why have I Developed High Blood Pressure at 40 while my Parents had it in their Late Fifties?

It is a common question when you know that your high blood pressure is due to the fact that it runs in the family. This can be partially explained by the fact that our parents probably didn't have a high level of stress, lived in joint families, had routine physical activity/exercise and obesity was less common. Their life used to be less competitive and they were satisfied with their achievements. Cycling used to be part of their daily life and was a common mode of transport while it is replaced today by motorcycles and cars. The message should be that even if my parents had high blood pressure doesn't mean that I am going to have it too. I shall be more vigilant and will take better care of myself.

What can be Done to Prevent Hypertension?

One should practice simple things in our day to day life. Just adopt a healthy lifestyle such as, increase the intake of seasonal fruits, vegetables and toned milk. Simultaneously increase the amount of daily physical activity for at least an hour apart from your daily routine. The daily intake of salt should be reduced; and salted nuts, *namkeens* and fried foods should be consumed occasionally. Maintain an ideal weight and reduce excess weight, if any. A sedentary lifestyle is the biggest culprit and should be avoided. Say no to tobacco in any form. Practice yoga and meditation (Table 12.2).

Table 12.2: Recommended Lifestyle Modifications From American Heart Association For High Blood Pressure for Its Prevention and Management

Lose weight and maintain ideal weight.
Limit alcohol intake - 60 ml of whisky, 200 ml of wine and 650 ml of beer.
Increase aerobic exercises - 30-45 minutes per day.
Reduce salt intake and consume not more than 6 gms of salt per day.
Maintain an adequate intake of potassium (fruits).
Consume enough calcium (mild and milk products).
Say NO to tobacco consumption and smoking.
Reduce intake of saturated fat.

What is Bothering us Today?

Today, high blood pressure can be diagnosed with little effort and can be effectively treated with cheap medicines. In spite of all this, it is still on the rise in India. Few factors given below are a cause of concern today and are bothering us despite all the advancement in the field of diagnosis and treatment for high blood pressure:

1. The blood pressure is not measured if one consults a doctor for minor health problems.
2. Lack of proper education and awareness among patients, paramedics and even physicians to an extent.
3. People are either ignorant or know very little about the risks attributed to high blood pressure.
4. The majority are not aware of the benefits of controlling blood pressure.
5. Young individuals do not adopt a healthy lifestyle so that the disease can be postponed or prevented for the next generation.
6. Little is thought or done to take steps to assist patients adhere to antihypertensive, lifestyle and drug therapies.
7. Poor adherence to antihypertensive therapy is a major barrier in the treatment and control of hypertension and prevention of hypertensive complications.
8. Patient adherence can be improved by awareness and education.
9. The name of the drug is written in English. For better drug compliance, it should be written in the local language also on the strip.
10. Myths associated with high blood pressure and the allopathic medicines attain less attention.
11. A false belief that a salt-free diet can cure the disease.
12. Cost of the medicines is a major hurdle, as the majority of Indians cannot afford them for longer periods as it has to be taken lifelong.

Hypertension at a Glance

1. High blood pressure is a common condition and increases with age.
2. High blood pressure is an important, modifiable risk factor for cardiovascular events.
3. Systolic blood pressure rises steadily with age and diastolic blood pressure tends to fall amongst adults older than 50 years in a normal population.
4. Approximately, one half of the adult population is hypertensive by the age of 60.
5. One in every five adults suffers from hypertension and the burden is increasing.
6. Mortality due to hypertension increases by almost 21 %.
7. Hypertensive disorders during pregnancy are the third leading cause of maternal death.
8. What is more alarming is that a large population is still unaware of their hypertensive condition.
9. The higher the blood pressure, the greater is the risk and the lower the blood pressure, the lower is the risk.
10. Blood pressure in all adults should be measured routinely by trained healthcare professionals using standardized techniques at all medical visits.
11. Lifestyle modifications are the cornerstone and equally important for the management of high blood pressure.
12. Steps for lifestyle management such as, low sodium (salt) in diet, increased consumption of fruits and vegetables, no use of tobacco, weight reduction and exercise are important to curb high blood pressure.
13. Awareness about high blood pressure is very poor and requires patient and population based education.

14. *Poor adherence to antihypertensive therapy is a major barrier for the treatment and control of hypertension and prevention of hypertensive complications.*
15. *Costly drugs and frequent dose schedule should be avoided.*
16. *All efforts should be directed on the patient's adherence to lifestyle modifications and antihypertensive therapy.*

Chapter 13

Diabetes Mellitus

Diabetes mellitus is the most common non-communicable disease worldwide and its prevalence has increased at epidemic rate in many developing countries. At the onset of twenty first century, there were about 194 million adults worldwide with diabetes and 314 million adults with impaired glucose tolerance. These numbers are projected to increase to 472 million diabetes patients by the year 2030, corresponding to almost 8 % of the world's population.

Just like CVD, diabetes is emerging as one of the fastest growing disease of twenty first century. Almost 70 % of people with diabetes live in low and middle income countries and the brunt of the disease will be borne by the developing countries. According to International Diabetes Federation, currently 4 out of 5 people with diabetes live in developing countries. It affects the working adult population and thereby imposes an immense financial burden on the country. In developing countries, the majority of people with diabetes are in the 45-64 years of age in contrast to developed countries where the majority are at or above 64 years of age. According to WHO, India and China, the two most populous nations in the world will bear the maximum burden and will lose national income equivalent to almost 900 billion US dollars between 2005 and 2015 to diabetes and cardiovascular disease. It is further emphasized that much of the loss is preventable. The number of people with diabetes in the world will be more than double from 2000 to 2030 and the greatest increase will occur in South Asia, Middle Eastern crescent and sub-Saharan Africa. The absolute increase in the number of people with diabetes will be maximum in India followed by China. However, Africa is catching up fast and is expected to record the highest relative increase in the number of individuals with diabetes in the next few decades.

The top ten countries estimated to have the highest number of people with diabetes by the year 2025 in order will be India, China, USA, Brazil, Pakistan, Mexico, Russia, Germany, Egypt and Bangladesh. Indonesia and Philippines are not far behind. Except the US and Germany, all the remaining countries fall in the category of low or middle income group. Since majority of diabetics die from cardiovascular diseases, the increasing prevalence of diabetes will result in an increasing proportion of deaths from CVD in these countries.

Today, in India, there are 41 million diabetes patients and this number is projected to be 70 million by the year 2025, more than any country in the world. By 2025, India will have the dubious distinction of being recognized as the capital of this deadly disease. The prevalence of diabetes in urban India is more than the rural area. The prevalence is rising at a rapid pace and the disease which was 2.3 % in the year 1971 is now 12-16 % in urban area. The increase in prevalence is more because of environmental factors such as unhealthy food choices and sedentary lifestyles. A thrifty gene which is inherent in our population may explain the low birth weight and development of diabetes in adulthood.

Diabetes and Health

Diabetes mellitus is a major concern today as it is linked with disability and death and affects all parts of the body at all ages. It is a major contributor to heart disease, stroke, renal failure, blindness, foot ulcers, gangrene and skin diseases. In India, diabetes affects the younger people more than the elderly that is, it occurs during the productive years of life and poses a considerable financial burden on the individual.

Sinister Fate

He was referred to me by one of my surgeon colleague regarding complaints of burning sensation in his upper abdomen, profuse sweating with uneasiness lasting for a few minutes early in the morning. He was an assistant general manager in one of the nationalized bank and was suffering from long standing diabetes, obesity and led a sedentary lifestyle. When I examined him, his blood pressure was slightly raised but all other parameters were normal. His ECG revealed 'Right bundle branch block', a common finding in the elderly which may be normal in up to 15 % of healthy individuals. No previous ECG was available at that time and the last check-up was done quite some time back. His blood sugar levels were also raised. Since there were no previous records to rule out any changes in the recent ECG, due to angina or a normal variation, I advised him hospital admission so that he could be monitored for the next few days and more tests could be done to rule out any heart problem. He was reluctant and tried to convince me that this was all because of some gas problem. He insisted on diagnosis. I explained that I had examined him for the first time today and with these ECG findings, I could only say at present that there is no heart attack but angina or an impending heart attack could not be ruled out. Hence, serial ECG and certain blood tests were obligatory which can help in establishing the diagnosis. He ignored my suggestions and continued, 'Doctor, in my opinion it is all because of gas (abdominal upset). I have had it a couple of times earlier also. I have an important and urgent meeting in Lucknow and since I belong to Lucknow I shall get myself checked there. Despite repeated persuasion and explanations by me and by his colleagues, he left the chamber with the medicines and promised me to get himself checked at Lucknow. After five days he was again brought to the OPD with similar complaints. This time the problem had started in his office. His colleagues revealed that he had attended the meeting and since next day was Sunday he came back to Varanasi as the month of March is crucial in the banking sector. It was also decided among the family members that he will undergo a thorough check up at New Delhi where his son was employed. This time his complaints were of moderate severity and he was uncomfortable. The uneasiness extended to his chest and back also. It was associated with two bouts of vomiting. The ECG revealed frank changes suggestive of a massive heart attack along with low blood pressure. He was admitted, treatment started and family members in Lucknow and New Delhi were informed. Unfortunately, he succumbed to his illness in a few hours, before the arrival of his near and dear ones.

I know death is destiny and is inevitable but precautions are of utmost importance. It is more so in patients with diabetes who can have life threatening illness with little or no complaint. The fault can be from either side, patients feel it is unnecessary or they postpone to get tested for minor problems either because of family or office engagements and physicians sometimes fail to correlate the subtle nature of complaints to serious illnesses.

What is Diabetes?

Diabetes is a disorder of metabolism of glucose which is an important source of energy in the body. Most of the food we eat is converted into glucose which is the main form of sugar in blood. Insulin is a hormone secreted by the pancreas, a linear organ sitting below the stomach. It is responsible for the shifting of glucose circulating in the blood into the cells and the production of energy. Inadequate insulin secretion by the pancreas or resistance to its action can lead to deficiency of insulin in blood. Without sufficient insulin, glucose is not transported to the cells and remains in the blood. Abnormally high level of glucose in the blood is termed as diabetes mellitus.

What are the Types of Diabetes?

There are two common types of diabetes: Type 1 and Type 2.

Type 1 diabetes results from partial or total loss of insulin secretion from the pancreas and is associated with acute onset of complaints related to high sugar in the blood such as increased hunger, thirst and/or urination. It may also present with unexplained rapid weight loss. Type 1 diabetes is commonly seen in childhood or adolescence but can occur at any age. These patients are typically lean and usually present with acute complications related with high blood sugar and ketoacidosis. It requires lifelong insulin therapy for proper control of diabetes.

Type 2 diabetes is an insulin-resistant form in which insulin is either produced in an insufficient quantity or is in an ineffective form. It accounts for 90 % of the diabetic population in India and is the commonest form of diabetes all over. It is more prevalent during adulthood. The development of this type of diabetes is strongly linked with obesity, especially abdominal obesity. In this type, the disease process is gradual. It may be associated with little or no complaints and it goes undiagnosed for many years. Type 2 diabetes is often diagnosed on routine blood sugar estimation. This type of diabetes can be controlled on diet, lifestyle measures and/or oral drugs. However a few of the Type 2 diabetics may require insulin therapy for better control of blood glucose.

How should Diabetes be diagnosed?

Diagnosis of diabetes is just a simple estimation of glucose or sugar level in blood. Elevated level of sugar beyond the normal clinch the diagnosis. The test is performed either after fasting or after taking meals or the glucose challenge. The blood estimated for sugar after 8-12 hours of fasting in the morning is termed as **fasting sugar**. The estimation of sugar in blood after 2 hours of meals or 75 gm of glucose dissolved in 200 ml of water is termed as **post prandial** and **glucose challenge sugar estimation** respectively. A fasting level of more than 126 mg% and post prandial level of more than 200 mg % is diagnostic of diabetes. A fasting level of sugar less than 100 mg /dl and post prandial level of less than 140 mg/dl are considered normal. A casual or random blood sugar level of more than 200 mg/dl should raise the suspicion and fasting and post prandial sugar should be estimated before declaring a diagnosis of diabetes.

What are the Symptoms or Complaints of Diabetes?

Both types of diabetes have similar symptoms and are related with abnormally high blood sugar levels in blood. Kidneys retain the essential elements including sugar, however, this property of the kidneys is lost if the sugar level is persistently higher than 180 mg/dl in blood. Then the kidney can no longer retain the sugar in the blood and is filtered through the kidneys in the urine. To eliminate excess of sugar in urine, a large amount of urine is formed and is manifested as excess of urination or increase in frequency of urine discharge called **polyuria**. This feature is more pronounced and noticeable in the night referred to as nocturnal urination. To compensate this loss of fluid in urine, a diabetic person starts consuming an excess of fluid and water and it manifests as an increase in thirst or **polydypsia**. Excess of sugar present in the blood is not utilized properly to produce energy needed for the body and to compensate it, people eat more. This is called **polyphagia**. This triad of excess eating, thirst and urination is the hallmark of diabetes. Since glucose is lost in the urine, and protein and fat of the body is utilized in place of sugar to produce energy for day to day activities, this results in weakness, loss of muscle mass and weight. A sudden and unexplained weight loss should raise suspicion of diabetes. Symptoms are more pronounced and common with Type 1 diabetes than Type 2, in which either there are no symptoms or symptoms are vague and overlooked for many years. Some people may present with complications of diabetes as the only complaint, which may include - partial or total blindness, tingling or a sensations of numbness in the arms or feet, non-healing ulcers, wounds or even chest infection such as tuberculosis.

What is Glycosylated Haemoglobin (HbA1c)?

It is the most talked about blood test nowadays, especially in the urban set up of India. This test helps us in knowing the blood sugar level and control for the preceding 8-12 weeks. When the beta chain of haemoglobin is exposed to a high level of blood sugar, glycation of haemoglobin (a process in which sugar is attached to this protein molecule) occurs resulting in the formation of glycosylated/glyacted haemoglobin. The process of glycation of haemoglobin is irreversible and the end product that is, glycosylated haemoglobin remains in the blood for 2 to 3 months. This time period is equivalent to the normal life span of red blood cells in the body. This test alone should not be used for diagnosis of diabetes.

How the Estimation of HbA1c Helps?

The estimation of HbA1c is getting popular globally as its level is recommended for the better management and goal of diabetes treatment by various scientific bodies. The results are not influenced by daily fluctuations of glucose, diet or exercise, and therefore are more reliable.

What are the Various Levels of HbA1c?

The result is reported in percentage and given below are the various levels in the blood:

< 5-6%	Normal
6-7%	Good control
7-8%	Fair control
8-10%	Unsatisfactory control
>10%	Poor control

Who can Get Diabetes?

Anyone can get diabetes. It affects both men and women alike. It is believed that heredity plays an important role. A person having diabetic parents or other family members are at high risk of developing diabetes. An obese person is more likely to get diabetes as insulin-glucose activity is interfered by central obesity. Physical inactivity also makes you prone to the development of diabetes. However, 'eating too much sugar can make you diabetic' is purely a myth.

Who Requires Screening for Diabetes in India?

An individual with or without any compliant who has crossed the age of 18 years, is obese or overweight, leads a sedentary lifestyle and has a family history of diabetes, should undergo screening tests for diabetes mellitus. People undergoing major or minor surgical procedures, or a wound taking an unduly long time to heal despite proper treatment, or people having any major disease of the body should also be screened for diabetes.

What is Pre-diabetes?

Pre-diabetes is a condition in which blood sugar levels are higher than normal but not high enough to be termed as diabetic. Pre-diabetic state is considered as a precursor of diabetes. Not all, but a majority of the people will develop overt diabetes in the coming years. These people should be identified and advised to maintain ideal body weight and perform a moderate degree of exercise to either prevent or postpone the development of diabetes. This is common with Type 2 diabetes. Pre-diabetics are more prone to develop heart disease or stroke compared to non-diabetics. These people with pre-diabetes have fasting blood sugar level of 101-126 mg/dl and/or blood sugar level of 140-200 mg/dl after 2 hours of glucose challenge.

Who can be Pre-diabetic?

There are certain individuals, who are more prone to develop diabetes. They require aggressive preventive measures to reduce or postpone the early development of the disease. These individuals are those who are either obese, have high blood pressure, have a sedentary lifestyle, have an impaired glucose challenge test or whose parents or first degree relatives are suffering from diabetes. Women whose pregnancies are complicated with diabetes, termed as gestational diabetes, are also prone to develop diabetes in the future. Certain specific ethnic groups such as African Americans, Native Americans or Asians fall under the umbrella of pre-diabetics.

Why should I Bother about Diabetes?

Glucose is an essential source of energy which is required by all the cells of the body. Therefore, an impairment in its utilization drastically affects the normal functioning of the body making you as well as the body's defence mechanism that fights against infection weak. In turn, it makes a person susceptible to infection. In developing countries, the most common disease is tuberculosis. It can also cause infections to last longer resulting in delayed or slow healing of wounds. Diabetes is a common cause of visual impairment and blindness, and can lead to heart, kidney, brain, skin or foot problems. Very few people are aware of these threats and ignore the disease which in the long run may prove fatal. You should know that patients do not die due to diabetes but die because of its complications.

What are the Various Complications of Diabetes?

Diabetes can affect each and every cell and organ of the body. The complications of diabetes are related to either the disease itself or are because of the treatment. Complications can be classified as acute, occurring within a very short span of time and chronic, developing in the due course which may take several years. Common acute complications include hypoglycaemia that is, lowering of blood sugar below a limit which is harmful or detrimental to the normal functioning of the body or hyperglycaemia that is, a very high level of sugar. Other acute complications can be stroke, heart attack and sudden loss of vision. Chronic complications include involvement of various organs of the body such as the brain, eyes, heart, kidneys, nerves, arteries and skin.

What is Hypoglycaemia?

An abnormally low level of glucose in the blood is termed as hypoglycaemia. It is a common complication resulting from the treatment of diabetes by either insulin or oral anti-diabetic drugs. The nervous system of the body, including the brain is dependent on glucose for their proper function. It requires a continuous supply and if this is hampered or interrupted for a few minutes, it can result in impairment of brain function causing a decrease in alertness, headache, blurred vision, confusion, drowsiness and/or impairment in judgment. If it persists for a longer period it can cause fits or even coma. It may also lead to excessive sweating, giddiness, weakness, tiredness, irritability, racing of the heart (palpitations) or hunger. This situation occurs because of an imbalance between the diet and the drugs taken for control of diabetes. The fear of hypoglycaemia is the commonest cause for improper blood sugar control in India. Common situations where hypoglycaemia is precipitated are wrong diagnosis or over judicious use of drugs. It is also precipitated by ingesting the drug twice either by confusion or by mistake. Hypoglycaemia can be precipitated if the diet is reduced either because of fever or during fasting or other medical conditions and routine doses of drugs are continued.

How to Treat Hypoglycaemia?

Every diabetic and responsible family member should be aware of the complaints related with hypoglycaemia for if they persist, they can lead to brain damage or death. If any of the above problems occur, a sweet candy or sugar should be taken immediately to avoid complications of hypoglycaemia. Some of the long acting drugs of diabetes may cause hypoglycaemic symptoms for longer periods. Elderly people and children with diabetes should be more vigilant as they frequently fail to recognize the symptoms of hypoglycaemia. Very low level of sugar or hypoglycaemia is an emergency and patients are advised to get their sugar levels checked and consult the doctor urgently. This is the only complication of diabetes which responds instantly to treatment and gives dramatic improvement. If a patient does not respond after ingestion of glucose or sweets or the response is partial, he should consult his doctor urgently.

What is Hyperglycaemia?

Abnormally high level of sugar in blood is termed as hyperglycaemia. Diabetic ketoacidosis is one of the commonest life threatening complications of hyperglycaemia. In this condition, blood sugar is usually more than 250 mg /dl (not all people having >250 mg will have ketoacidosis). Though the blood sugar levels are very high, the cells cannot utilize it for energy production. Then the body starts utilizing fat as an alternative source of energy. Fat is broken down and ketones are produced as an end product and as an alternative source of energy. Since excess ketones make the blood acidic, this condition is known as ketoacidosis. It manifests as increased thirst, urination, nausea, abdominal discomfort and difficulty or rapid breathing or a combination of all. Deep and rapid breathing is common, a compensatory effort on the part of the body to correct the acidic environment in the blood. Excessive urinary output and rapid breathing causes quick loss of fluids and results in dehydration. Diabetic ketoacidosis is an emergency requiring prompt medical attention. The patients are usually in a very bad condition with low blood pressure, rapid breathing and pulse, often dehydrated, drowsy or sometimes unconscious. This situation is precipitated if a person misses the doses of insulin or oral drugs, is having a fever and infection or is under certain stressful conditions such as after a heart attack, stroke or surgery. This is commonly seen with people suffering from Type 1 diabetes.

Diabetes Mellitus and the Role of the Physician in India

Diabetes mellitus is a well established, independent risk factor for cardiovascular disease development and is an important contributor of a growing number of related problems all over India. The increase in cardiovascular diseases, especially heart attack and stroke in the Indian population can be explained by the increase of diabetes. In India, diabetes is mainly treated by physicians and rarely by specialists. The help of an endocrinologist is only sought once the disease gets uncontrolled or there are complications related with diabetes. Heart attack and stroke are the two common acute and life threatening complications needing the immediate attention of cardiologists and neurologists respectively. These complications are closely linked and are managed separately by two teams of doctors. Therefore, it requires better management and patient education to prevent the complications of CVD. The role of a physician becomes very important not only in the treatment and education of the patient but also in the prevention of the complication. Physicians are required to refer the patients to a specialist at the earliest so that the problem can be diagnosed, treated and complications are averted in time. This is true with heart related problems as diabetics have vague complaints and it must be diagnosed reliably before catastrophic events like heart attack or sudden death occur. This coordinated and comprehensive strategy will not only improve the overall quality of care but will reduce the burden of CVD in our society.

Diabetes and Coronary Heart Disease

Diabetes is traditionally a metabolic disease but it is now considered as a vascular disease as well. This is based on the fact that most patients who have diabetes develop cardiovascular complications which are responsible for 80 % deaths in diabetic patients. Cardiovascular disease, especially coronary heart disease is the foremost cause of death and disability in diabetic patients. Diabetic individuals die more of heart related complications than any other complications related to diabetes. The risk of development of coronary heart disease is 2-4 times higher than in non-diabetic persons. Diabetes is referred to as coronary equivalent; it means, your risk of having a heart attack is the same as someone without diabetes who has already had a heart attack earlier. Women with diabetes are more at risk than men for the development of CHD and having diabetes cancels the protective effects of oestrogen which safeguards women before menopause from the development of heart disease. In diabetics, the heart attack occurs at an early age and is more serious. Complications and death rate is high when compared to non-diabetic individuals. People with diabetes who have also suffered a heart attack, have a higher risk of getting a second attack. Not only is the disease severe but even the complications related with the treatment such as, PTCA and CABG are higher in diabetics as compared to non-diabetics.

Diabetes and Atherosclerosis

Diabetes in itself causes early promotion and progression of the atherosclerotic process. The cardiovascular system of the body is affected badly by the multiple processes which include early endothelial dysfunction, lipid abnormality, various inflammatory and oxidative stresses and increased thrombotic complications which cause blockage of blood vessels supplying to the heart, the brain and other parts of the body. It can affect both the larger and smaller blood vessels. Many of the scientific bodies consider that having diabetes is equivalent to having two or three major risk factors for coronary atherosclerosis. Diabetics are more prone to high blood pressure and abnormal cholesterol levels which are not only independent risk factors but also contribute to the increased process of atherosclerosis.

What is the Effect of Coronary Involvement?

Atherosclerosis, a key process in the development of CHD is enhanced in diabetic individuals leading to the development of premature atherosclerosis of coronary arteries which supply blood to the heart. It affects both large and small coronary arteries of the heart. When the large coronary blood vessels are affected, it can result in various manifestations of heart attack including sudden death. When only smaller blood vessels are affected, the heart muscles can get damaged, making them weak and resulting in severe dysfunction of the heart - a condition known as diabetic cardiomyopathy which causes heart failure.

What are the Symptoms which should Prompt a Person to Consult a Doctor?

As mentioned earlier, symptoms in diabetes are mild or vague and a person should be alert. Symptoms may come and go. A complaint of chest pain on exertion, following stress or emotional outburst, unexplained and persistent breathing difficulty, sweating, nausea or upper abdominal or persistent back pain may be the warning signals that indicate to you that your heart is getting affected. It should not be ignored in a diabetic person and a consultation with your family physician is required immediately. Fortunately, there are certain tests such as stress ECG (treadmill test) and stress echocardiography which can be helpful in diagnosing the heart disease before its manifestations and complications. Transient loss of vision, double vision, difficulty in speaking, headache and confusion, loss of balance which may last for a few seconds to minutes are signals that something may be wrong with the blood vessels of your brain and you need attention and proper care urgently. These symptoms can lead to a paralytic attack or stroke if ignored. Numbness, tingling and pain in legs, especially calf muscle pain during walking suggests involvement of lower limb arteries. Patients often describe it as pin pricks or a burning sensation in the limbs and soles.

How Safe is Coronary Bypass Surgery in Diabetics?

It is a common concern that patients and family members are afraid of infection and the outcome of surgery. The safety of bypass surgery depends upon the control of diabetes and the condition of the heart. Bypass surgery in a controlled diabetic with good heart function is quite safe and the risk of surgery is even less than 1 %. However, if the heart function is poor or depressed and there are incompetent heart valves, especially mitral valve then the risk of surgery is high depending upon the severity of heart damage. Post-operative surgical complications, especially infection is definitely a matter of concern in diabetics. However, with a better control of blood sugar, use of appropriate antibiotics and isolation of the patient in an intensive care unit, it is no longer a matter of concern today. New advances and techniques such as off pump surgeries or surgeries performed on beating hearts have further reduced the risk of heart surgery. Therefore bypass surgery or even any surgery in diabetics is safe today if the sugar level is controlled.

Hypertension and Diabetes

Hypertension or high blood pressure and diabetes frequently coexist and are independent risk factors for cardiovascular disease. Both represent an important health problem as the combination of the two disorders is common and carries significant death and disability risks. The prevalence of hypertension in diabetic patients is twice as in the non-diabetics. Diabetes in itself is a major risk for cardiovascular disorders and the presence of hypertension increases the risk by 4-5 folds. Since hypertension is a major determinant it should be detected and dealt promptly in diabetic patients to avoid complications and adverse outcomes. Hypertension in diabetes can coexist but can be due to complications of diabetes itself such as secondary to involvement of kidney (diabetic nephropathy) or part of the metabolic syndrome. However despite simple methods of detection and cheap treatment for hypertension, high blood pressure in diabetic individuals is not under control in a majority of cases. The goal of treatment for diabetic patients is to keep their blood pressure below 130/85 mmHg.

Lipids and Diabetes

Lipid or fat abnormality is common among diabetes mellitus patients. Abnormal level of lipids is an independent risk factor for CHD. Common lipid abnormalities associated with diabetes are a high level of triglycerides, a low level of HDL and a high level of small dense LDL. This abnormal triad is a lethal combination in the presence of diabetes and is common in Indians. This may or may not be associated with elevation of total cholesterol. Obesity, especially central obesity which is found in almost 60-85 % of Type 2 diabetes contributes to an abnormal level of lipids. Lipid levels should be aggressively managed in diabetic patients.

Sudden Death and Diabetes

Sudden death is defined as death occurring within 24 hours of symptoms and the commonest cause is heart disease. Diabetic patients are more prone to die suddenly because of silent heart attacks and the development of lethal abnormal rhythms of the heart such as, ventricular tachycardia or fibrillation. In this type of heart rhythm, the lower chamber of the heart that is, ventricle starts beating erratically and contributes to no ejection of blood from the heart or cessation of heart function, resulting in brain death as the brain cannot survive more than 3-5 minutes without blood. It is characterized by loss of consciousness, seizures and death in a few minutes.

What is the Treatment of Diabetes?

Once diabetes is detected, the treatment requires participation of the physician as well as the patient. Physicians should educate the patient about the disease, its future course and complications. All patients should be made to understand the role of diet, exercise and to avoid smoking, which are equally important as medicines. Along with diet and lifestyle modifications, the majority of Type 1 diabetes cases will require insulin and Type 2 diabetes can be controlled by oral drugs. However, a few patients of Type 2 may also require insulin therapy alone or with oral drugs. Patients should realize that this disease is chronic in nature, is going to stay and that the patient himself is equally responsible for the control and care of the disease. Whether you make the disease a friend or foe is entirely your choice. It should be emphasized to all that it is the complications of diabetes that makes your life hell and not the disease itself. Therefore, you have to take charge of your diabetes so that the complications are either prevented or postponed. The mantra of diabetic care is, it is harmless if cared for and fatal if neglected.

Exercise in Diabetes

A diabetic patient needs to know the importance and essential component of exercise programs. They should be made aware that exercise will not only help in controlling their sugar level but will also help in controlling weight and high blood pressure besides delaying the disease related complications.

Stress and Diabetes

Stress is a condition which is encountered daily by everyone. However, many people live with more stress which can be due to environmental factors such as office or household work or it may be due to an illness such as fever or heart attack. It is true that stress is a part of life. However, if prolonged it is unkind to the body and diabetes. When one is stressed, a large dose of sugar is released so that the person can deal with the situation. In diabetics, this extra sugar released in the blood remains so as proportionate amount of insulin is not released simultaneously resulting in high blood sugar levels. Most of the stressed people do not get proper sleep, eat inappropriately and even exercise less. All these factors contribute to increase in the blood sugar. Stressed people become more careless, often neglect themselves and get their blood sugar level checked infrequently, further complicating the status of diabetes. Even uncontrolled sugar levels in itself is a stressful condition. If stress is transient or temporary, it may not affect much, but a persistent or prolonged stressful condition is definitely detrimental to diabetics and their health in the larger perspective. Each and every patient of diabetes responds individually to stress and patterns of sugar rise vary from person to person. Be honest and good to yourself in stressful conditions. Try to avoid stressful conditions if possible or face it with a positive attitude that it will pass with time. Try to figure out a solution by yourself or take the help of someone who understands you well and is ready to help you in this situation. Take a walk, play with children, go for entertainment or take a short vacation - they all help. Even costly medicines or too many pills prescribed for the control of diabetes or its complications may cause stress. So talk to your doctor and discuss all points that might cause stress to you. This is especially applicable to the elderly people.

Weight and Diabetes

There is a strong relation between the development of Type 2 diabetes and central obesity. Weight control is an integral part of treatment for all types of diabetes. It not only helps in controlling diabetes but it also helps in reducing the risk of development of new cases. Weight control can be achieved by realistic changes in eating habits and physical activity. Do not indulge yourself in long periods of starvation or unpalatable dietary schedules. Try to fix a modest goal for weight control. Even a small reduction in weight can drastically change the outcome in diabetics. Losing 10 % of your existing weight can confer positive health and boost your confidence. Very obese people can take the help of medications or surgery meant for weight control, but only after consulting their physician and with a proper diet and exercise protocol. Maintenance of ideal weight after loss is very important. Therefore, adopt and continue the diet and exercise protocol which can be followed and practiced life-long.

Diet and Diabetes

Diabetes is a metabolic disorder characterized by high blood sugar. It is linked with the abnormality of carbohydrate metabolism due to insulin deficiency. Considering this, diet is the integral part of treatment for diabetes. Carbohydrate is the cheapest source of energy and food. It forms the bulk or staple diet for the majority. The aim of a diet is not only to control the elevated level of blood sugar but it should also be appropriate for the prevention of hypertension, obesity if any, lipid abnormality, heart disease and kidney problems. One diet pattern cannot fit into the menu of all, therefore it should be personalized, giving due care to each individual's choice of foods and family dietary patterns along with various factors such as age, sex, activity level, ethnic and cultural preferences. Cost and availability of food should also be considered before making any suggestions. The aim should be to create a better balance of nutritious food with good physical activity to provide the best possible quality of life.

The energy is supplied by carbohydrates, fats and proteins in one's diet. Carbohydrates are the major source of energy in an Indian diet supplied by rice or wheat. Sugar and milk are other sources of carbohydrate in the Indian diet. The age old practice of saying no to rice as a major staple diet of a majority of Indians is no longer practiced and 60 % of the energy should be provided by the carbohydrate. It is not the type of cereal which is important, it is the amount, that is consumed which is important. Fat is the second common source of energy in diabetics and the choice is such that it should also take care of the lipids in the blood. Saturated fats such as butter, ghee (clarified butter), vanaspati oil and coconut or palm oil should be avoided. Oil rich in monounsaturated fats such as mustard oil, groundnut oil, canola, olive oil are preferred over oils rich in polyunsaturated fats such as sunflower, safflower or corn oil. Gingelly (til) oil and rice bran oil are rich in both mono- and polyunsaturated fats are also preferred. It is advisable not to stick to any particular oil but change it from time to time. Protein in diet should be such that it provides 15-20 % of the total energy requirement. Plant sources of protein such as legumes and pulses should be preferred over animal proteins. However, fish consumption once a week is beneficial. Diabetic individuals with kidney disease should take care of their protein intake. Table 13.1 summarizes the practical food guidelines for patients suffering from diabetes mellitus.

Table 13.1: Food Table Guide for Patients Suffering From Diabetes Mellitus

Food	Preferred	Restrict	Avoid
Carbo-hydrate	Wheat, bran rice, ragi, maize, bajra	White or polished rice, maida or refined flour, whole milk and its products	Simple sugar, honey, sweets, pudding, cakes, pastry, fruit juices and shakes

Fat or oil	Canola, corn oil, olive oil, groundnut, rice bran, gingely, sunflower oil, safflower oil, mustard oil	Palm oil, coconut oil, hard margarine, cheese	Butter, ghee, *vanaspati*, deep fried foods like wafers, *samosas*, *tikki*, etc., high fat salad dressings which use cream, mayonnaise, etc.
Protein	Vegetable sources such as legumes and pulses, fish, mushrooms, egg white	Chicken and lean cuts of red meat, yellow part of egg	Organ meats such as brain, liver etc., fried meat items
Vegetables	All green leafy vegetables, beans, gourd, cucumber, lady finger, onion, garlic, cabbage, broccoli, tomato, etc.	Carrot, beetroot, peas, double beans	Potatoes, turnip, tapioca
Fruits	Apple, papaya, guava, pear, watermelon, sweet lime, jamun (jambu fruit)	Oranges, grapes, mangoes, jack fruit, natural fruit juices, fruit salads	Fruit custards, puddings, fruit punch and shakes, fruit juices with sugar
Sweets	Limited amount of chikki or groundnut with a little jaggery, marie biscuits (with more of fibre and less sugar)	All sweets	Cakes, pastry, *halwa*, *kulfi*, *kheer*, custards, refined sugars, honey, jaggery, jam and jellies
Beverages	Tea or coffee without sugar, butter milk, rasam, jaljeera, clear vegetable soups	Small quantity of fresh fruit juices	Sweet *lassi*, sweet curd or *misthi doi*, carbonated drinks

Alcohol	Not more than 30-60 ml per day on a regular basis		Alcohol, do not start alcohol if you do not consume alcohol
Nuts	Groundnut, chestnut, cashew nut, almonds, walnut- 50 gm, twice a week	Roasted and salted nuts	Raisins, dates, currants, rancid nuts

What is Glycaemic Index?

The glycaemic index measures how fast a food is likely to raise your blood sugar. Foods with low glycaemic index increase the blood sugar gradually as compared to foods with high glycaemic index. Food items with a high glycaemic index may be injurious to health, especially for diabetic persons, as it has no or little nutritive value and increases the blood sugar level sharply. The glycaemic index is a number which is given to a food item. Glucose is the fastest absorbing carbohydrate and raises the blood sugar level instantaneously. It is given an arbitrary number of 100 and the rest of the food items are given numbers relative to it. The lower the number, the slower is the rise of blood glucose and the higher the number, the faster is the rise in the blood sugar. It is difficult to remember the various numbers and it is wise to consume food items which taste less sweet to your taste buds and avoid those which taste sweeter.

What Precautions are to be Taken while Fasting?

All over the globe both fasting and feasting are common and frequent. Fasting is linked with religious sentiments while feasting with joyful occasions. Diabetics should be cautious in both situations. Fasting should be avoided if possible especially where sugar is not under control. If it is unavoidable due to reasons such as marriage of daughter or religious sentiments, it is better to omit the drug on the day of fast and restart later. In the month of Ramadan, the drug should be taken when the fast is broken and avoid sweets if possible during this period. During this period, short acting drugs with low chances of hypoglycaemia should be preferred. It is in the interest of patient and for their well-being that fasting should be avoided. Always keep some sugar with you and inform a responsible family member about the drug used to control diabetes and the extent of days of fasting. Elderly patients are more prone to complications and should take extra precautions. Long acting drugs should be avoided in the interest of the patient.

I am a Diabetic.
How should I Keep myself Healthy?

Inculcate Healthy Eating Habits

1. Follow a healthy meal pattern which suits you and take the help of a dietician or your family physician who will guide you according to your age, sex, activity and food pattern prevalent in your culture and family.
2. Eat frequent and small meals; skipping meals and fasting is not advisable.
3. Eat more fibre and less of fat and salt. Choose whole grains, beans, green vegetables to increase your fibre in diet.
4. Avoid foods rich in simple carbohydrates which have a high glycaemic index, such as - sweets, sugar, jaggery, honey, sweetened beverages, alcohol and deep fried foods.

5. Avoid very sweet fruits such as mango, banana and *sappota*. One can take a limited amount of apple, papaya, pear, *jamun*, guava according to seasonal availability.
6. Green salads which include lettuce leaves, tomatoes, onions, radish and carrots are good for health.
7. Rice is a staple diet for the majority of Indians. Therefore, its consumption may be continued with other cereals and you should learn how much to take and how to replace it with other cereals such as wheat, maize, *jowar*, *ragi*, etc.
8. The choice of food is yours and successful adherence is your responsibility for a healthy life. Your dietician and physician only can guide you. Do not hesitate to ask your questions about meals at every visit to your physician as it is an integral part to your medical care.
9. If you use tobacco, stop it immediately.
10. Moderate consumption of alcohol (1 or 2 pegs per day) is beneficial. It should be taken with meals, but it is better not to take it for other harmful affects linked with alcohol drinking.

Be Physically Active

Physical activity is an essential part of treatment and is as important as diet and medicines. Be physically active every day and maintain regularity. It can be performed at any time of the day, but choose the cooler parts of the day. Regular exercise not only controls sugar but it also lowers blood pressure and cholesterol.

Take Care of your Eyes, Feet, Heart and Kidneys

1. Take care of your feet by checking them daily, especially between your toes and look for cuts, sores, redness, swelling or blisters. Keep your feet clean and dry.

2. Do not walk barefoot. Prefer wearing comfortable shoes or slippers with no metal ends. Avoid shoes and slippers that are tight fitting.
3. Get your eyes checked every six months along with an estimation of protein in your urine, kidney profile and various cholesterol components in blood.
4. Get a resting ECG, a stress ECG, X-ray of chest and an echocardiography annually for early detection of heart problems.
5. Aim for a healthy weight as weight loss helps not only in the control of diabetes, it also helps in reducing cholesterol and blood pressure-two common conditions existing with diabetes.

Monitor your Sugar Frequently

1. Take a blood sugar test as often as your doctor suggests. It is better to get it checked at home with the help of a glucometer, a device which can estimate your capillary blood sugar level instantaneously. Keep a record of your blood sugar done at home, as it helps your doctor. Do not rely or monitor your sugar by urine estimation.
2. You should know your blood sugar goals. American Diabetes Association recommends fasting or blood sugar levels before meals of 90-130 mg/dl, after meals <180 mg/dl and at bedtime 111-150 mg/dl. Rely on fasting and post prandial blood sugar estimation and avoid random sugar estimation.
3. You should know about HbA1c or glycosylated haemoglobin level, as it tells you your average blood sugar control for the last two to three months. You should know that a level of HbA1c of 7 % or less is a better predictor of your control of diabetes. It may be performed every 3 or 4 months.

Stick to your Treatment

Always take your medicines as has been prescribed by your physician. Do not increase or decrease the dose on your own. Habit of changing the dose schedule according to your size of meals is a common practice which should be discouraged. Insulin therapy is feared by a majority of Indians. You should know that it is governed by the type of diabetes and status of control of diabetes. It is not an individual's choice. There are certain conditions where it is mandatory to take insulin for the proper control of diabetes. You should learn about the safe storage of insulin, how to read the units to be injected (a diabetic with an eye problem may require the assistance of a family member) and the place where it has to be injected. The first dose should be administered under the supervision of your health care personal. Keep a close watch on your weight when you are on insulin therapy.

It requires a little effort but a lot of determination to keep your diabetes under control. It is better to take charge of your diabetes immediately as diabetics die frequently as a result of the complications rather than the disease itself.

What is Bothering us Today?

General physicians today who are responsible for the treatment of diabetes at large are overburdened. Less time is devoted towards educating the patient, and they often find it difficult to manage complications. The picture is further complicated by the tendency of patients. In the initial years of the disease, because of the lack of symptoms, patients try to evade the fact that they are having the disease and avoid physicians or rely on indigenous medicines. There is a widespread misconception in society that the long term use of modern medicines will damage kidneys and other parts of the body. To avoid allopathic medicines, a few patients give lame excuses that it causes weakness or it does not suit them. All these have been propagated by lack of awareness, poverty, unqualified physicians who are readily available in rural and semi-urban setups, and the false belief that indigenous medicines are safe. The asymptomatic status of the disease in the initial few years and lack of awareness make the situation worse. Also the patients do not get their blood sugar checked or consult a doctor. The majority of them rely on urine sample estimations and no or trace reports give them satisfaction, ultimately resulting in inaction. Dietary restrictions are not taught properly and the patient's apathy complicates the issue. Random blood sugar tests are performed more frequently than fasting and post prandial samples. Still HbA1c estimation is not popular and quiet costly, so it is avoided by both patients and doctors, especially in rural and semi-urban setups. In developing countries including India, apathy, ignorance, poor awareness, costly treatment, fear of drugs to be taken life long and asymptomatic status enhances the number of uncontrolled patients and so the complications. Insulin therapy is avoided by a majority, either because of the fear of a pin prick or the belief that the disease is at the terminal stage and insulin is to be taken life-long. Physicians often complain of non-cooperation and patients complain of how to carry out the physician's instructions regarding taking an insulin injection successfully. Things have changed in the twenty first century as better understanding of the disease, large numbers of seminars and conferences for physicians, newer drugs and awareness programmes for patients are stressed and available. Today the key issue is to deal with the disease effectively and to prevent the progression of complications by effective relations among physicians and patients. The population at large should also be encouraged to combat the growing threat of diabetes by increasing the level of physical activity, choosing healthy eating habits and ideal weight levels.

Diabetes at a Glance

1. *Diabetes is a common problem. Type 2 diabetes has reached an epidemic proportion in developing countries including India.*
2. *It is no more a disease of the rich or obese only. It is also a disease of sedentary people with unhealthy diet habits.*
3. *India will have the maximum number of diabetic patients by 2025 and every fifth diabetic will be an Indian.*
4. *Today, India occupies the second position with respect to the number of subjects with impaired glucose tolerance (IGT).*
5. *Prevalence of obesity and being overweight due to urbanization is increasing the number of diabetic patients.*
6. *Urban housing architecture and the automobile revolution promotes physical inactivity and new diabetic patients.*
7. *Everyday 3600 new cases of diabetes mellitus are diagnosed.*
8. *Diabetes is no more recognized as a metabolic disease. It is now widely accepted as a vascular disease.*
9. *Diabetics have a 2-4 fold increased risk for the development of cardiovascular disease.*
10. *The epidemic of diabetes has led to an excess of cardiovascular disease in India.*
11. *Cardiovascular diseases are the main cause of death and disability in diabetes.*
12. *Almost two thirds of diabetics die of a heart attack, heart failure, stroke or silently due to sudden cardiac death.*
13. *Only controlling blood sugar will not reduce the burden of cardiovascular disease. Control of obesity, high blood pressure,*

abnormal cholesterol levels, increased physical activity, cessation of tobacco and alcohol abstinence are all of paramount importance.

14. *Patients should know that the disease is chronic and will remain with them. Making diabetes a friend and treating it with utmost care is obligatory.*
15. *Patient's education and awareness should be a part of the treatment and prevention.*
16. *Society, schools and social organizations should be actively involved in the awareness and prevention of diabetes.*

Chapter 14
Metabolic Syndrome

Metabolic syndrome is a major public health problem worldwide. It represents a constellation of metabolic derangements in the body at the same time which include central obesity, glucose intolerance or insulin resistance, lipid and fat derangements and hypertension (high blood pressure). People with metabolic syndrome are at high risk of developing diabetes mellitus and cardiovascular disease as well as increased death rate from heart disease. The recognition of metabolic syndrome provides early identification of people with increased cardiovascular risks and warrant prompt intervention to all risk factors. The genetic and environmental factors both play an important role in the genesis of metabolic syndrome. The various risk factors which make a person prone to metabolic syndrome include age, obesity and family history of diabetes.

Many names have been given to this entity. Some of the common names are insulin resistance syndrome or syndrome X. Whatever be the name, this particular entity is of utmost importance as far as Indians are concerned. This partially explains the rapid surge of diabetes mellitus and heart disease in India. In the last two decades not only has there been a steep rise in the number of diabetics but the prevalence of metabolic syndrome has also been increased tremendously. The cost of medical treatment required by sufferers of metabolic syndrome places an enormous burden on the health care system, and will increase further as the prevalence of the syndrome is on the rise.

Cardiovascular Risks and Metabolic Syndrome

All the components of metabolic syndrome are also the risk factors for cardiovascular disease and increase the risk for development of atherosclerosis and coronary heart disease. According to the INTERHEART study which evaluated risks for the first heart attack in 52 countries including India, 26 % people had metabolic syndrome and when diabetes, high blood pressure and central obesity were added to this, the risk rose to almost 50 %. The presence of metabolic syndrome is highly predictive for the development of Type 2 diabetes as the basic defect in Type 2 diabetes is insulin resistance. The risk of development of new diabetes is 4 fold and heart disease is 2 fold in metabolic syndrome.

Metabolic Syndrome and its Global Prevalence

Metabolic syndrome is a major public health problem worldwide. Various studies have shown the prevalence of metabolic syndrome ranging from 8-24 % in men and from 8-46 % in women. Increased obesity due to lifestyle changes has led to an increase in the metabolic syndrome. The prevalence of metabolic syndrome increases with age. In adolescents it is 7 % in contrast to adults where it is as high as 50 %. In addition to age and sex, another factor that influences the prevalence of metabolic syndrome is ethnicity.

High Prevalence in India

The Asian population has a propensity for central obesity and high prevalence rates of metabolic syndrome have been noted in the Indian subcontinent. This is more common in the urban population as compared to the rural population and is more frequent amongst women than men. Almost one third of the urban Indian population suffers from metabolic syndrome. However, limited information is available regarding the prevalence of metabolic syndrome in India. Various studies have shown that the prevalence of metabolic syndrome ranges from 8-24 % in men and from 4-46 % in women. In addition to age and sex, the other factor that influences the prevalence of metabolic syndrome is ethnicity. Why Indians are at a higher risk for developing metabolic syndrome, the exact reason is not known. However, the main risk factor for the development of metabolic syndrome in India may be attributed to:

1. Lack of physical activity.
2. High consumption of fried and refined foods.
3. Unhealthy lifestyle due to urbanization and industrialization.
4. Central obesity common in Indians (genetic).
5. Lipid abnormality or dyslipidaemia is common.

Diagnosis

There are currently five major definitions or criteria for the diagnosis of metabolic syndrome. The criteria given by the World Health Organization, National Cholesterol Education Program and International Diabetes Federation vary slightly. The definition proposed for Asian Indians is very much closer to the definition recommended by International Diabetes Federation (IDF). The basic idea is to follow a definition which can identify many of the individuals of metabolic syndrome in the given population. The common practice for diagnosis of metabolic syndrome is that an individual should have at least 3 of the 5 following criteria:

1. Central obesity (waist circumference; male > 90 cm and female > 80 cm).
2. High blood pressure (> 130/85 mmHg).
3. High triglycerides in blood or bad cholesterol (> 150 mg/dl).
4. Low level of good or HDL cholesterol (males < 40 mg/dl and females < 50 mg/dl).
5. Insulin resistance, leading to impaired glucose tolerance (fasting blood glucose > 100 mg/dl).

Therapy

The value of increased physical activity and restriction of calorie intake is well established in metabolic syndrome. Weight reduction is the treatment of choice. It can also influence the other components of metabolic syndrome. However, drug treatment is frequently required for specific components. Generally, the individual diseases that comprise the metabolic syndrome are treated separately such as, medicines for high blood pressure. Medicine may also be used to lower LDL cholesterol and triglyceride levels, if they are elevated, and to raise HDL cholesterol levels if they are low.

Prevention

To prevent the development of metabolic syndrome it requires simple measures such as regular physical activity and reduction in the consumption of calorie rich foods. Decreasing sodium intake will reduce the blood pressure. Low fat dairy products which are rich in calcium can further reduce blood pressure. Avoiding simple sugars and sweets along with an increased intake of vegetables and fresh fruits can improve lipid abnormality. Consumption of fish and monounsaturated oils in the diet can also be helpful in controlling lipid levels. Excess use of saturated and trans-fats should be avoided. Exercise and moderate calorie reduction can promote weight loss and decrease central obesity. Quitting smoking and increasing physical activity will reduce triglyceride and increase HDL cholesterol.

Metabolic Syndrome at a Glance

1. *Metabolic syndrome is highly prevalent in the Indian subcontinent and the prevalence is increasing, especially among the urban and female population.*
2. *It is a known fact today that individuals suffering from metabolic syndrome are at a high risk for the development of diabetes mellitus and heart disease.*
3. *Obesity, particularly abdominal obesity which is common amongst Indians is strongly associated with metabolic syndrome.*
4. *The good part of metabolic syndrome (MS) is that all the components of metabolic syndrome are reversible and recognition of metabolic syndrome provides an opportunity to reduce risks in high risk patients.*
5. *All the components of metabolic syndrome can be improved by simply reducing the weight and increasing the level of physical activity and it remains the treatment of choice.*
6. *It is expected that once people have been given knowledge of or diagnosed with metabolic syndrome, they are much more willing to accept modified foods and would be willing to change their*

lifestyle.
7. Recognition and tackling their metabolic syndrome early will reduce the burden of diabetes and heart disease in individuals.

Chapter 15
Cholesterol and Fat

Cholesterol is a soft, fat-like waxy substance found in the blood stream and in all parts of our body. The majority of cholesterol is made in the liver. Only a small amount is required in the diet. Dairy products, cream, butter, red meats, fish, egg and saturated oils are rich sources of cholesterol in diet. The cholesterol consumed in diet or manufactured in the liver, is stored in various organs of the body and underneath the skin. It is normal to have cholesterol, however, presence of too much cholesterol in blood is harmful and a major risk for coronary heart disease and stroke. When there is excess of cholesterol in blood, the condition is known as hypercholesterolaemia.

Convenient Ignorance

It is said that doctors are the worst patients. The saying was proved when one of my senior colleague had a heart attack. He used to argue each and every part of treatment and cause for his illness. He was more cautious about the side effects of medicine than the benefits and was always afraid that he may be overdosed. He was not only concerned that the recovery was slow but simultaneously worried that even every minor discomfort in the body was related to his heart problem.

He was addicted to chewing tobacco, a habit he developed after quitting smoking. He was a college level volleyball player but had left the physical activity after he settled in his private practice. He never had time to think about himself in the rat race of practice. He was also ignorant about the advances in the other fields of medicine. It was really difficult for him to accept that he could suffer from a heart attack. Now his illness had confined him in his house. He had enough time to realize the wrongs done in the previous years. Even after the angioplasty, which he received promptly after the attack had only benefitted him partially. He was not very comfortable and felt weak and fatigued all the time. His heart function was below normal and was short of breath even while doing his routine household activities.

For an active person like him, it was not only frustrating but a cause of concern for future life. His wife, who herself was a doctor used to enquire about the role of cholesterol components in blood and its relation with tobacco consumption. When they were told that in his case these were the probable causes for his condition along with a sedentary lifestyle, it was hard for both of them to accept that tobacco consumption can lead to such a severe heart disease even when his total cholesterol, LDL cholesterol and triglycerides levels were normal in blood. I told them about the role of HDL cholesterol which is protective and was less than 30 mg/dl in his case. I also explained that apart from sedentary lifestyle, tobacco consumption is the commonest cause of low HDL cholesterol and it was one of the probable reasons for his illness. Both of them realized late even though they were in medical profession neglected their body and had very little knowledge about the role of various cholesterol components. They were also living in a false impression that it is the high cholesterol level alone which is mainly responsible for a heart attack. He never imagined that tobacco chewing with bêtel leaf (pan), which he rarely ingested can alter the cholesterol levels in blood, especially HDL cholesterol to such an extent that it can affect his life adversely.

Role of Cholesterol

What is the Role of Cholesterol in General Health?

In the body, cholesterol plays a vital role. It maintains the membrane of all cells. It is a good source of energy and supports growth. It helps in making prostaglandins which regulate many body processes including inflammation and blood clotting. Another requirement of fat in the diet is because it helps in the absorption of fat-soluble vitamins A, D, E which are present in food. Fat is essential for normal brain development during infancy and early childhood. However, in adult life only a small amount of fat is required on a daily basis and an average Indian diet provides more than what is required. The excess of fat in diet results in the accumulation of excess cholesterol or fat in the body.

A high level of cholesterol which circulates in the blood is in itself a serious risk factor for many. It is a prerequisite for the development of atherosclerosis - a process in which cholesterol is deposited on the walls of blood vessels making them stiff and obstructing the lumen in the long run. This process is slow and continues, lasts lifelong starting early in the childhood. The development of atherosclerosis does not produce any symptoms but greatly increases the risk of development of heart disease and brain stroke.

Is Cholesterol a Risk Factor for Heart Disease?

An increased level of cholesterol in the blood is associated with increased cardiovascular disease burden. This relationship is consistent with the large body of epidemiological data and data available from clinical trials of cholesterol lowering therapy. These data suggest that for every 30 mg/dl decrease in low density lipoprotein cholesterol (LDL-c a bad cholesterol) the risk of coronary heart disease is reduced by about 30 %. This is true for both developed and developing countries including India which is no different.

Why is High Cholesterol Considered a Silent Killer?

An excess of circulating cholesterol in the blood can injure blood vessels (arteries), especially the coronary arteries that supply blood to the heart, or the brain to which blood is supplied by cerebral arteries. This leads to accumulation of cholesterol in the vessel linings, resulting in the formation of cholesterol rich blocks (plaque) in the inner wall of blood vessels. Subsequently it grows in size and later on this cholesterol rich plaque can quietly clog or choke your arteries, blocking the flow of blood to your brain and/or heart, causing strokes and heart attacks respectively. Both the conditions come without warning and may be disastrous for health. Therefore, high cholesterol can silently kill you.

Why we, in India, should be Bothered about Cholesterol?

Most Indians are vegetarian while the remaining are non-vegetarians consuming meat or meat products occasionally. So why should we bother about our cholesterol? The irony is that despite being vegetarians, the incidence of heart disease and stroke is increasing in India. Figures speak differently from what we assume, the average cholesterol levels of Indians has increased from 160 mg/dl to 200mg/dl from 1960 to 2000. These figures in themselves support the growing concern regarding heart disease in India and the role played by high cholesterol in blood.

What are the Other Diseases Linked with High Levels of Cholesterol?

Excessive fat intake can also lead to obesity, high blood pressure and colon cancer, besides being linked to a number of other disorders as well. All these are contributing factors for significant diseases, disabilities and even death. To understand how fat intake is related to these health problems, it is necessary to understand the different types of fats available and the ways in which these fats act within the body.

What is Fatty Acid?

The main components of all fats are fatty acids. There are three major categories of fatty acids-saturated, polyunsaturated and monounsaturated. These classifications are based on the number of hydrogen atoms in the chemical structure of a given molecule of fatty acid. As far as the health of the heart is concerned, saturated fats along with trans-fats are harmful and polyunsaturated and monounsaturated fats are beneficial.

What is the Effect of Saturated Fats on the Body?

The liver uses saturated fats to manufacture cholesterol. Therefore, excessive dietary intake of saturated fats can significantly raise the blood cholesterol level, especially the level of low density lipoproteins (LDLs) or 'bad cholesterol.' Guidelines issued by the National Cholesterol Education Program (NCEP) which are widely supported by most experts, recommend that the daily intake of saturated fats should be kept below 10 % of the total calorie intake. However, for people who have severe problems with high blood cholesterol or heart disease, even that level may be too high and the saturated fat intake should be reduced to less than 7 %. Saturated fat intake is the strongest dietary determinant of blood cholesterol.

What are the Sources of Saturated Fat or Fatty Acids?

Saturated fatty acids are found primarily in animal products, including dairy items, such as whole milk, butter, fat, cream, ice cream and cheese, and fatty meats like that of goat, pork, beef, lamb, ham and chicken with skin. Egg yolk is also a rich source of saturated fats. Plant oils such as coconut, palm, kernel oils are rich in saturated fats. Coconut oil is extensively used as a cooking medium in South India and Sri Lanka. Fast foods are a rich source of saturated fats and salt. Vanaspati ghee and desi ghee (clarified butter), common in India are also rich sources of saturated fats.

What are Monounsaturated Fatty Acids?

Monounsaturated fatty acids are found mostly in vegetable and nut oils such as those obtained from olive, peanut, mustard and canola. These fats appear to reduce blood levels of LDL cholesterol. It has no effect on the HDL cholesterol level. However, this positive impact upon LDL cholesterol is relatively modest. The NCEP guidelines recommend that intake of monounsaturated fats should be kept between 10 and 15 % of the total calorie intake.

What are Polyunsaturated Fatty Acids?

Polyunsaturated fatty acids are found in abundance in corn, soya bean, safflower and sunflower oils. Certain fish oils are also high in polyunsaturated fats. Unlike the saturated fats, polyunsaturated fats help in lowering of total blood cholesterol level. However, large amount of polyunsaturated fats in the diet has a tendency to reduce high density lipoproteins (HDLs) also. For this reason and because, like all fats, polyunsaturated fats are high in calories the NCEP guidelines state that an individual's intake of polyunsaturated fats should not exceed

10 % of the total calorie intake. The two major categories of polyunsaturated fat are omega 6 and omega 3 fatty acids.

Essential Fatty Acids

Out of the three fatty acids, saturated and monounsaturated fats are not necessary in the diet as they can be made in the human body. However, two polyunsaturated fatty acids (PUFAs) that cannot be made in the body are alpha-linolenic acid (omega 3 fatty acids) and linoleic acid (omega 6 fatty acids). They must be provided in diet and are known as essential fatty acids. Within the body both can be converted to other PUFAs such as arachidonic acid or eicosapentaenoic acid (EPA) and docosahexaenoic acid (DHA). Omega 6 and omega 3 fatty acids are best consumed in a ratio of about 3:1- three omega 6 for one omega 3.

Understanding Omega 3 and Omega 6 Fatty Acids

Omega 3 Fatty Acid

As mentioned, it is a polyunsaturated fatty acid and is beneficial for health. It increases the level of HDL cholesterol, decreases triglycerides in blood and prevents blood clot formation. It helps in increasing metabolism, in regulating the blood sugar level and lowering the risk of obesity and diabetes. Omega 3 fatty acids are beneficial for the heart and are available in food items such as fish and fish oils. Vegetarians can get omega 3 fatty acids from flaxseeds (linseeds), mustard seeds, pumpkin seeds, soya bean, walnut oil, green leafy vegetables, broccoli, grains and spirulina. Fish is not the only source of omega 3 acids. Flaxseed oil contains twice as much as is found in fish oil.

Omega 6 Fatty Acid

Linoleic acid is one of the most essential fatty acids. Excess of omega 6 fatty acids can cause water retention and raise blood clotting. Safflower is the richest source of omega 6 fatty acids. Sunflower, sesame, corn, nuts such as walnut, cashews, almonds, pumpkin are other food items rich in omega 6 fatty acids.

Although most foods, including some plant derived foods contain a combination of all three types of fatty acids, one of the types usually predominates. Thus, a fat or oil is considered 'saturated', when it is composed primarily of saturated fatty acids. An example is coconut oil. Such saturated fats are usually solid at room temperature. Similarly, a fat or oil composed mostly of polyunsaturated fatty acids is called 'polyunsaturated,' while a fat or oil composed mostly of monounsaturated fatty acids is called 'monounsaturated.' If the goal is to lower cholesterol levels, polyunsaturated and mono unsaturated fats are more desirable than saturated fats or products with trans-fatty acids. In other words, oils used if solid at room temperature are bad for health. It is also important that your total calories from fat should not constitute more than 20-25 % of the daily calorie intake.

About Trans-fatty Acids

One other element, trans-fatty acid, plays an important role in blood cholesterol levels. It is also called trans-fats and is manufactured when polyunsaturated oils are altered through hydrogenation, a process used to harden liquid vegetable oils into solid foods. Trans-fatty acids raise LDL cholesterol levels, behaving much like saturated fats. Simultaneously, the trans-fatty acids reduce HDL cholesterol readings. Deep frying is a common practice, however, few know that deep frying results in spontaneous hydrogenation and formation of trans-fats.

Because of financial reasons, left over oil is not discarded and reused again which further deteriorates its nutritive value and makes its dangerous for health. Trans-fats should constitute less than 1 % of the total calorie value. All fast foods and junk foods are a rich source of trans-fats. Commercially available food items are rich in trans-fat as it is the cheapest oil in India and used extensively as cooking oil.

What is Lipid Profile?

Lipid profile is a blood test and is frequently ordered by your doctor. The test estimates various cholesterol components present in blood. Cholesterol can't dissolve in blood. It is transported in the blood with the help of protein particles known as lipoproteins so that it can be utilized, stored in excess or excreted from the body. The various cholesterol components which are measured in the blood are, total cholesterol (TC), low density lipoproteins (LDL), triglycerides (TG), very low density lipoproteins (VLDL) and high density lipoproteins (HDL). Out of all five components, only HDL is the good cholesterol and protects the body. Lipoprotein [Lp(a)] is also included in this list by some labs. Lipid profile is done in the serum obtained from blood. Blood should be collected after 10-12 hours of fasting as estimation of triglyceride, an important component of lipid profile is influenced by diet.

What are the Major Lipid Disorders in the Body?

Abnormal levels of various lipid components can be present in the body alone or in combination. Increased level of LDL cholesterol alone is a strong predictor of heart disease and stroke. In India, increased level of serum triglycerides (TG), increased VLDL, and increased level of small dense LDL cholesterol along with low level of protective or good cholesterol that is, HDL is more frequent. A large population of the developing world including Indians suffer from diabetes mellitus. A low level of HDL and high level of TG is frequent with diabetes mellitus and both result in the development of heart disease or coronary heart disease. In Indians, high triglycerides levels, high Lp(a) along with low levels of HDL is considered a deadly combination and is detrimental to health.

What does the Cholesterol Number Mean to Health?

The total cholesterol count should be less than 200 mg/dl and if it is more than 250 mg/dl then it should be a cause of concern and requires urgent attention. Between 200 – 250 mg/dl is borderline, requires dietary and lifestyle modifications and should be monitored closely. In India, usually LDL is not too raised, a count of more than 130 mg/dl is considered high and should be monitored. If one is suffering from diabetes mellitus or heart disease, LDL should be kept at less than 100 mg/dl. The good cholesterol (HDL) count is important for everyone's health. It is the only cholesterol count which should be kept high. Unfortunately in Indians it is lower in a majority of cases. It should be above 40 mg/dl and 50 mg/dl for men and women respectively. Sedentary habits and tobacco use influence the HDL level in blood and anything lower than 40 mg/dl should be a cause for concern, as this type of cholesterol actually protects you from heart disease and stroke. Triglycerides are another type of fat in the blood, that are also usually measured when a cholesterol count is done. Triglyceride levels that are less than 150 mg/dl are good for health and any number which is above 250 mg/dl should make you alert. As against western standards, Indians tend to have higher triglyceride levels than LDL cholesterol.

What is Bad Cholesterol?
LDL cholesterol is regarded to be harmful as it causes build up and potential blockages in your arteries. It is thus responsible for increased chances of heart disease and stroke. Because of this link with the cardiovascular disease process LDL cholesterol is regarded as bad cholesterol.

What is Good Cholesterol?
For every 1 mg/dl increase in HDL, the incidence of adverse cardiac event decreases by 2 % in men and 3 % in women. The mechanism by which it protects us against heart disease is not very clear. It is hypothesized that HDL can remove cholesterol from fatty build ups (atheroma) within blood vessels. The removed cholesterol is transported back to the liver either for excretion or re-utilization. Thus HDL cholesterol clears the other cholesterol components. A low level of HDL-c rather than high level of LDL-c is currently the most common abnormality in patients with CHD in the Indian subcontinent. High prevalence of low HDL-c may play a role in the development of early or premature CHD.

What is Triglyceride Cholesterol?
Triglyceride is a form of fat which is commonly raised in Indians and is manufactured in the body. Excess of triglycerides in blood is termed as hypertriglyceridaemia. Several clinical studies have shown that people with above normal triglyceride levels (greater than or equal to 250 mg/dl) have an increased risk of heart disease. High level of triglycerides in blood is often associated with obesity, smoking, alcohol consumption, sedentary lifestyle, diet rich in carbohydrate and diabetes mellitus. All is common amongst Indians. National Cholesterol Education Program (NCEP) classified the triglyceride levels in blood (Table 15.1) and proposed drug treatment once it is

high and very high with statin alone or in combination with other cholesterol lowering drugs. Borderline high triglycerides should be treated with lifestyle modification alone.

Table 15.1: NCEP Classification for Triglyceride Levels

Less than 150 mg/dl	Normal
150-199 mg/dl	Borderline high
200-499 mg/dl	High
More than 500 mg/dl	Very high

What is Lp(a) Cholesterol?

Lp(a) is a sub-fraction of LDL (bad) cholesterol. A high level of Lp(a) is a significant risk factor for the premature development of fatty deposits in arteries. Age, sex, diet and environmental factors do not have any influence on its level. Lp(a) isn't fully understood, but it may interact with substances found in artery walls and contribute to the build-up of fatty deposits.

What is Xanthelasma and Xanthomas?

Various lipid disorders which result in excess of cholesterol in blood can manifest as deposits of fat beneath the skin. It can be deposited around your eyes which is yellowish in colour and is considered a marker of high cholesterol levels in the body and is called as xanthelasma. When it is deposited around tendons (structure which joins muscles to bone) and along the creases of your palm it is termed as xanthomas. Presence of these may be a sign of high cholesterol in blood and alert you to get your cholesterol level checked. However, presence of xanthomas is more specific and correlates more with hyperlipidaemia as compared to xanthelasma.

What are Cholesterol Guidelines and how much should I Know?

The Report of the National Cholesterol Education Program (NCEP) Expert panel on detection, evaluation and treatment of high blood cholesterol in adults (adult Treatment Panel III (ATP III) provides evidence-based recommendations on the management of high cholesterol and related disorders. NCEP guidelines are usually based on the available scientific data published and are revised from time to time. Differences in approach have existed between US and European guidelines. The former focused on banding risk according to LDL cholesterol and had a low target of below 100 mg/dl for those at high risk (that is, secondary prevention) or 70 mg/dl for very high risk groups, while the latter emphasized the importance of global risk assessment and used a moderate LDL goal. Noteworthy features in the recent guidelines are as follows:

1. First the definition of low HDL is < 40 mg/dl. This can increase substantially the number of subjects who broach risk criterion, and this is very important in the context of India where HDL cholesterol is low.
2. Second, physicians are encouraged to assess the global risk of a coronary event using the charts developed from the Framingham epidemiological study. Other medical conditions and diseases should also be taken into account. A higher risk person should be targeted aggressively.
3. Third diabetes is considered a 'CHD equivalent risk'. There is now substantial data to support the view that a patient with diabetes who has not had a heart attack is at approximately the same risk of a future adverse heart (coronary) event as a non-diabetic patient with established CHD. Since rates of diabetes are very high in Indians, the disease further contributes to heart disease risk in this population.

4. Fourth, the particular constellation of risk factors comprising the 'metabolic syndrome' is recognized as identifying individuals at risk of CHD in the absence of elevated LDL. In India, there is a growing trend towards metabolic syndrome. This syndrome is a deadly combination of hypertension, diabetes mellitus, heart disease and abnormal lipid levels or dyslipidaemia due to abdominal obesity. The cause of this is both bad genes and bad environment. Coronary risk factor profiles in the various population survey conducted has confirmed the high frequency of central obesity, low plasma HDL cholesterol, high plasma triglycerides and hyperinsulinaemia. This is more amongst urban population than rural population.

What is Bothering Indians?

National Cholesterol Education Program Adult Treatment Panel III (NCEPATP III) guidelines establish the acceptable 'normal' level of triglycerides as < 150 mg/dl. In Indians, this level is usually > 150 mg/dl. The HDL level is also low and is usually < 40 mg/d. In Asian Indians, living in the US, it was found that 54 % of the men had HDL below 40 mg/dl, and 68 % of women had levels below 50 mg/dl. The cardio-protective effects of HDL depend on the size of the HDL particle. Large HDL particles are associated with a lesser risk of atherosclerosis as compared to small HDL particles. Thus, small HDL particles give less protection against atherosclerosis and increase the progression of atherosclerosis. At a given level of cholesterol, the concentrations of large HDL cholesterol (HDL2) were lower and concentrations of small HDL cholesterol (HDL3) were significantly higher in Indians. It is not only that total HDL concentration which is low but the overall HDL particle size is smaller in Indians as compared to people living in Europe and Americas. These abnormalities may represent dysfunctional HDL that is not ascertained by the conventional lipid profile.

Lp(a) also is a major risk factor in Indians, which could explain the high incidence of early myocardial infarction in this population. Elevated Lp(a) is a genetic risk factor that has been shown to at least double the risk of heart attack. Although Lp(a) levels more than 30 mg/dl are generally considered the threshold at which the risk of premature CHD increases rapidly, levels below 20 mg/dl are considered optimum, particularly in Asian Indians. Furthermore, small LDL particle is a risk factor in any population, but it is particularly prevalent in Indians. Small, dense LDL particles can be more easily oxidized and they penetrate the artery wall much more efficiently than larger LDL particles, a key step in the initiation of atherosclerosis.

What is the Desirable Level of Different Cholesterol Components?

The latest recommendations suggest that adults with no heart disease or diabetes mellitus should have LDL level less than 130 mg/dl and triglycerides below 150 mg/dl. The optimal level for HDL should be more than 40 mg/dl and 60 mg/dl in men and women respectively. The total cholesterol should be less than 200 mg/dl (Table 15.2).

Table 15.2: Desirable Levels of Various Cholesterol Fractions in Blood

Cholesterol	Level mg/dl
Total cholesterol	< 200
LDL cholesterol	< 130 in health and < 100 in CHD
Triglyceride (TG)	< 150
HDL cholesterol	> 40 in male, > 60 in female
Lipoprotein Lp(a)	< 20

How to Manage Cholesterol Abnormalities?

In practice all the lipid abnormalities are managed together. All measures should be adopted so that bad cholesterol such as LDL, triglycerides and total cholesterol (TC) are below the target level and HDL is above the target level.

What Are the Management Strategies for High Cholesterol?

The principle of management is to educate people and encourage them to adopt healthy eating habits and lifestyles. If the lifestyles and diet measures alone are inadequate then drugs may be started. The management strategies adopted are as follows:

1. Lifestyle changes include exercise, reduction in weight, quitting tobacco consumption and moderate consumption of alcohol.
2. Diet is the next most important aspect. Diet should be such that it should have not only the desired calories but it should be low in saturated fats, trans-fats, cholesterol and refined sugars.
3. Cholesterol lowering drugs should always be used in conjunction with diet and lifestyle changes.

How Much Fat Should be Taken Daily?

Total fats in diet should be restricted to around 20-25 % of total calories. If the fat content is more than 30 % then it is not possible to limit the intake of saturated fats to maintain a low level of LDL-c and triglycerides. Saturated fat intake should be limited to less than 10 % of total calories and remaining fat should be substituted with unsaturated fats. Excessive of fat intake is associated with excessive consumption of calories resulting in obesity. On the other hand, if the total fat content is less than 25 % triglycerides can rise and the HDL levels can decline. Thus, very low fat diets may be harmful. A very low fat diet or a fat-free diet is deleterious for health and should not be practiced.

What are the Dietary Precautions?

Dietary modifications are the cornerstone of prevention and treatment of lipid disorders. Its purpose is to reduce the risk for CHD by limiting the intake of saturated fat, maintaining a nutritious diet and an appropriate calorie level. The principles for treatment are:

1. Total fat intake should be restricted to one fourth of the total calorie intake.
2. Ensure correct essential fatty acids (EFA) intake with near optimal omega 6/omega 3 ratio; it should be 3:1 (w6/w3).
3. Foods rich in saturated fat and trans-fat should be avoided.

The practical guide is to consume:

1. Seasonal vegetables and fruits should be consumed in plenty and regularly.
2. Cooking oil should be rich in monounsaturated fats with less of polyunsaturated and saturated fats.
3. Egg intake should be restricted to one per day and the yellow portion should be avoided.
4. Fish consumption should be encouraged followed by lean meat and poultry.
5. Organ meats (brain, liver, etc.) and sea foods such as shrimps, crabs and lobsters should be reduced as they are rich sources of cholesterol.
6. Skimmed milk and its products should be a part of the daily diet and consumption of whole milk, butter, cheese, ghee should be avoided. Prefer cow's milk as it contains half the fat content of buffalo milk.

7. Avoid simple sugars in diet such as sweets; replace it with fruit desserts.
8. Fried and fast foods should be avoided. Instead, food should preferably be grilled, steamed, boiled or micro waved.
9. Extreme dietary modifications and a fat-less diet are injurious to health and should be avoided

What is the Role of Fish Oils in Diet?

Fish oils are rich in polyunsaturated fatty acids such as omega 3 fatty acids which are associated with the reduction in occurrence of heart disease. It has been proved that the habitual intake of oily fish appears to offer protection against heart disease. Intake of two portions of oily fish once a week is associated with a reduction in heart disease. Commercial fish oil preparation is available as a capsule and can be taken with food with similar benefits. It is quite safe, however, in a few cases it may cause gastric upset. It should not be prescribed to people suffering from bleeding disorders or who are taking blood thinning drugs or anticoagulants.

How can Vegetarians Get the Benefit of Omega 3 Fatty Acids?

A majority of Indians are vegetarian. Considering this, consumption of nuts, flaxseeds (linseed), mustard seeds, pumpkin seeds, soya bean, walnut oil, green leafy vegetables and rapeseed (canola) will provide enough omega 3 fatty acids in diet. It is advisable to consume 50 gm of nuts, especially walnuts twice a week. Apricot is also rich in omega 3 fatty acids.

What is the Role of Garlic?

Regular use of garlic (a routine ingredient of Indian food) helps to reduce cholesterol levels in blood. It can be eaten raw or with food and one or two cloves of garlic a day is sufficient. It has antiviral and antibacterial properties also.

What is the Role of Smoking and Alcohol?

Smoking decreases the level of good HDL cholesterol and modest regular consumption of alcohol that is, 2 or less than 2 pegs per day increases the HDL cholesterol. Tobacco consumption should be discouraged in any form and alcohol should not be consumed to increase the level of HDL as there are other healthy ways of increasing HDL levels. The best way is through regular physical exercise.

What are the Cholesterol Lowering Drugs?

Statins, fibrates, resins and ezetimibe are the drugs which are often used for the treatment of lipid or cholesterol abnormalities. Niacin is the only drug which helps in increasing the level of good cholesterol that is, HDL. However, this drug can cause gastric upsets, flushing and rashes (red spots). Fibrates are the drugs which lower triglyceride levels. Statins can lower LDL, triglycerides and total cholesterol. Therefore, it is the most widely prescribed drug for lowering cholesterol in the body. Statins are the most popular drug all over the globe for lowering cholesterol levels.

How do Statins Work?

Statins inhibit the enzyme hydroxyl-3-methylglutaryl coenzyme A (HMG CoA) reductase. This is the rate limiting enzyme in the cholesterol synthetic pathway. Inhibition of the enzyme causes a reduction in cholesterol synthesis which thereby reduces the total cholesterol and LDL cholesterol.

Where should Statins be Used?

The drug is used to control high levels of total cholesterol and LDL cholesterol. It can also be used to reduce high levels of triglycerides. It can also increase the level of HDL cholesterol. This reduces the process of atherosclerosis, inhibits the growth of atheromatous plaque and helps in reducing the disease burden linked with high cholesterol.

When should Statin be Started and in what Dosage?

It should be started as early as possible. The dose of statins varies from 10-80 mg per day and will be decided by your doctor.

When should Statins be Avoided?

This drug should not be administered in individuals who have liver disease. It should also not be given during pregnancy and breast feeding. Porphyria is another condition where this drug should not be used.

What are the Adverse Effects of Statins?

The safety profile is excellent with statins and the majority of patients tolerate the drug well. Adverse effects leading to discontinuation of this drug are rare. Gastric upset, weakness, headache and muscle pain may occur in a few cases. The most serious adverse effect with statin therapy is myopathy or serious cramps. It is a very rare complication and characterized by painful muscles. Myopathy resolves completely once the drug is discontinued. Patients are advised to stop the drug if they develop severe muscle pains and to consult their doctor immediately.

Is the Treatment Different for the Indian Subcontinent?

Indians have slightly different cholesterol composition than their western counterparts. High triglyceride levels and low HDL levels are more common than high LDL cholesterol levels. Therefore, for Indians, the aim of the treatment is to think beyond LDL control.

How to Treat High Triglyceride Levels?

For triglyceride levels below 250 mg/dl, the importance of therapeutic lifestyle changes are stressed and practiced. Few essential aspects of lifestyle changes are weight control, increased physical activity, cessation of smoking and restriction of alcohol. For triglyceride levels between 250-500 it is better to start drugs with lifestyle changes. The primary drug is statin along with fibrates, niacin and/or fish oil. Statins lower triglyceride level by 7-30 %, fibrates by 20-50 %, niacin by 20-50 % and fish oil by 20-45%. Statins are usually preferred with fibrates or fish oil as niacin is associated with more side effects. Apart from this, niacin in larger doses that is, more than 2 gm per day can worsen the glucose level in people with diabetes or insulin resistance. This must be taken into consideration while treating triglyceride abnormality in diabetics.

How to Treat Low HDL?

Low HDL cholesterol is a problem and a common abnormality in Indians. It is postulated that low levels of HDL is a powerful predictor of CHD risk, even more so than elevated LDL or total cholesterol. Causes of low HDL include, a high level of triglyceride, Type 2 diabetes, physical inactivity, smoking or use of tobacco, very high carbohydrate diet (> 60 % of total calories), obesity and genetic. All these are highly prevalent in India. Weight loss, cessation of smoking, exercise and diet high in omega 3 fatty acids, all raise HDL. Moderate alcohol consumption also raises HDL but is not recommended for this purpose. Drugs such as statin can be used with fibrate to increase the level of HDL. Therapeutic lifestyle changes raise the HDL cholesterol by 5-39 %. Niacin is a very effective drug in raising HDL levels by 15-35 %. Statins and fibrates raise it by 5-15 % and 10-35 %, respectively. Oestrogen, a female hormone, can increase the levels of HDL but it simultaneously increases the level of triglycerides as age advances.

Woman and Cholesterol

In women, over their life span, you will be surprised to know that the total cholesterol composition is not the same and changes with age. During childhood, HDL cholesterol and LDL cholesterol concentration remains the same in both sexes. During puberty, HDL levels fall in men while they remain the same in women. Till women attain menopause, they usually maintain high HDL cholesterol and low LDL cholesterol levels. However, after menopause, LDL cholesterol levels are higher in women than in men of the same age. Hence, after menopause, the LDL cholesterol levels rise in women, so does the risk of CHD.

Premenopausal women are usually protected from ill effects of LDL cholesterol because of the female hormone oestrogen. Oestrogen tends to raise HDL cholesterol levels. The various cholesterol levels tend to increase as the age advances and the protective effect of oestrogen is lost after menopause. Diabetes mellitus in women is one condition which is often associated with lipid abnormalities. In our country, women, especially after menopause are less active and gain weight which can increase the cholesterol levels in blood. If you are approaching menopause or suffering from diabetes or hypertension, it is better to have your cholesterol checked and talk to your doctor regarding your options as it is no more a man's problem. Many women with high cholesterol levels are at coronary heart disease risk, yet their abnormal lipid levels are largely undetected in India, leaving considerable risk for future events. If your cholesterol levels are normal, even then it is important to eat a heart healthy diet, stay physically active, maintain an ideal weight and avoid tobacco.

Cholesterol and Kids

Until recently, tracking cholesterol in children was unheard of, and health risks associated with high cholesterol levels, such as heart attack and stroke were of little concern. That is not the case today and weight related medical problems are increasingly common among obese children. Many see the foreshadowing of a generation of teens and adolescents with cardiovascular disease. Obesity in children easily puts them on track for high blood pressure, risk of diabetes, heart problems and other serious health issues. Studies revealed that children with elevated levels of triglyceride, a common problem in Indians may be at an increased risk of cardiovascular disease events in early adulthood. Elevated paediatric triglyceride level is an exceptionally strong, independent risk factor for early onset of cardiac events. Cholesterol estimation may be necessary especially for obese kids with or without a family history of heart disease. Statin the most widely prescribed drug to lower cholesterol levels should not be used below 8 years of age.

What is the Cause of Concern Today?

People are not aware of the role played by cholesterol on health. Screening and aggressiveness of treatment for high cholesterol levels are often overlooked even though it is a major risk factor for CHD. Getting lipid profile estimation lags behind the estimation of sugar levels because the test is costly and people are more aware of Diabetes mellitus. Since high cholesterol is a number and results in no complaint it is often neglected. These disparities may reflect either a traditional emphasis on sugar management in diabetic patients that outweighs emphasis on other cardiovascular risk factors or a slow adoption of lipid management guidelines. Even though effective drug therapy is available, it is prescribed less frequently by the physicians either because of high cost of the therapy or because of lack of knowledge.

Cholesterol at a Glance

1. *Cholesterol or fat is a wax-like substance and is essential for health.*
2. *A small quantity of fat in diet is necessary for body functions and absorption of fat soluble vitamins.*
3. *In adults, only a small quantity is needed in the diet as large quantities is manufactured in the liver itself. One requires only 200 mg of cholesterol daily which is equivalent to consuming an egg.*
4. *Fats are made up of fatty acids which are mainly saturated or unsaturated.*

5. *Excess consumption of saturated fats is bad for health. Saturated fat is present in whole milk and its products, coconut or palm oil and fatty meat cuts. These are all bad for health.*
6. *Monounsaturated fat is a type of unsaturated fat which is good for health as it reduces LDL cholesterol. It is mainly found in olive, canola, peanuts and mustard oils.*
7. *Polyunsaturated fat is again a type of unsaturated fat. It lowers total cholesterol. However, in large amounts it reduces HDL cholesterol also. It is found in safflower, sunflower, corn and soya bean oils.*
8. *Omega fatty acids are a type of fatty acids which are essential for health and are not manufactured in the body.*
9. *Intake of fish which is rich in omega fatty acids, once or twice a week can protect you against heart disease.*
10. *Walnut is rich in omega fatty acids. 50 gms, twice a week for vegetarian Indians is enough to provide the necessary quantity.*
11. *Trans-fats which are obtained by hydrogenation of vegetable oils is bad for health and should be consumed less than 1 % per day.*
12. *There are five types of cholesterol components in blood. High level of cholesterol is called hypercholesterolaemia and is a major risk factor for CHD.*
13. *Low density lipoprotein cholesterol and triglycerides are bad for health as they deposit against artery walls and increase the risk of heart disease (bad cholesterol).*
14. *High density lipoprotein cholesterol is known as good cholesterol and protects from heart disease.*
15. *In India, high triglyceride levels and low levels of HDL cholesterol is common as compared to high LDL cholesterol level which is prevalent in the west.*

16. Physical inactivity and excessive tobacco consumption decreases the levels of HDL. Diabetes mellitus, excessive intake of whole milk and its products along with red and organ meat increase the levels of triglycerides in Indians.
17. All components of cholesterol and their level can be estimated by a simple blood test known as lipid profile.
18. Statin is the most prescribed and preferred drug for controlling high levels of cholesterol components in blood. However, it may be associated with severe muscle pain or cramps in a few cases.
19. Women have high levels of HDL cholesterol till menopause as compared to men. However, after menopause, the level decreases and increases the incidence of CHD in women.
20. In India, childhood obesity resulting from physical inactivity and unhealthy food habits is causing low levels of HDL and high levels of triglycerides. All this increases the future risk of CHD which can lead to premature development of heart disease.

Chapter 16

Smoking and Tobacco Use

Smoking and tobacco use is a major health problem worldwide and more so in developing countries. Today, there are almost a billion smokers in the world out of which 70 % are in developing countries. China tops the list of smokers in the world. WHO estimates that tobacco use kills 5.4 million people every year and the epidemic is worsening, especially in the developing world where more than 80 % of tobacco-caused deaths will occur in the coming decades. A total of 100 million people lost their lives in the twentieth century and if the same trend continues and if no urgent measures are taken, one billion people will die worldwide from tobacco use in the twenty first century, despite the fact that it is the leading cause of preventable disease and death in the world. A firm determination and habit of saying NO to tobacco consumption can save millions of people each year from tobacco linked lung and heart diseases. Increased initiative at different levels has led to positive results and a decrease in the number of smokers in developed countries. Developing countries including India have to make a lot more effort, where the consumption of tobacco is increasing by 3.4 % annually.

Global tobacco epidemic not only affects the health of millions of people but is also a major economic threat that costs huge amounts of money in health expenditure and other economic losses each year. Tobacco use hurts the poor more than the rich and digs into the pocket, deepens poverty by misusing money needed for basic necessities such as food, shelter and education. The tobacco habit kills wage earners in the prime of their lives. We Indians are no different. The total economic burden of major diseases due to tobacco use in India runs in thousands of crores of rupees or billions of dollars. It is also a social threat as the majority of tobacco users also consume alcohol, heroin, cocaine, *ganja or bhang* (cannabis) and are associated with household and community violence.

When you burn a cigarette or *bidi*, the heat breaks the tobacco into various toxins resulting in lethal consequences. It not only burns your lungs but breaks your heart along with the heart of your beloved ones.

It is not worth it

'I am just 39 and a school teacher. Our lives were shattered and changed forever, when I lost my husband, a chain smoker, to a massive heart attack. It was the severest blow of my life. We all had lost a dear one-a caring father and a loving husband. Initially I was under the impression that smoking is inherently not good but now I have realized that it is a dangerous habit. It was then that I really learnt the importance of our body. I teach my children, who are 14 and 16, that we may be young but our body will age with us and it will age faster if we don't take care of it. Our bodies are amazing tools, a marvellous gift of nature given to us and we should learn to treat our body the way nature cares. I can only urge my children to take a pledge in the name of their late father that they will not spoil their body with the smoke of tobacco. Never start smoking.'

Is Tobacco Use Common Among Indians?

Yes. Tobacco use in various forms including smoking and chewing has been always the integral part of community life in India. In India, tobacco was introduced by the Portuguese during 1600 AD in Karnataka. Smoking a bidi (Indian cigarette) is the commonest form of tobacco consumption in India and accounts for 40 % of the total tobacco use. *Bidi* smoking is common amongst the rural population because it is cheaper compared to cigarettes. Cigarette smoking is the next commonest addiction of tobacco in urban India. Hookah is also another form of tobacco use and is restricted to a few rural pockets in India. Cigar and pipes are an uncommon form of tobacco use and is prevalent in high socio-economic groups. Smokeless tobacco in the form of chewing tobacco alone (*khaini* or *surti*, sun dried tobacco grounded well with lime) or gutka (tobacco, areca nut and other flavoured substances sold in powder or granulated form in attractive small pouches) is common both in rural and urban India. The rapid surge in the use of *gutka* among young Indians is a matter of concern. Betel leaves with pieces of areca nut, tobacco (*zarda*) and slaked lime is a common practice as it is assumed to remove bad breath. Apart from being a breath freshener, it is also believed that it can help in digestion. Tobacco used as snuff (*gul*) is less common than chewing tobacco. Use of tobacco as toothpaste is another form of tobacco addiction. Electronic or e-cigarette is now sold in India and is growing in popularity among elite class of young Indians.

Burden of Tobacco Use in India

Smoking and tobacco chewing are very common in both urban and rural India. The cause of concern is that people start this addiction from a very early age and continue with it life-long. In the last decade, chewing tobacco in the form of pan masala has become extremely popular among the youths across India.

It is estimated that 250 million people above the age of 15 years consume some form of tobacco. It is also estimated that about 150 million people smoke tobacco, while 100 million used as smokeless form of tobacco. Death associated with tobacco use is estimated to be one million every year in India and it is projected that it will rise to 1.5 million by 2020. In the traditional Indian system, the habit of tobacco consumption varies between socio-economic groups and between genders. Prevalence in men is more (51 %) as compared to women (20-25 %) since smoking is not widely accepted amongst women in the Indian society. The consumption of tobacco is more in rural areas as compared to urban areas and almost 70 % of the people in rural India smoke bidi or use other tobacco products regularly.

State Level Variation

The use of tobacco products vary significantly among different states of India. The education level and religion has a vast influence over tobacco consumption. Punjab has the lowest level of tobacco consumption because its consumption is prohibited by the Sikh religion. The poor and weaker sections of society consume more tobacco products as compared to the higher income groups. Chewing tobacco is more common in the Central, Eastern, Western and North Eastern states, compared to Northern and Southern states. In these states tobacco smoking is more common probably due to high income and literacy rates.

What is a *Bidi*?

Bidi is also known as Indian cigarette. It is very common in rural India. Bidis are made of tobacco, hand rolled in *tendu or temburni (Diospyros melanoxylon)* leaf. The *bidi* is typically tied on one or both ends with a colourful string and is unfiltered. They usually cost less than regular cigarettes, and its use is frequent both in men and women in rural India.

Bidi packs contained no health warning labels that traditional cigarettes did till 2006. The recent move to make pictorial warnings on tobacco products mandatory is yet another step towards curbing the tobacco epidemic in India.

Is *Bidi* Smoking Different from Cigarette Smoking?

No, *bidis* appear to have all the same health risks as regular cigarettes. Though the *bidi* contains less tobacco than regular cigarettes, it is more harmful than a cigarette as it contains three times more nicotine and five times more tar. Also it is unfiltered. *Bidi* smokers take a deep and frequent puff to prevent it from getting extinguished. *Bidi* smokers are more susceptible to the risks of heart attack, chronic bronchitis and some cancers than non-smokers. Studies in India, where *bidi* smoking is common, have shown that the death rates of *bidi* smokers are as high as those of cigarette smokers and much higher than those of non-smokers.

The problem is further worsened by the sheer number of people who smoke *bidis*. There are twice as many *bidi* smokers as compared to cigarette smokers in India. *Bidi* smokers do not get the same attention and priority, as the majority belongs to rural area and low economic group. Low literacy rate, lack of awareness about the dangers of tobacco and poor health facilities among *bidi* smokers make the problem worse.

What is a Hookah?

Hookah smoking started in the Middle East but some believe that its birth place is in India. This unique gadget has many names and has a long history. It is called a hookah in India and Pakistan, *Shsiha* in the Middle East, *Nargila* in Turkey, *Kalian* in Egypt and *Chillum* in Uzbekistan. One can simply call it a smoking water pipe. A majority of user burn flavoured tobacco and inhale the smoke through a long pipe. The smoke of tobacco is drawn through water to cool it. It has been popular in different parts of the world and people use to smoke different herbs, roots and leaves of plant for curative purposes. A coconut or an earthen pot serves as a vessel and a long flexible pipe is attached to it. It is usually placed on the floor or a low table. It is believed that the hookah should be smoked after a full meal and in a sitting or reclining position on a mattress or sofa pillows or cushions are added to make the surroundings cosy. Traditionally, it should not be smoked with alcohol. Hookah smoking is usually a social event that allows the smokers to spend time together and talk as they pass the pipe around. The use of hookah from ancient times in India was not only a custom, but a matter of prestige. The rich people and landlords would smoke hookahs. Offering a hookah was a gesture of respect and regard to guests and clients. Tobacco is smoked in hookahs in many villages as per their traditional customs and is a community affair. The person who shares his hookah with others indicates his equality with the other members. Molasses in hookah is also used by youths today. Various forms of hookah are served in some bars, coffee shops and road side restaurants *(dhabas)* in modern India. It has also found a place in some five star hotels.

Is the Hookah Safe?

It is believed to be a safe alternative to cigarettes because the percentage of tobacco in the product smoked is low due to the passage of smoke through water. This claim for safety is false and it is not true. Water does not filter out many toxins. In fact, hookah smoke contains more toxins such as nicotine, carbon monoxide, tar and other hazardous substances than cigarette smoke. Several types of cancer have been linked to hookah smoking. Hookah use is also linked to other unique risks not linked with cigarette smoking. For example, infectious diseases such as tuberculosis can be spread by sharing the pipe or through the way the tobacco is prepared.

What is Smokeless Tobacco?

Smokeless tobacco products consist of tobacco or a tobacco blend that is chewed, kept in the mouth, inhaled or sucked on rather than being smoked. The use of smokeless tobacco is increasing at an alarming rate amongst the youth. It is becoming increasingly popular amongst women, both in rural and urban India. In India, it is available in three forms:

1. **Chewing Tobacco:** A type of smokeless tobacco in which tobacco is chewed in the form of a dried leaf with lime. *Surti, khaini or sada* (tobacco leaf and lime mixture), *zarda, mawa or mishri* with or without betel leaf are common forms of smokeless tobacco and are highly prevalent in rural areas. *Gutka or pan masala* which are industrially manufactured tobacco contain areca nut, tobacco and other ingredients. It has become extremely popular amongst young Indians in the recent times.

2. **Snuff or *Gul*:** This is available as a dry or moist form of tobacco leaf which comes in pouches. A pinch of snuff may be placed and inhaled through the nostrils.

    Tobacco toothpastes (*noora*) are applied in the oral cavity to get strong and healthy teeth.

3. **Betel Quid:** Betel leaves *(Piper betle)* with pieces of areca nut, tobacco *(zarda)* and slaked lime are routinely consumed by both men and women alike. Offering and serving betel quid with or without tobacco to guests is a

common practice in social gatherings and marriages as a sign of hospitality. Varanasi or Banaras is famous for its betel quid or *'Banarasi pan'*. People who consume tobacco with betel, live in the false belief that it is not absorbed into the blood, since they do not ingest the tobacco and spit it out.

What are the Myths Attached with Tobacco Use in India?

In India, tobacco users have many reasons and excuses to either start or continue tobacco use. Some of the false beliefs in India are:

1. Those who use tobacco look more attractive and smart.
2. People who smoke are more successful.
3. Tobacco users think that tobacco helped people feel more comfortable and relaxed.
4. Tobacco users feel that tobacco helps in relieving toothaches and constipation.
5. A few believe that tobacco use and smoking helps in losing weight.
6. Long distance drivers think that its use helps them to remain more alert and awake.
7. Tobacco users feel that the tobacco habit is difficult to quit.

How Common is Tobacco Use Among School Students in India?

The prevalence of tobacco use in school going students is not only alarming but a matter of serious concern. It is very high in a few states such as Bihar and North-Eastern India. The use among boys range from 50 to 74 % and in girls it is 32-56 %. The reason for such high prevalence may be due to the fact that students are not aware of the harmful effects of tobacco use as it is neither taught in school nor at home. Peer pressure from friends, easy availability, low cost (gutka pouch costs a rupee only) and advertisement by celebrities, youth targeted advertisements are few of the reasons for early initiation of tobacco use in school going children. Global School Personnel Survey (GSPS) is a school based survey of school personnel. It collects data on the prevalence of cigarette and other tobacco use, a tobacco free school policy, attitude on tobacco control issues and training to prevent youth tobacco use by school personnel. Their survey revealed astonishing facts. Some of the major findings were:

1. As per the survey, an alarming proportion of over 33 % of school personnel used tobacco in some form.
2. Most schools do not have a 'tobacco-free school' policy.
3. Teaching materials on tobacco control are not available in a majority of the schools and hardly any training on the subject is provided to school personnel.
4. Those who start at an early age usually belong to the low socio-economic strata, are victims of a broken family and by the time they realize the risk and hazard, they are addicted to it.

What is the Role Played by the Tobacco Industry?

Approximately 100 countries produce tobacco in the world and India is a major player in the international tobacco trade. It is the second largest producer and eighth largest exporter of tobacco in the world. It contributes to 6 % of the total tobacco trade of the international market. The *bidi* industry is the largest manufacturer of tobacco products in India. You will be surprised to know that a few of the *bidi* manufacturers are the top tax payers of India.

The burden of smoking related illnesses falls disproportionately on those belonging to the lower socio-economic status. The tobacco companies prey especially upon the poor, uneducated and the most vulnerable population, the NATION'S YOUTH. The tobacco industry's advertisements and other promotions for its products are another big influence on our society. Youth-targeted media advertisements and sports sponsorships influence this attitude. Sports sponsorship by tobacco companies influence the minds of children and helps initiate smoking in India. *Gutka* and *pan masala* are one of the most highly advertised products in almost all media and surrogate advertisements are popular to defy the law. Tobacco is the only commercially available product that has no benefit and is unequivocally hazardous to human health. Many of the large tobacco companies regularly donate huge sums of money to the national political parties. The role of the tobacco industry is very clear – they increase their revenue by decreasing your life span.

What is the Role of Government Agencies?

The fight against tobacco has been initiated from various quarters. It is estimated that at least 30 % of the future burden of cancer cases is potentially preventable through tobacco control. Government has tried to control tobacco use by passing various laws and regulations, despite stiff resistance from the manufacturers. Key provisions of the law include prohibition on direct and indirect advertisements of tobacco products, prohibiting the sale of tobacco products to minors, prohibition of smoking in public places and prohibition on the sale of tobacco products near educational institutions. Provision for heavy taxes on cigarettes, *bidis* and other tobacco products along with allocation of separate funds for tobacco control have been made. Recent provisions related to mandatory display of the pictorial (scorpion, X-ray of diseased lung or gangrene over limb) health warnings on tobacco product packs are cost effective ways of increasing the public awareness regarding the serious health risks of tobacco. These efforts may trigger a more intense response and may generate a greater degree of motivation and an intention to quit tobacco products. These efforts are more helpful for people with low levels of literacy or among the uneducated and the young vulnerable population. The laws, provisions, bans are welcome moves. They can save several hundreds of lives if well implemented and enforced properly. However, the best option is to ban the use of tobacco products altogether as various laws, provisions and bans have often been difficult to enforce and in practice, these are widely flouted.

What are the Harmful or Toxic Substances in Tobacco?

There are approximately 4000 chemicals in tobacco or cigarette smoke and 3000 chemicals in smokeless tobacco, many of them are toxic and harmful for the human body. Also, there are over 60 known cancer-causing chemicals in tobacco smoke. A few common toxic chemical substances present in tobacco smoke are nicotine, tar, carbon monoxide, nitrogen oxides, hydrogen cyanide, free radicals, metals, radioactive compounds and ammonia. You will be surprised to know that few toxins present in tobacco smoke are also used as rat poison (arsenic), preservation fluid with a strong odour (formaldehyde), radioactive material (polonium 210), fuels and toilet cleaning acids.

How do these Toxins Affect the Human Body?

The toxins present in tobacco smoke come in direct contact with the various organs of the human body such as mouth, throat, lungs, heart, and stomach and adversely affects the normal functioning of these organs. The defence mechanism of the body is damaged by these toxins and the capability to fight against infection and inflammation is compromised and lost in due course. The person becomes prone to minor and major infections such as sore throat, bronchitis and tuberculosis. Various toxins and gases produced by burning cigarette get quickly absorbed in the blood and circulate throughout the body. Therefore, the destruction caused by tobacco use is extensive and profound. The toxins also trigger various changes in the body which are fatal in the long run. Various ill-effects of the important toxins present in cigarettes can be summarized as:

1. **Nicotine:** This is the most important addictive chemical substance found in tobacco smoke. It is rapidly absorbed in the blood stream. It reaches the brain in a few seconds and has a powerful effect on the nervous system. In small doses it is a stimulant and causes alertness and mood elevation. However, in large doses it is poisonous and can cause nerve and muscle paralysis. Nicotine can kill people by paralyzing the muscles which help in breathing.

2. **Carbon monoxide:** It has greater affinity than oxygen for binding haemoglobin. Thus, carbon monoxide gets attached to red blood cells more quickly than oxygen so red blood cells carry less of oxygen resulting in a decrease in the oxygen carrying capacity of the blood. Carbon monoxide also damages the alveoli, fine honeycombs like structure of the lung which helps in the exchange of gases from the atmosphere and thereby hampers the gaseous exchange in the lung. Both mechanisms result in a decrease of oxygen saturation in the blood.

3. **Hydrogen Cyanide:** Lungs contain tiny hair-like structures called cilia that help in keeping the lungs clean by constantly moving foreign substances out in the atmosphere. Hydrogen cyanide present in smoke damages this clearance system of the lungs. It prevents it from working properly and causes an accumulation of poisonous and irritant chemicals inside the lungs. This facilitates various infections inside the lung and is responsible for a chronic irritating cough or smoker's cough.

Tobacco smoke also contains cancer-causing agents such as arsenic, cadmium and lead. These agents damage the genes which control the growth of cells, causing them to grow abnormally and rapidly. Tobacco smoke is also rich in certain radioactive substances which are known to produce cancers.

What Factors Affect the Damage to the Body?

The damage in the body starts with the first single use. Subsequent use makes the person addicted to it. The harmful effects of tobacco are dose dependent and the number of years it has been used. The ill-effects and damage to various organs of the body is influenced by a number of factors. Some of them are:

1. Number of cigarettes/*bidis* smoked per day.
2. How deep it is inhaled.
3. How long you smoke or keep the tobacco in mouth.
4. The number of years you have been using tobacco products.
5. The type of tobacco used.

Is Tobacco Addictive?

Yes. The nicotine found in tobacco causes addiction. Nicotine, like heroin and cocaine is also a strong addictive drug. When tobacco smoke is inhaled, the level of nicotine in the blood rises very rapidly and by the time the entire cigarette or *bidi* is smoked it is estimated that 90 % of the nicotine present in the inhaled smoke is in the blood circulation. Nicotine is absorbed more slowly when tobacco is chewed. Since tobacco chewers keep tobacco in their mouth for a longer period, nicotine absorbed in this manner is sufficient to attain a significant level of nicotine in blood. Nicotine absorbed in the blood crosses the blood-brain barrier and reaches the brain. In the brain, nicotine binds and acts on nicotine receptors. Nicotine binding generates a sequence of events in the brain which include increased alertness and dependence by initiating a complex reinforcing effect on the nervous system leading to physical dependence. Nicotine is absorbed so quickly that even one cigarette can get you hooked to it.

Why People Start Tobacco Use?

Most people begin smoking in their teens, usually because of curiosity and peer pressure from friends or colleagues. People with friends and/or parents who smoke are more likely to take up smoking than those who don't. Almost 90 % of the adult smokers started at or before the age of 19. This is a matter of concern, since the younger the children start using tobacco, the more likely are they to become addicted and suffer from tobacco related diseases. It is seen in India that tobacco products are widely available (in every street and corner) and the youth has no difficulty in buying tobacco products despite their young age, indicating that laws restricting sale of tobacco to minors are not working. Hookah and tobacco with betel leaf *(pan)* are offered as courtesy or to show respect at various ceremonies in urban and rural India. Lack of knowledge about the harmful effects of tobacco and surrogate tobacco advertisements also influence or make a person initiate tobacco use.

How Does Tobacco Affect the Heart?

It is a heart breaking habit and it increases the risk of heart disease. Its use causes a decrease in HDL cholesterol (good cholesterol) and simultaneously increases the level of LDL cholesterol (bad cholesterol) in blood. In addition, it constricts (narrowing) the blood vessels and decreases blood flow and oxygen to various vital organs and parts of the body including the heart itself. The chemicals released from tobacco damage the inner protective lining of blood vessels known as endothelium, making them raw and sticky. This damaged raw and sticky surface attracts cholesterol and various factors present in the circulating blood increasing the risk of clot formation which clogs the arteries and raises the risk of a heart attack and other such related problems. Tobacco use is also linked with the release of certain hormones such as adrenaline and nor adrenaline. These hormones are known as 'stress hormones' and result in an increase of the heart rate and high blood pressure which in turn increases the risk for heart related problems.

Is Tobacco Use Associated With CHD?

Smoking is a major risk factor for CHD. There is a clear dose response in terms of smoking. Even passive smoking is associated with an increased risk for CHD. It is an extremely common and modifiable risk factor amongst individuals. Researchers have found that smoking between 1 to 5 cigarettes a day increased the risk of heart attack by about 40 %; a pack/day quadrupled the risk, and two packs a day increased the risk by a factor of 9 folds. In India, heart attacks and related diseases were the problem of wealthy people a few decades earlier. However, its prevalence has increased in the recent past in rural India and amongst the low socio-economic population. Today, smoking and tobacco use is regarded as the single biggest risk factor responsible for increased prevalence of heart disease in young and rural India.

What are the Cancers Caused by Tobacco Use?

Smoking is well established as the leading cause of lung cancer. Use of tobacco in any form is linked with cancers of the mouth, pharynx (throat), larynx (voice box), oesophagus (swallowing tube), stomach and pancreas, urinary bladder, cervix and kidney. The occurrence of these cancers in smokers is 3 times more common than in non-smokers, and tobacco-related cancer contributes to 40-50 % of all cases in India.

Use of *gutka* in India is a major concern as it causes sub-mucosal fibrosis in the mouth, a disease which develops very early, and is a precursor of oral cancer with no known cure. Sub-mucosal fibrosis results by replacing the normal elastic tissue by dead fibrosed tissue which prevents the proper opening of the mouth and destroys the taste buds

Is there Anything Beyond Lung Cancer?

There is enough evidence and data to suggest that sustained use of tobacco causes a large spectrum of diseases. Damage to the lungs begins early in smokers, and all cigarette smokers have a lower level of lung function than non-smokers. This continues to worsen as long as the person smokes. Cigarette smoking causes many lung diseases such as emphysema, smokers cough and chronic obstructive lung diseases (COPD) - all can be just as dangerous as lung cancer. It affects all parts of the body and can cause stroke, vascular diseases especially deep vein thrombosis, lower limb gangrene, cataract, gum and tooth diseases, gastric upsets, infertility, hearing loss or even osteoporosis.

How to Inform People about the Ill-effects of Tobacco?

In India, knowledge about the various ill-effects of tobacco use is very poor and it is estimated that less than 10 % of people are aware of the dangerous effects of tobacco use. Illiteracy, ignorance and lack of knowledge along with poverty prevents many from even reading the warning notes written on the products they consume. The majority of smokers share cigarettes or even purchase one or two pieces and since the warning note is written on the packets, that too in fine print, they are not reminded of the injurious nature of tobacco use against health. An effort from the government to make pictorial warning signs mandatory on the packets of tobacco products will help a lot in the near future in educating people about the adverse effects and health hazards linked with tobacco use. The education in India regarding the health hazards associated with tobacco use can be imagined with the result of a survey conducted among third year medical students from 15 medical centres in India. The individuals included in the study population were highly educated and will be responsible for the future health of the society. The results were not only appalling but eye opening. A few major findings of the study were:

1. High prevalence of tobacco use and passive smoking among students in medical colleges of India.
2. Poor enforcement of smoking ban in medical schools.
3. Desire to quit among most tobacco users but poor availability of cessation services in medical schools.

4. Non-existent formal cessation training in medical schools of India.

Is there any Safe Cigarette?

Public hue and cry and concern has forced many cigarette manufacturers to introduce cigarettes with low tar and nicotine content. This is again not safe as smokers compensate for decreased nicotine yield and take more frequent and deeper puffs of these so-called safe products. With a false belief, smokers tend to smoke a greater number of cigarettes per day and thereby increase their health risk. This approach is promoted by the tobacco industry but it does not reduce the risk and so are neither safe nor recommended.

What is Herbal Cigarette?

Herbal cigarettes are cigarettes that do not contain nicotine. Even though they do not contain tobacco their inhaled smoke is rich in tar, carbon monoxide, benzene and other substances which are equally dangerous to health. Herbal cigarettes contain natural ingredients such as rose petals, marshmallow leaves, red clover flowers which are perceived as a safe alternative to regular cigarettes. The message should be clear that inhalation of smoke of any kind is not safe and smoking even herbal cigarettes will lead to lung cancer and heart problems.

What is E-cigarette?

Recently, electronic or e-cigarette has been introduced as an alternative to conventional smoking and promoted as safe as it contains only nicotine. It is a battery operated electronic device which delivers nicotine in the form of vapours. The e-cigarette resembles a ball pen and consists of a led light cover, heating element know as atomizer, cartridge of nicotine referred as mouthpiece and a rechargeable lithium battery with an electronic circuit. The nicotine liquid is contained within the cartridge and is a few millimetres away from the atomizer. When the device is turned on, the atomizer element heats up and the heat generated vapourizes the liquid nicotine present in the cartridge which is inhaled by the person. Most of the e-cigarettes are reusable devices.

Is E-cigarette Safe?

Nicotine is a powerful, toxic and highly addictive substance which cannot be considered healthy. Dependence on tobacco use is related to the action of nicotine on the brain. Nicotine is also rapidly absorbed in the blood. Therefore, it cannot be recommended as safe and all efforts should be to remove it from our lives and society. In some countries, its sale is promoted solely for medical purpose that is, for the stop smoking mission. Marketing companies argue that the e-cigarette contains only nicotine and that too is less than what is present in the nicotine replacement therapies, which are already in use. They also promote it as a substitute for smoking, but whatever be the argument, since it is a highly addictive substance, the aim should be to get rid of nicotine at the earliest and completely.

E-cigarettes are not a healthy substitute to smoking and should not be encouraged as a long term replacement for tobacco as promoted by the manufacturers. Using e-cigarette for few weeks to months as a stepping stone to become nicotine free may be a wiser choice but continuing it indefinitely may harm the body and can invite various cancers.

What is Passive Smoking?

Passive smoking, second hand smoking or environmental tobacco smoking are various terms that are used to describe the smoke that is exhaled by smokers or that burns from the end of a cigarette, pipe or cigar and is then involuntarily inhaled by non-smokers. The smoke lingers in the air for several hours after the smoker stops smoking, especially in closed spaces. Smokers do not realize that their habit of smoking affects even those around them. Research has proved beyond doubt that passive smoking can lead to serious health problems. Non-smokers who are exposed to passive smoking have 25 % more increased risk of heart disease as compared to non-smokers who are not exposed to passive smoking. In a democratic society one can argue that smoking is their right and they can do whatever they like and please their body but simultaneously, they should also realize that the health effects of passive smoking are as serious and debilitating as smoking itself and they cannot play with the rights of other people who want to live in a smoke free-environment. The commonest place where non-smokers are exposed to a large amount of passive smoke is in their own home or the house of their friends. It not only leads to health or social problems in the family but encourages children to take up the habit of smoking. About 43 % of US children are exposed to cigarette smoke by household members. Childhood exposure to passive smoking has been shown to cause asthma, bronchitis, pneumonia and ear infections. Passive smoking is a major reason for an increase in the risk of still births, spontaneous abortions and low birth weight babies. Low birth weight in itself is a major and serious health problem which contributes to the already high number of infant deaths in this country. Some other common places where passive smoking can occur are public places such as railway stations or platforms, restaurants, rest rooms, bars, sporting events and social gatherings. Though the law in India prohibits smoking at public places, it still continues unabated.

How to Minimize the Effects of Tobacco which have Already Occurred?

Stop the use of tobacco immediately as it is never too late to benefit from stopping. Benefit starts almost immediately, as all carbon monoxide from the blood is removed in 24 hours and nicotine in the next 48 hours. Next, the blood pressure and the heart rate returns to normal and so does the blood flow in the body. After 5 years of quitting, your risk of getting a heart attack is reduced to half and by 10 years, your risk of developing the disease is equivalent to that of the non-smokers.

If I Quit Smoking can I Take Smokeless Tobacco?

This is a common question from individuals who are asked to quit smoking. Smokeless tobacco is as harmful as smoking and using smokeless tobacco can cause serious health problems, from white patches, sub-mucosal fibrosis to oral cancer.

How to Quit Smoking?

Unfortunately, smoking is not a disease that can be treated. Instead, it is a hard habit known to kill people. Deciding how to quit smoking can be one of the most crucial and difficult decisions a person can make. Most people wrongly assume that smoking does not cause dependence or addiction. Trying to quit smoking is easier said than done because it is habit forming and addictive in nature. Stopping to smoke is one of the most important and most challenging lifestyle changes an individual can make. It is important to create awareness among smokers that they need both social and medical help to quit smoking because nicotine is a highly addictive substance.

Considering the numerous health, social and economic benefits of quitting, it is in the smoker's best interest to quit urgently. Quitting smoking is difficult, and some people try many times before succeeding. Since there is no single best way to quit, it requires many different approaches and attempts to overcome this habit. Talking to and convincing the person several times is important. One should emphasize that it is very important and urgent for you to leave this habit for the sake of your health and for your family because they need you more than the tobacco you need. They should be assured that everyone is with them and will help them in quitting tobacco. For success, one should talk to their physician. One way is to try and fix a quit smoking day. We live in a God fearing society; a promise to say a big NO to tobacco can be made at the place of worship. Always take the help of your friends, family members or sometimes even from NGOs. To fight against this killer addiction of tobacco nowadays, nicotine replacement therapy or smoking cessation products are helpful and available commercially. Before making all these efforts, ask yourself why do you smoke and why you want to quit? You will have no success trying to quit if you really don't want to quit. Helping someone quit smoking when they really don't want to is nearly impossible.

What is the Role of the Family Physician?

The role of physicians is crucial not only in helping their patients to stop this bad habit but also in explaining to them the health hazards. It should be a common practice to ask every patient about the use of tobacco status and persuading them to get rid of this habit at the earliest. They should be helped, motivated and encouraged to stop tobacco use. Majority of the people know that tobacco use is harmful but are unaware of the true risks and health hazards. They should be explained that it will not only affect their health but it will also affect the health of their near and dear ones, who live with them. Many patients do resist with their lame excuses but sometimes the physicians should be emphatic in explaining the matter to them in front of their children. Also tell them that there is a greater chance of your son or daughter starting the habit if they continue with it. It is a hard truth that none of the parents in India want that their habit should be practiced by sons or daughters and will give it a second thought to quit themselves.

What is Nicotine Replacement Therapy?

There are two major types of therapies available in the market, nicotine replacement therapy (NRT) and other pharmacological therapies. Nicotine replacement therapy comes in a variety of delivery modes, transdermal patches, chewing gums, inhalers, nasal sprays and lozenges. The modes of action of these products differ. It provides small amounts of nicotine to prevent nicotine withdrawal symptoms.

Nicotine replacement therapy works on the brain and the nervous system to curb nicotine dependence. Pharmacological therapy includes bupropion and is available in India. These therapies should be taken under the supervision of qualified physicians. These therapies help by reducing the severity of withdrawal symptoms and cravings in patients abstaining from tobacco. Nicotine replacement therapies have been shown to double quit rates compared to placebos.

What are the Withdrawal Symptoms?

Withdrawal symptoms are those experiences and events which are generally known to occur in nicotine dependent people trying to give up smoking. Symptoms of nicotine withdrawal vary among individuals, but in general they are unpleasant and sometimes intolerable. It includes anxiety, nervousness, irritability, insomnia, increased appetite, impaired concentration and sometimes decreased heart rate. All these features last no more than one week and during this period, a person requires multiple assurances and medical support if required to assist him in quitting smoking. Once these symptoms are overcome, a majority of people leave the habit of consuming tobacco. However, reuse after a few months is common in some or switching from one form to another has also been observed. To overcome this problem, one may be encouraged to develop some healthy alternatives such as, use of chewing gum, cardamom *(elaichi)* or aniseed *(saunf)*.

If you ask smokers why they are unable to quit smoking, the answers might be – I love smoking and it gives me pleasure. It elevates my mood, gives me energy, relaxes me and relieves my constipation. So I crave cigarettes and I am addicted to them. A majority of them admit that it is impossible for them to leave smoking despite the fact that they are aware of its injurious and deadly effects on health. They can be encouraged by incorporating certain healthy habits such as:

1. Smoking is a deadly problem so hang up 'No smoking' signs in your bedroom and office.
2. Every effort should be made to quit smoking and help from others should be sought.
3. Physical withdrawal symptoms last about 1-2 weeks. Hang on! And take the help of medicines if required.
4. Destroy all tobacco products and ash trays.
5. Avoid people who smoke and smoke filled places like bars and restaurants.
6. Do not wait for a catastrophic event which will force you to quit. Instead quit yourself.
7. If there is difficulty in quitting, cut down gradually. Smoke fewer cigarettes, smoke only half or one third and inhale less smoke.
8. Have a strong will power and urgency in you to quit.

A Dozen Reasons NOT to Start Tobacco Use

1. I want to reduce the risk of heart attack which is double in smokers.
2. I do not want to get affected by cancer of lungs, mouth and larynx.
3. I do not want to suffer from lung diseases such as a hacking morning cough, (smoker's cough), bronchitis or tuberculosis.
4. I want to maintain my physical ability and performance which is reduced in smokers.
5. I want my great artery that is, the aorta to remain healthy as unusual dilatation and rupture, which is known as aortic aneurysm is 6 times more common in smokers.

6. I do not want to limit my walking distance by narrowing the blood vessels of my legs which is a common problem amongst smokers (peripheral arterial disease).
7. I do not want to shorten my life span (smoking one cigarette reduces life by 5 minutes).
8. I want to be a role model for my children and society by not smoking.
9. I want to save money spent on cigarettes for a better cause.
10. I do not want to annoy my spouse or children due to bad breath.
11. I know tobacco kills 2 Indians every minute and I do not want to be one of them (tobacco kills 2,500 Indians everyday).
12. I want to give my fellow citizens a clean environment as passive smoking is also harmful.

Tobacco Use at a Glance

1. *Tobacco is the only commercially available substance which can lead to grave health hazards.*
2. *It is the leading cause of preventable diseases and death in the world.*
3. *In India, tobacco is responsible for an estimated 8 lakh deaths annually.*
4. *Treatment of tobacco related diseases and the loss of productivity costs India almost 14000 crores of rupees annually.*
5. *Use of tobacco and its product in India is increasing, especially in young Indians. This is a cause of concern.*
6. *Bidi is smoked twice as much compared to cigarette.*
7. *In the last few decades, the consumption of smokeless tobacco and chewing tobacco has been on the rise.*

8. Smoking causes lung cancer and tobacco chewing, cancer of the oral cavity.
9. Heart disease is twice more common among tobacco users. It is the prime cause of rapid surge of CHD in rural and low socio-economic strata of society.
10. Apart from cancer and heart disease, smoking causes irritating cough, chronic bronchitis, emphysema, tuberculosis and chronic obstructive lung diseases which have no or little cure.
11. Herbal cigarette, electronic cigarette or safe cigarettes are all promoted as safe alternatives to smoking, but all are deleterious to health.
12. Tobacco use is not a disease, rather it is a dangerous habit that should be given up at the earliest.
13. Quitting tobacco use is not an easy task. It requires multiple efforts, but if you are determined to quit, you have every reason to be successful.

Chapter 17

Obesity

'You go from being chubby to overweight, to obese, to morbidly obese and then there is disability which can lead to disease and death. Only losing weight can save people from this ugly fate.'

Obesity is a disorder in which excess body fat is acquired to such an extent that it affects the total health condition of an individual. Most people will agree that obesity and excess fat can compromise the gains in life expectancy and kill people prematurely. Today, it is the most common nutritional disorder and is defined as generalized accumulation of fat, both beneath the skin and all over the body. The prevalence of obesity has reached epidemic proportions in developed countries, with about one in three people being obese, and another one in three people are overweight and at the risk of developing obesity. The onset of obesity may occur at any age. Prevalence of obesity amongst youth and children is increasing rapidly. It has become an important public health problem, particularly in developed and developing nations. A dramatic increase in obesity prevalence is noticed in those countries which are undergoing rapid industrialization, urbanization and economic transition and it is true for India, especially urban Indians. Obesity has no sex predilection and everyone of all ages is susceptible to it. It knows no boundaries, thus it has become a global problem. What is alarming is that the problem is not stagnating but increasing year after year. If this trend persists, the health consequences of obesity will have a tremendous impact on the future burden on health costs and loss of work hours. Today in India, obesity is accepted more as a cosmetic problem and people fail to recognize that excess weight is a major risk factor for chronic diseases and other medical complications.

Never Too Late to Realize

'I am in bed and cannot use the right side of my body. Immediately after I came to know that I had had a paralytic attack, I was frustrated, depressed and extremely worried. I have been informed that recovery takes a long time and is affected adversely by my obesity and high blood pressure. I was shocked and puzzled trying to understand how a drastic event such as a stroke had happened to me. I have been keeping myself active, working eight hours in my college and taking medicines regularly to keep my high blood pressure under control. Recently I had been working overtime as admissions were taking place in the college where I was the principal and was hard pressed for time. My husband had been constantly reminding me to visit my doctor as irritability had started dominating me. I brushed it off assuming that it was all due to the work pressure of the new session and busy schedule at college and postponed the doctor's visit for a later date. I was taken by surprise when I learnt that my job is classified as a sedentary job and a majority of the problems are linked with my obesity. I know I am obese and this has persisted for so many years but it has never hampered my ability and capacity in discharging my duties. I have tried my level best, but could not succeed in shedding the extra kilos which I used to achieve with diet and exercise. It was all because of my work pressure. I know it all started after my children were born and subsequently years passed by in raising the family and building my career while making a perfect balance between home and workplace. I am in the hospital.

I now realized the wrongs that had been committed and am deeply concerned about my health.

My doctor told me, that though I have been active in my college but my exercise level was not sufficient to burn off the extra calories which I have accumulated over the years. Moreover, a habit of taking tea along with colleagues or in meetings while in college has contributed in adding up more calories than I had thought. I used to convince myself I don't eat much, only two slices of bread or cornflakes with milk at breakfast, a fruit or glass of fruit juice and two chappatis with vegetables at lunch and then same with a little rice at dinner. I could not resist taking sweets often for which I was warned many times by my husband and children. I was living under a false impression, consuming numerous cups of tea, often with biscuits, munching, mingling in between meals was never perceived by me as a source of extra calories, and I regret it now. Though I was active in college, I had little physical work at home as we were living in a joint family. Recently, because of pain in my left knee I developed a habit of avoiding stairs.

They warned me that my recovery will take time. I have a small blood clot in my brain and it will dissolve in a few weeks-time. My physician was worried about the complication of bed sores and deep vein thrombosis due to prolonged bed rest and immobilization. It was causing tension in me too. I knew, to prevent all these complications, my position had to be changed frequently and I can't do it myself. I needed someone's help. This is the first time that I have felt a sense of guilt in me when I found out that at least two people were necessary to move me in bed.

Health Burden

Although obesity is an individual clinical condition, it is an independent risk factor for early death and disabilities. It is estimated that obese people are 3 times more likely to die prematurely than their healthy weight counterparts. Apart from being an independent risk factor, most of us will also agree that excessive body weight is strongly associated with a number of serious medical conditions. A few common diseases strongly linked with obesity are diabetes mellitus, metabolic syndrome, hypertension and high cholesterol which are all risk factors for heart disease. The distribution of fat in the body is also important as far as disease prevalence is concerned. Disease prevalence is high where fat is distributed more around the abdomen resulting in apple obesity as compared to fat accumulation around the waist (pear obesity). Indians are prone to apple obesity and high prevalence of apple obesity partially explains the increased surge of diabetes mellitus and heart disease in India over the last few decades. Other medical illnesses such as stroke, gall bladder stone, cancers of colon (part of large intestine), breast and cervix (female reproductive organ) are increased in the presence of excess weight. Excess weight is like carrying extra weight of a bag full of fat along with the usual body weight. This also has to be borne by the skeleton of the body. With advancing age, the body framework succumbs under its pressure and may lead to mechanical problems such as low back pain and arthritis of weight bearing joints, especially knee joint. All these lead to chronic pain, dependency and disability. By the time we recognize the adverse effects of obesity, especially in perimenopausal women, it is too late. It is more so in India where female obesity is more common than their male counterpart. Low calcium is common in females around menopause and these mechanical problems frequently lead to impaired physical performance, painful and poor quality of life and prevent one from enjoying good health.

Sleep apnoea syndrome is another mechanical problem which results in both respiratory and heart disease. People with this syndrome temporarily stop breathing many times at night. A drop in oxygen sends an emergency signal to the brain that briefly wakes the sleeper and he or she gasps for air. During this period, adrenaline - a stress hormone is released which makes the heart beat faster and increase blood pressure. This repeated process can damage your blood vessels and increase the tendency of blood to clot - a root cause of heart attack and stroke. It is also known as Pickwickian Syndrome named after the fat boy Joe, a character of 'Pickwick Papers', a novel by Charles Dickens who had some of the features of this syndrome.

Obesity per se is not responsible for psychological problems but depression, low esteem, insomnia and poor sexual performance leading to psychological impotence is common with morbid obesity.

Obesity and Heart

One of the first medical consequences of obesity to be recognized was cardiovascular disease (CVD) but it was named a major modifiable coronary risk factor only during the last few decades. Obesity, however, carries a broader cardiovascular risk though this has not been fully explored in any society. Neither the full range of cardiovascular problems related to obesity nor the complete burden, as measured by both fatal and non-fatal events, has been quantified in detail. Obesity raises the risk of CVD by influencing the other risk factors such as hypertension, high cholesterol, diabetes mellitus and glucose intolerance. The harmful cardiovascular effects of obesity extend beyond coronary heart disease though, numerically, coronary events (heart attack) account for the greatest proportion of all cardiovascular events. Stroke (paralytic attack), heart failure and thromboembolism are the next most frequent adverse cardiovascular outcomes after coronary heart disease. In India, prevalence of obesity is increasing dramatically in the recent years. However, the magnitude of change in heart disease risk factors among the growing proportion of the overweight and obese Indians remains unknown. It is beyond doubt that the prevalence of obesity places a rapidly growing burden of coronary heart disease on both individuals and society.

Non-medical Consequences of Obesity

Besides an increase in the risk of diseases and mortality, there are other implications of obesity. Some of the non-medical consequences include:

1. Sizable overall economic burden and escalating medical cost attributed to obesity.
2. Decreased work productivity because of absence from work and feeling of lethargy or run down.
3. These people have a problem in adjusting themselves in the economy class of flights and of course, cannot enjoy wearing western outfits.

How Common is Obesity?

The prevalence of obesity has reached unprecedented proportions. Amongst the developed countries, the United States has the highest rate of obesity. From 1980 to 2002, obesity has doubled in adults and overweight prevalence has tripled in children and adolescents. An estimated 1.6 billion adults worldwide are either obese or overweight. Nearly one-third of Americans are obese. It is estimated that there are up to 200 million obese citizens in the recently expanded European Union. The obesity epidemic has also afflicted the developing countries. There is appropriate concern that this alarming trend will have major public health consequences globally.

India

As a result of the booming economy, increased average incomes, a large population of urban India recently adopted a more sedentary lifestyle and at the same time began consuming more calorie-rich foods. The recent automobile revolution in India has further increased the sedentary habits of Indians and contributed to excessive weight. From 1991 to 2004, in less than 15 years, there has been an increase in the percentage of adults who are overweight or obese from 4 % to 27 %. In India, the prevalence of obesity is linked with economic prosperity. States with high level of prosperity have greater prevalence of obesity as compared to states with less prosperity. Among all states, Punjab tops the list of obese people followed by Kerala and Goa. Today urban women are more prone to obesity and almost 30 % of women and 20 % of men are obese. Abdominal obesity complicates the issue further which is again very common in women. Almost 40 % of the women have abdominal obesity in the middle and high income group of urban India. It is predicted that the prevalence of obesity in India would further increase in both sexes in the coming years and it will be more marked in urban dwellers as compared to rural dwellers. Indians also tend to have excess of body fat around the abdomen. The irony is that the prevalence of obesity in India continues to rise in spite of the fact that one third of India's population is still below the poverty line.

Cultural and Social Significance

Not all cultures disapprove of obesity. There are many cultures which are traditionally more approving of obesity, especially African and Middle East countries. Indian culture is no different. Here, obesity is considered a symbol of health, wealth and social status.

In the Indian society, obesity is creeping up at a fast rate in urban children and at a slow rate in their rural counterparts. Today, it is a major public health problem because of its increased prevalence and the associated cost burden. The current environment produces risk factors for decreased physical activity and for increased calorie consumption. Lack of physical activity, lower relative cost of foodstuff, increased marketing and fast food restaurants, changing work force and hours, and double income households are few factors that have contributed tremendously towards the rising prevalence of obesity in the Indian culture and society. Thus, the rising trend of obesity in India is attributed to both environmental and social wealth. In the two and a half decades since 1980, growth rate of obesity in India has accelerated markedly. Today, almost half of the urban Indians are unhappy with their body shape and size.

Measurement of Obesity

Obesity is the only entity in the medical field which can be measured reliably at home and by anyone. It requires simple, cheap tools and no complicated skill or training. A measuring inch tape and a weighing machine are all we need.

Body Mass Index (BMI)

Body mass index, popularly known as BMI is a simple and most widely used method for estimating obesity in the population. BMI is a mathematical formula based on height and weight. It is calculated by measuring the person's height in meters and weight in kilograms. Then that total body weight is divided by the square of height in meters. That is,

BMI = kg/ m².

For example, a person who is 1.7 meters tall and weighs 70 kg has a BMI of 70 divided by square of 1.7 (70/1.7²) that is 24.2.

Having high body mass index is a useful indicator of overall obesity. However, evidence shows that BMI alone may not accurately predict a person's risk of obesity and heart disease but it works pretty well for most adults. WHO proposed a classification of obesity based on the calculation of body mass index.

WHO's Definition of BMI Regarding Obesity

- A BMI less than 18.5 is *underweight*
- A BMI of 18.5-24.9 is *normal weight*
- A BMI of 25.0-29.9 is *overweight*
- A BMI of 30.0-39.9 is *obese*
- A BMI of 40.0 or higher is *severely (or morbidly) obese*
- A BMI of 35.0 or higher in *the presence of at least one other significant co-morbidity is also classified by some bodies as morbid obesity.*

Waist Circumference

Waist circumference (WC) reflects the magnitude of abdominal adipose tissue (fat) deposits as well as total fat mass and thereby complement body mass index in the evaluation of obesity associated cardiovascular disease risk by providing a measure of body fat distribution. It is measured at the midpoint between the lowest rib and the highest point of iliac crest or hip bone. Studies have shown that the waist circumference, a simple and useful anthropometric measure, is complementary or superior to BMI in assessing the CVD risks.

International Diabetes Federation (IDF) has given a criteria for waist circumference which is as follows:

- Europeans   M > 94 cm, F > 80 cm
- South Asia M > 90 cm, F > 80 cm
- Chinese   M > 90 cm, F > 80 cm
- Japanese   M > 90 cm, F > 80 cm

For United States, the criteria are different; waist circumference should be greater than 102 cm and 88 cm for men and women respectively. For other ethnic groups of the world such as central and South Americans, the criteria laid down for South Asians are followed. However, for Eastern Mediterranean, Middle East (Arab) and sub-Saharan African population, European recommendations are used.

Waist to Hip Ratio (WHR)

With the help of a measuring tape, the circumference of the waist and hip are measured at the smallest and widest point respectively. To calculate the waist-to-hip ratio, the measurement of waist circumference is divided by hip circumference. For example, a waist measurement of 33 and a hip measurement of 44 give a ratio of 0.75. It is superior then BMI or waist circumference alone and is a better predictor of the risk factor assessment for heart disease, hypertension and Type 2 diabetes. A waist-to-hip ratio greater than 0.9 for men and 0.85 for women indicates increased health risks.

The current recommended cut-off points for waist circumference in Indians is the absolute waist circumference (>90 cm in men and >80 cm in women) or waist-hip ratio (>0.9 for men and >0.85 for women), and both are used as measures of central obesity.

Body Fat Measurement

An alternative way to determine obesity is to assess the % of body fat. Men with more than 25 % body fat and women with more than 30 % body fat are considered obese. However, it is difficult to measure body fat exactly. Two simple methods for measuring body fat are the skin-fold test, in which a pinch of skin is precisely measured to determine the thickness of the fat layer underneath the skin. The skin fold thickness measurement provides a fairly good estimate of the body fat. It is dependent on the skill of the observer and can be subject to the inter observer variations.

The second method is through the use of sophisticated instruments. In bioelectric impedance method, a small alternating current is passed through the body to assess the total body water, from which the body fat percentage is derived.

Both the methods are not used routinely and are meant for specialized clinics or research purposes. The development of sophisticated imaging techniques such as magnetic resonance or computed tomography or dual energy X-ray absorptiometry (DEXA) has made it possible to distinguish, with high level of precision, intra-abdominal or visceral fat depot from subcutaneous abdominal fat. DEXA is widely used because of its high precision and simplicity. It can also measure bone mineral mass.

Causes and Mechanisms of Obesity

What results in obesity is not very clear but it is influenced by various factors. There are a number of handful medical conditions which are responsible for excess of body weight but they can only be the tip of the iceberg. Genetic factors also play a part to a certain extent but the most important contributory and causative factor remains the imbalance between the excessive energy consumption and less utilization. Knowledge about the cause of obesity is important as it helps to provide a rational approach for subsequent treatment.

1. Behavioural and Environmental Factors

Various studies have proved beyond doubt that the combination of an excessive nutrient intake and a sedentary or easy going life are the main cause for the rapid acceleration of obesity in various societies. This trend gained pace at the end of the last century and continues in this century as a result of the burgeoning economy. Thus, lifestyle changes such as sedentary habits, increased income, calorie rich foods and psychosocial stress are some important factors which have led to generalized or central obesity. This is simple mathematics and we have to understand that if energy consumed is more than what is needed, the excess is stored as fat in the body and when this habit continues it results in weight gain and ultimately obesity. You will be surprised to know that consuming just 100 calories a day beyond what is burned leads to a weight gain of 4-6 kg a year. Subsequently, it may lead to an average 15-25 kg gain in 10 years. It is a result of the imbalance between expenditure and small average daily consumption of calories.

There is a saying that 'you are what you eat' but let us elaborate and reframe it in today's context 'you are what you eat and burn'. This, to a greater extent explains the increased prevalence of obesity in developed countries and the increasing trend in developing countries.

2. Urban India Factor

Today, food is cheaper and one can consume a large number of calories by spending little money. An increasing number of fast food chains are adding inches to the individual's waist. Trans-fat a cheaper option of cooking oil is used extensively. Also, deep frying is a common practice for preparing food in India. Both these factors are hazardous to the health of the heart and body. Outdoor activities are reduced. Exercise is less and irregular, as children watch more television and spend a lot of time on the computer resulting in childhood obesity and adult obesity. Shrinking playgrounds and parks, little time for children by working parents, attitude of neighbours and degrading social values force the children to remain indoors.

3. Genetic Factor

As with many medical conditions, the caloric imbalance that results in obesity often develops from a combination of genetic and environmental factors. Genetic factors may influence a wide range of metabolic and behavioural characteristics that together determine an individual's susceptibility to obesity. While it is thought that a large proportion of the causative genes are still to be identified, much obesity is likely to be the result of interactions between multiple genes. Non-genetic factors are also important.

4. Medical Illness

Certain physical and mental diseases and some pharmaceutical substances may predispose an individual to obesity. Medical illnesses that increase obesity risk include several rare congenital syndromes. Some of the common diseases which can cause obesity are hypothyroidism, Cushing's syndrome and growth hormone deficiency. Quitting smoking may also lead to moderate weight gain, as nicotine suppresses the appetite. Certain medications such as steroids, psychotic drugs, insulin therapy and other hormones may also make people susceptible to weight gain.

Distribution of Body Fat and Disease

Distribution of fat in the body is an important factor in determining your health risks. Fat which is stored around the waist is associated with an increased risk of certain health problems such as diabetes, heart disease, high blood pressure and metabolic syndrome. This type of fat distribution is more problematic and termed as apple obesity or central obesity or abdominal obesity. Fat distributed around the hip is termed as pear shaped obesity and is associated with less disability. Peripheral obesity poses CVS benefits due to secretion of adiponectin, which has anti-inflammatory, insulin sensitizing and anti-cholesterol (atherogenic) effects in addition to an association with lower body fat content. The fact is that the subcutaneous body fat is relatively 'inert' and possesses fewer health hazards. However, whether it is central or peripheral obesity, it is in the best interest of the person to reduce weight and maintain a healthy weight pattern.

Treatment

The aim of treatment is to maintain an ideal body weight. It is easier said than done. Treatment strategies include a combination of diet, exercise, drugs and/or surgery. Sometimes a combination of all treatment modalities may be required, especially in morbid obesity. The basic principle in obesity management is to learn about calorie consumption and calories burned.

What is the Diet Therapy for the Treatment of Obesity?

The principle of diet therapy is to adjust your diet in such a way that it contains fewer calories and it should also be slightly less than your needs. Diet therapy involves instructions on how to adjust a diet to reduce the number of calories eaten. Reducing calories moderately is essential for achieving a slow but steady weight loss, which is also important for the maintenance of body shape. Strategies of dietary therapy include teaching about calorie content of different foods, food composition (fats, carbohydrates and proteins), reading nutrition labels, types of foods to buy and how to prepare foods. Fats are a concentrated source of energy and contain double the calories per gram compared to carbohydrates and proteins. The unfortunate part is that a majority of food stuffs available in India, lack information about their calorific content. Fried food items, sweets and simple sugar are rich in calories and are easily converted into fat in the body. Vegetables and fruits are poor in calories. Processed food items in any form are not good for health. Thus, food stuffs in their natural form help in reducing weight.

For many people, it may be beneficial to reduce their calorie intake by eating less and eating more healthily. It is not necessary to go for a crash diet schedule. This usually ends with the person either getting weaker or giving it up completely in frustration.

Some Practical Tips to Avoid Extra Calories

Is your eating habit eating you? Find out those food items which are rich in calories in your diet and evolve methods to reduce their consumption yourself. One should introspect eating habits once every six months. One may take the help of a dietician or physician. One should not indulge in dieting which is not only harmful for the body but cannot be practiced life-long. Hence, it is appropriate to follow a healthy eating pattern instead of frightening slogans such as dieting. This will not only help in curtailing the calories in your diet but give, you an opportunity to enjoy your food. This habit of choosing healthy food options is not only practical but can be practiced for a longer period. You should realize the truth that you have gained weight over years and you cannot reduce it in a few days. Crash dieting leads to weakness, avulsion to food, lack of interest making a majority give up all efforts in desperation.

Eating is a personal, cultural and emotional experience. Therefore, one diet plan does not fit all. You have to know your eating pattern, food items and the value of food items in terms of fats, carbohydrates, proteins and calories. It looks complicated and may be impractical for a majority. You should learn to say no to simple sugars, fried food stuffs, fast food items, cheese, butter, whole milk and meat with fat, as all these are rich in both calories and fat. Whole grains, fresh vegetables and fruits are rich in vitamins and fibre, low in fat and calories. Every opportunity should be sought to add them in your diet. Apart from knowing the food content, you should also count how much and how many times you eat. Some of the following tips may help:

1. Drink plenty of fluids even if you are not thirsty and use an excess of water instead of juices.
2. Eat more of home cooked food and avoid fast foods and restaurants.
3. Base your diet on seasonal fruits, vegetables, whole grains and legumes.
4. Eat less lunch and dinner than usual and have smaller portions of the food you enjoy.
5. Take a glass of water, *jal jeera* or clear vegetable soup before your meal. It will reduce your total intake of food.
6. Eat slowly to give your brain time to signal when you are full.
7. Avoid a second helping at dinner.
8. Avoid snacks between meals, which may have become a habit.
9. Many cultures and religions prohibit leaving food and regard it as humiliation to food. So it is advised to start with small portions and if required, go for a second serving.
10. Remove all the eatables from your dinning-table once you are done and use small size serving plates.
11. If you are fond of sweets take the smallest possible bite and remind yourself that your stomach is not a dustbin.
12. Cut down on beer and alcohol.

All these things will influence your health in a positive way.

Exercise

It is simple calculation-calories in must be less than calories out otherwise you will gain weight. Calories are provided from food and are burnt by activity and exercise. Thus, the best way to a sustainable, permanent weight loss and management is regular exercise and an active lifestyle. Remember, without adequate exercise you will never succeed in reducing weight.

Exercise regularly and look for ways to increase your daily activity because burning calories is also important for reducing weight and general well-being. Grab every opportunity for physical activity. In India, people argue that they perform enough day to day activity in their homes or offices and they do not require more exercise. These daily physical activities are usually not enough to burn calories consumed in excess and this imbalance becomes crucial in the effort to weight loss. Every person should adopt extra activities for at least half an hour daily other than routine chores. Once you have decided that you want to reduce weight, you have to increase this to an hour or more. It should be emphasized that a healthy weight is complemented with smooth running blood and a disease free heart and body. Aerobic exercises in any form should be the integral part of weight control. The message conveyed is that the leaner the frame the better the body.

Drugs and Surgery

Certain drugs help in reducing weight. However, these drugs are associated with a lot of side effects and therefore are not used routinely. Drugs are reserved for people who cannot do physical activity due to morbid obesity. It may be prescribed for the initial few months as initial loss of weight encourages them and helps in increasing their exercising capacity and duration. Drugs cannot be used indefinitely as these are associated with abdominal disturbances, depression and development of certain cancers. Operations or surgical options are for those who have morbid obesity that is, BMI > 40 or BMI > 35 with other medical diseases. Gastric bypass, gastric banding, gastroplasty and biliopancreatic diversion with duodenal switch are a few procedures popular to reduce obesity. They are grouped as bariatric surgery for obesity. These surgeries are costly and beyond the reach of common people in India. However, the decision regarding drug therapy and surgical option for controlling obesity should be left to your treating physician.

When to Consult Your Doctor?

It is advised that you should consult your physician urgently if any of the following events happen in your life:
1. When weight gain occurs in a short span of time.
2. When weight gain is due to some medicines.
3. When you need advice regarding eating or exercising.
4. When there is no loss of weight despite enough exercise and cutting down your calories.
5. When you are suffering from some illness.
6. When you feel your body is swelling.

Benefits of Weight Loss

'I am healthy and am not having any disease. Why should I worry about my weight?'– this is a false belief in which we all live today. This is a common reaction once you try to convince others about the significant health benefits of reducing extra weight. This approach is a type of convenient ignorance, as it is difficult for adults to modify their eating and exercise habits. The majority will say that they do not have enough time for physical activity or dieting meaning they will be devoid of their favourite food or they have to live on only unpalatable food items. Every overweight person should be taught that obesity is a serious medical condition associated with a considerable burden of ill health. In India, knowledge about heart disease, diabetes, high blood pressure is negligible. However, people understand the mechanical complications of obesity easily because it hurts them daily in the form of knee joint pain and chronic back pain. They should realize that if they lose weight they will be free from these painful conditions and will be able to squat and bend properly in their daily routine. It should be stressed that you have to start at the earliest because once these mechanical complications set in, you will not be able to walk also, and you will not succeed in losing weight by only improving your diet as it contributes to weakness and lethargy. The experiences of people who have lost weight successfully and have maintained themselves should be shared rather than listening to the sermons of medical professionals or dieticians alone. In one study, a 10 kg loss of weight in a 100 kg subject showed 20-30 % reduction in death, significant lowering of blood pressure and cholesterol in blood and a reduction in new onset of diabetes mellitus. It also helped in building physical and psychological well-being. Short term weight loss and again gaining weight is not associated with any medical benefit. It should be discouraged. Losing weight in established cases of hypertension or diabetes helps in reducing the number of drugs or in some, drug therapy may be stopped if the weight loss and other precautions are continued successfully. It is practical to lose and maintain at least 10 % of your existing weight in 6 – 12 month's time, which is associated with a lot of health benefits and can be maintained lifelong.

Childhood Obesity

In 1998, WHO declared obesity as a global epidemic. Increasingly, this epidemic is becoming more pronounced among children and adolescents and is considered a public health crisis. It is estimated that 10 % of the world's school going children are carrying excess body fat and one quarter of these are overweight. For America, Europe and the Middle East the figures are much higher. More than 30 % of school going children in America and approximately 20 % in Europe are overweight. Some of the African countries have the lowest prevalence of childhood obesity that is, in the tune of 2 % or less. Childhood obesity has numerous potential medical complications. A majority of medical complications including CVS are effects of childhood obesity that tend to persist into adulthood.

Childhood obesity was considered a problem of affluent countries. However, today the problem has started appearing in developing countries also. In India, it is every mother's desire and dream to have chubby babies and kids. Many of us live in the false belief that this childhood fat will disappear as the baby grows older. But the fact is that 50-80 % obese children will continue into adult obesity. Thus, effective prevention of adult obesity will require the prevention and management of childhood obesity. WHO has emphasized the urgent need of understanding the prevalence, factors contributing and developing strategies for effective prevention. In India, childhood obesity has grown like an epidemic in the last three decades and has become an important health problem, especially in urban India. School surveys have shown that almost 30 % of adolescents in our cities are obese. Though it has gained a tremendous amount of attention in the past few years, especially in cities, the problem is still on the rise. There is a paucity of nationwide data on the prevalence of childhood obesity. However, studies from different states of India suggest that childhood obesity ranges from 7-16 %.

Rising standards of living, increase in per capita income, double income in the family, more family outings, more fast food joints and commercials on television raise the risk of obesity in children. Today children have more money to spend then their parents did and more eatables and joints are available at their disposal than the past. Numerous environmental factors that limit physical activities and facilitate obesity have been identified. Urban housing designs and land use, scarcity of parks and playgrounds (shrinking green space), 24 hour cartoon channels and other television serials, new computer games and play stations, all influence their physical activity. Nuclear families, both parents working and long and exhaustive working and commuting hours, leave no option for children but to remain at home, glued to the television screens. Video games and computer 'screen time' has grown phenomenally. Fierce academic competitiveness promoted by both school and parents leave children with no option and force them to remain indoors. With life reduced to shuttling between coaching and schools, students have hardly any time to enjoy. Time to play or exercise is a rare habit and physical education has practically disappeared from schools.

The good news with childhood obesity is that childhood eating and exercise habits are more easily modified than adult habits. It should not be made a child issue only, rather it should be a family concern. It is the duty of parents to practice what they preach by setting good dietary and exercise examples. The idea is to install healthy eating habits which the whole family can follow. Parents should understand that the family history of obesity associated with a lack of physical activity and consuming high energy foods completes the triad of important factors which influence childhood obesity. Today the increasing prevalence of childhood obesity has become the most common and serious nutritional disorder in upper and middle class in India. Childhood obesity is associated with 8 fold rise in high blood pressure and 3-6 fold increase in high cholesterol levels in blood. Other consequences of childhood obesity include respiratory problems, physical inactivity and joint problems. It is a potential precursor to Type 2 diabetes, a disease of which India will be the global capital by 2025. As these children reach adulthood, they will add to the already existing number of diabetes, heart problems and hypertension sufferers.

Prevention of Obesity

It is high time to ask ourselves a burning question - are we raising an overweight and out of shape generation of children for a prosperous India? Or should we have a dream where everyone should have healthy bodies to enjoy a long, happy and disease-free life in a prosperous India? To achieve this, one should have an ideal body weight. All these require preventive strategies against obesity which should be started from childhood and be continued life-long. Prevention of obesity means, adopting measures which will help to maintain an ideal weight or to prevent weight gain in lean subjects. Preventive measures should also be extended to those who are obese or overweight or informally obese people who have successfully lost weight.

Increased consumption of seasonal fruits, vegetables and cereals along with fish, white of egg, white meat without skin and a decrease in the intake of dietary fat, whole milk and its products, simple sugars, sweets and red meat will all help to reduce the risk of obesity. Increase in physical activity has shown to be a key component in the prevention of obesity and its importance should be emphasized to all. The issue of physical inactivity in our day to day life should be addressed urgently and every effort should be made to improve it. An old saying of 'eat well and burn well' may not be applicable totally to Indians. In fact, in today's context, it should be modified to 'eat well and burn more'. Therefore, every Indian should perform aerobic exercises for at least 45 – 60 minutes daily. Besides balancing food intake and appropriate exercise, policy makers, family physicians, dieticians, teachers, parents and community social workers should be involved in comprehensive obesity prevention programmes. If early preventive measures are not adopted today, then in the coming years, increasing life expectancy, increasing income and increase in girth will increase the expenditure related with obesity.

Benefits of Weight Loss

1. Obesity is the most important risk factor in relation to the development of Type 2 diabetes. A weight loss of 5-7 % decreases the risk of development of diabetes mellitus and increases insulin sensitivity.
2. A 10 kg weight loss is associated with 30-50 % reduction in sugar level and 15 % reduction in HbA1c (glycosylated haemoglobin) level in diabetics.
3. Reduction of weight is associated with a reduction in blood pressure, the number of episodes of angina and/or heart pain.
4. It increases the exercise capacity by almost 30 %.
5. Weight reduction is associated with an increase in good cholesterol that is, HDL by 10 %.
6. Weight reduction of 10 kg is associated with a 30 % reduction in serum triglycerides, 15 % reduction in LDL cholesterol and 10 % reduction in total cholesterol.

7. Not only does it reduce the death rate by 20-30 %, it also decreases the number of tablets taken for other diseases.

Obesity At a Glance

1. Obesity is one of the major health disorders across the globe.
2. India is currently experiencing an increasing obesity epidemic.
3. Indians are genetically susceptible to weight gain, especially around the waist. Today approximately 5 % of the population suffers from obesity or are overweight in India.
4. Indians are prone to abdominal obesity. BMI assessment coupled with waist circumference measurement seems to be an appropriate guide to predict future health hazards.
5. Nearly a third of all men and more than half women belonging to the upper middle class in India are overweight and on the verge of obesity.
6. The state of Punjab tops the list of obese people in India.
7. Obesity is more prevalent in women than men in India.
8. A family history of obesity associated with a lack of physical activity and unhealthy eating habits are important causes for obesity.
9. Two third of children and adolescents eat junk food (noodles, chips, pizzas, burgers, pastas, pakodas, samosas, chaat and biscuits) daily as a part of snacks followed by regular dinner in metro cities.
10. People living in metro cities have the worst eating habits that is, they eat more restaurant food than homemade food.
11. This culture is fast percolating into the medium and smaller cities because of aggressive market advertisements and mall culture.

12. Indians are not fond of physical activity. Time constraints or inability to manage time, sedentary work habits and shrinking green space further contribute to physical inactivity and obesity.
13. Every two hours spent daily in front of television increases the risk of obesity by 23 %.
14. One hour of per day brisk walking (5-6 km/day) decreases the risk of obesity by 24 %.
15. Morbid obesity is associated with many serious and potentially deadly health problems apart from physical, social and psychological problems.
16. Avoiding consumption of foods rich in fats such as fatty meat cuts, organ meats, egg yolks, chocolates, junk foods, etc. help in reducing weight.
17. Dieting is not advisable and is detrimental to health. Use of pocket friendly green vegetables, fruits and whole grains are beneficial.
18. Many a times it is difficult to lose weight with diet and exercise. Remember you have gained weight in years and you cannot lose the same in days, have patience and perform brisk aerobic exercises regularly.
19. Weight reduction surgery can improve conditions such as sleep apnoea, diabetes, high blood pressure and high cholesterol but only a few can afford it because of its high cost.
20. Prevention of obesity requires a healthier lifestyle.

Chapter 18

Exercise

'Start the day with morning exercise and this will carry you through the day'.

Heart is a muscular organ and is the most active muscle in the body. It not only requires proper nutrition, but like any other muscles in the body it also requires regular exercise to tone it up and maintain it in good shape. Regular and moderate physical activity can improve the working capacity of the heart making it strong. Exercise also tones up the blood vessels and maintains its elasticity. Additional benefits of being physically active are that it gives you energy, boosts your self-esteem, keeps you fit and healthy, changes your look as well as your outlook towards life. Above all, it helps you relax and enjoy life, or in other words it not only adds years to your life but also prevents or delays the onset of heart disease in your golden years.

Is a Sedentary Lifestyle Associated with Heart Disease?

Sedentary lifestyle in itself is a major risk factor for heart disease. A heart attack is almost twice as common in a physically inactive person than in a physically active person. It has also been observed that people who are physically active have fewer complications or tolerate well the complications associated with heart diseases. The level of good cholesterol that is HDL is low and the level of bad cholesterol that is LDL and TG are high in sedentary persons. A novel way of increasing good cholesterol HDL is exercise. A study examining major risk factors of global and regional burden of heart disease confirmed that sedentary lifestyle as a major risk factor for death and disease in both developed and developing countries worldwide.

What Constitutes a Sedentary Lifestyle?

Today a majority of urban Indians are accustomed to leading a sedentary lifestyle. A large number of professionals such as office workers, computer operators, teachers, doctors, executives, retired professionals, peons, barbers, tailors, housewives all fall in the category of sedentary work. Exercise is something which many Indians are not fond of and is not practiced on a regular basis. We think that the daily work done at office or home is sufficient and there is no need to do extra physical work. Physical activity recommendations for sedentary people should include a regular moderate grade of exercise on practically all days for 30 – 60 minutes to be done over and above the regular day to day activities.

Innocent but Lethal Submission

Ask yourself how much time you spend on watching television, on a computer, going to a cinema, using a scooter, motorcycle or car, using a lift instead of stairs, or sitting in the office all day. Remember all this constitutes a sedentary lifestyle and is not a healthy approach towards life. It will definitely invite various diseases in your body and one of them is heart disease. This is the lifestyle many of us follow daily and we give lame excuses such as I do not get enough time for exercise or what is the need for exercise? One has to understand the simple rules of life, if you can spend a majority of your time for your job and family, you should be able to take out 45 minutes a day for yourself because if you are not fit then everything else is unfit, either today or tomorrow. Forty five minutes per day from your 24 hour schedule will make a lot of difference once you start it. It requires no money or sophisticated gadgets. It only requires a little thought, firm determination and rescheduling your daily routine.

Does Exercise Reduce the Risk of Heart Disease?

Various studies have demonstrated beyond a doubt that regular exercise can reduce the risk of heart disease and it helps you to fight against various risk factors associated with heart disease. Obesity and being overweight, hypertension, diabetes mellitus, high cholesterol and stress which contribute significantly towards the health of your heart can all be controlled with the help of regular exercise. Thus, physical activity takes care of not only the heart but also the associated risk factors. Exercise also tones up your whole body, relieves you from gastric upsets, hyperacidity and constipation. It improves your breathing and lung capacity, prevents or halts development of joint problems or arthritis and makes you new friends. Exercise helps in a positive manner and is a cheap, safe and powerful treatment option for your heart and body.

If your goal of exercising is to look like your favourite star then you are likely to fail but if you exercise to improve the quality of your life and get it in good shape you will feel comfortable and satisfied in the long run.

The Benefits of Exercise for a Healthy Heart
1. Lowers blood pressure.
2. Prevents new onset of diabetes.
3. Helps in lowering glucose.
4. Promotes weight loss.
5. Increases level of good HDL cholesterol.
6. Lowers bad cholesterol LDL and TG.
7. Lowers clotting tendency.
8. Improves endothelial function.
9. Improves self-esteem and reduces stress.
10. Tones up the heart muscles and maintains elasticity in blood vessels.

What Exercise is Best?

The best form of exercise is aerobic exercises. These exercises include walking, cycling, jogging, swimming which are feasible in our country and require little expenditure. These exercises do not require any special equipment or membership of expensive health clubs. Aerobic exercises require and consume plenty of oxygen. Mountaineering, rowing, skating, and skiing are other options but are not popular in developing countries including India.

How Frequently should one Exercise?

Regular physical activity for 30-45 minutes, either continuously or intermittently every day for at least 5 days a week is sufficient. It should exclude 5 minutes of warming up and cooling down period. The timing and frequency can be adjusted as per individual needs. If you have been sedentary, it is important that you should exercise frequently and do small sessions of exercise. It should be emphasized that physical exercise does not have to be arduously long to benefit you. Even short (10-15 minutes) sessions may also confer health benefits.

What should be the intensity of Exercise?

Slow and steady is the mantra for exercise. Vigorous exercise such as sprinting cannot be done at all ages and cannot be maintained for more than a minute. It is better to warm up or start slowly and build up the amount and intensity gradually so that it can be performed for 45-60 minutes. If you have a heart problem or any other disease, first consult your doctor before starting any exercise schedule.

How hard one should exercise can be decided by a simple talk test, that is you should be able to talk to a fellow person comfortably and should not get out of breath. If you are breathless during a conversation, you are probably exerting more and should reduce the pace. If you are walking and gossiping comfortably then again it is of no good to your heart. Walking with a speed of 6 km an hour or covering a distance of one kilometre in 10-12 minutes is considered fairly good walking exercise for adults. Maximum exercise benefits are obtained if one can achieve 60-90 % of their maximum heart rate. Maximum heart rate is calculated by a simple formula of 220 minus the age of the person. If you are of 40 years age, your maximum heart rate is 180 beats per minute (220-40=180) and you should exercise between 108-162 beats per minute. If you are healthy and free of any disease, it is advised to achieve 80-90 % of your predicted heart rate. However, people with heart disease and older people should achieve 60-70 % of their maximum heart rate.

When to Exercise?

For a majority, the best time to exercise is in the morning. Running and heavier exercises can be left for the evening, when the body is more adaptable to training. This is not practically possible for working people. A morning schedule for exercise may be more convenient and can be maintained regularly as evening engagements break the regularity and pollution is at a peak during the evening. Studies have confirmed the benefit of short bursts of exercise similar to a long period of exercise. Hence, exercising for even 10-15 minutes, 3 times a day will have a similar advantage. Exercise during extreme weather conditions and against the wind should be avoided.

What Exercise is Best at Home?

In case of unavoidable circumstances which do not permit you to go outdoors for a walk or the gym, you can always try skipping at home which is an excellent calorie burning activity. Other methods can be using an exercise bike or treadmill. If nothing is feasible, push ups, free hand exercises, fast walking on the roof top or corridors can be done. Mopping the floor, gardening, free hand exercises, sit ups, yoga, walking your pets, washing your car and/or scooter or motorcycle are other household physical activities which help in burning calories. Playing indoor games such as table tennis, basketball or badminton with children is also a good way to exercise.

How to Increase Physical Activity in Day to day Work?

First of all think of your daily activity and find out the opportunities to be active in your day to day activity. Common opportunities can be the use of stairs frequently. If you have to go to the twelfth floor then get down at the tenth floor and take two flights of stairs. You can do the same while going down. Go for shopping frequently and use a bicycle. At lunch time, if feasible, take a short brisk walk for 10 – 15 minutes. Take your kids to the park or a playground and play with them. Play badminton or table tennis or go for a swim with colleagues or children. Walking to your workplace also helps. Dancing to your favourite tune may be another option. It is advisable to pick every opportunity to keep yourself physically active.

What are the Risks of Exercise for Patients with CHD?

As the risks of physical activity are very low compared to the resultant health benefits, a majority of the uncomplicated patients do not require medical consultation before starting on an exercise programme. It should not be started just after a heart attack or chest pain which is occurring with routine household activity. Patients with multiple risk factors and with heart failure or serious heart rhythm disturbances should consult their doctor before starting exercise. The risk of serious cardiac events associated with exercise as a part of a cardiac rehabilitation programme is reported as very low.

When should Physical Activity be Resumed after a Heart Attack?

The patient may be allowed to choose his or her own form of exercise but walking is the most appropriate and safe exercise for a majority of patients. It is advisable to walk in your room for 5 minutes, 2-3 times a day in uncomplicated patients at the end of the first week. After 2 weeks, one can start limited walking and gradually increase the duration to 10 minutes, 2-3 times and add up the minutes with every walking schedule. After 2 weeks you can walk up the stairs slowly. In 3-4 weeks time, you can walk up to 45 minutes. Start slowly initially and gradually build a pace that is comfortable for you. Do not try to compete with someone or with time. The appropriate mode, frequency, intensity and duration of exercise schedule should be tailored to an individual's heart and medical condition.

What are the Rules of Exercise?

The following rules should be followed to make exercise enjoyable and trouble- free:

1. Warming up before any exercise is important and it can be done by slow walking for a few minutes before starting routine exercise activity. Similarly, walking slowly or stretching for a few minutes at the end of exercise is helpful to cool down your body.
2. Intensity of exercise should be such that you sweat or you feel your own breathing. In other words you should be able to converse during exercise but should not be out of breath.
3. If you are not fatigued and you have recovered from your exercise and you have no problem in conducting day to day activities, you can exercise daily.
4. Any problem faced during exercise, especially people having a heart disease should consult their doctor.
5. Always listen to your body. Reduce your exercise if you feel excessive weight loss, constant sense of fatigue, muscle aches, reduced appetite or sleep. Talk to your trainer or doctor.
6. You should not take heavy meals before exercise. It is advisable to exercise on an empty stomach. Water intake is important and it should be taken in adequate amounts 3-4 litres /day for a normal person as you lose a lot of water through sweating and breathing during exercise. Water should not be consumed immediately after exercise. Do not consume a lot of caffeine or alcohol to replace water as these beverages increase urination and in fact, reduce the water content of your body.
7. One should know how many calories have been burned in various indoor and outdoor activities. The exercise level and intensity should be tailored according to the age, sex and physical ability of the individual (Table 18.1).

8. Use appropriate, good quality shoes and comfortable clothing during exercise. Do not perform exercise on hard and uneven surfaces.
9. Safety tips for heart patients are the same but they should consult their physician or trainer before indulging in exercise. They should avoid weight training or isotonic exercises. This form of exercise increases the contraction of muscles thereby increasing the resistance in your blood vessels, ultimately imposing an extra burden on your heart.

Table 18.1: Approximate Calories Spent in Various Indoor and Outdoor Activities for a 60 kg man

Activities	Calories burned
Sitting, sleeping, relaxing in bed, standing, watching television, knitting, sewing, writing, reading, talking, car driving, desk work, computer work, studying, etc.	1-1.5 calories / minute
Household kitchen work, playing musical instruments, playing billiards or snooker or leisure walking (2 km per hour), shaving, brushing teeth, combing, cooking.	2-3 calories / minute
Playing badminton or table tennis, mopping the floor, cleaning windows, washing the car, walking 4 km per hour (social walking).	4-5 calories / minute
Playing competitive game such as badminton, table tennis, roller skating, digging in a garden, walking or jogging 6 km per hour (brisk walking), climbing stairs, cycling 15 km per hour, dancing, casual swimming, horse riding.	6-8 calories / minute
Running at 8 km per hour, playing vigorous games like basketball, swimming, volleyball, football, squash, handball or competitive swimming, hiking, mountain climbing.	8-10 calories / minute

Exercise Myths

A large number of exercise myths are popular among Indians. Some of them are:
1. Sit-ups will help you lose fat around your stomach.
2. If you're exercising and not losing weight, its a waste of time.
3. Weight training will make you muscle bound.
4. Its best and beneficial to exercise in the morning only.
5. Exercise turns fat into muscle.
6. Exercise will injure you.
7. You need extra salt after sweating heavily.
8. You should eat more protein if you're trying to build up muscles.
9. Exercise machines are more effective than free weights.
10. You need extra vitamins and minerals after exercise.

Simple Calculation

Weekdays

A morning walk for 6 days a week at a speed of 6 kms per hour or walking or cycling to the work place daily for 50 minutes (50 x 6 days x 6 calories/minute = 1800 calories).

Sundays

Washing your car or scooter for 10 minutes (10 x 5 calories/minute = 50 calories) + going to a playground with the children for an hour (60 x 5 calories/minute = 300 calories).

Over the week you have just burned 2150 calories which is merely enough to keep your heart healthy. So inculcate a habit of getting active wherever possible.

Chapter 19
Stress and Behaviour

Stress and emotions affect the heart directly or indirectly through the nervous system. An enlarged heart is a serious condition in cardiovascular disease while a big heart is an emotional compliment to generous people. Similarly, skipping of a heartbeat at the sight of your loved one is a joyful expression of emotions while a broken heart is the other side of the coin. Stress is normal to life and can be defined as a state of mental and physical reaction to certain external or internal stimuli. This reaction is difficult to predict and varies from person to person. It may include joy, fear, anger, depression, panic attacks, dejection or frustration. Stress in itself is not bad and is a part of life. However, persistent stress is a serious condition, and can lead to emotional, psychological and life threatening physical illnesses such as high blood pressure, heart attack, irregular heartbeats and stroke. In extreme cases, it may lead to chronic depression and sometimes suicide. It is said in India that everyone has some form of stress in their life except true saints and the insane.

Relationship Between Stress and Heart disease

The relationship between stress and heart disease or heart attack is not very clear. People with a higher degree of stress or prolonged stress conditions have higher blood pressure than normal and are prone to hardening and narrowing of arteries. Both the conditions can result in or precipitate a heart attack. Thus, stress can act as an independent external risk factor for atherosclerotic cardiovascular disease. Stress also influences other risk factors of heart disease such as cholesterol level, obesity and smoking, making them worse. Prolonged and uncontrolled stress increases the secretions of adrenaline and cortisol in blood exposing the body to increased levels of these stress hormones. Simultaneously, stress enhances blood clotting factors in the body. All these changes in the body during stress contribute to heart disease and stroke. In spite of all this information, much more research is needed to know exactly how stress increases the risk of heart disease.

Stress and Contributory Factors

During stress, pressure and strain exerted on the body adversely affects the life of a person. Willingly or unwillingly, stress has become a part of our daily life. Stress is good as long as it promotes healthy competition amongst all but it is precarious when it gets prolonged, and starts affecting the narrow gap between life and insanity. Positive stress motivates, excites and energizes people, and is good for mental and physical health.

Today life has become so strenuous and demanding that stress has become an integral part of our daily routine. As we can't escape from stress, we have to at best cope up with it and learn to live with it. Stress comes in all forms and types and is caused by physical, emotional or environmental changes in our life. Things which make one feel stressed are called stressors and success in life depends upon how one adjusts and responds to these factors. We, in India, readily get stressed and jealous of the wealth and fame of others as well as their lifestyle. Malicious approach has only increased the stress in one's life and is further building up the pressure. We are not satisfied with our own achievements, instead we readily get envious of others.

Stress Signals

Stress signals are usually vague and may not correlate well with the degree of stress. Headache, indigestion, muscular cramps, loss of appetite or sleep, a heartbeat that rings in the ears, feeling run down, weakness, feeling tense or anxious, eagerness to finish the work are some symptoms which are indicative of a stressful life. Prolonged exposure to stress causes severe mental damage, inability to concentrate, loss of recent memory, forgetfulness, depression, anxiety, irritability, loneliness, nervousness, mood swings and sudden or unexplained outbursts. In extreme cases it can lead to suicidal tendencies or even suicide. It is important to note that stress does not start from factors that come from another universe but from our own surroundings and day to day activities like changing of school, home, job, unfriendly atmosphere at the office or home, etc. It is important to identify these stress signals and factors and deal with them effectively and decisively.

Should Stress Signals be Ignored?

No. Your body is the best gift God has given you and when subjected to stress, recognize the warning signals promptly and realize that something is wrong. These warning signals may be in the form of physical, mental, emotional and behavioural changes that have to be understood. They should never be ignored or overlooked. Steps should be taken to take care of it properly. These signals indicate that you need to change your life's pattern or break up your life's pace, seek a change of surroundings, environment or place of work to sooth the agitated mind. If this is not done or the body is not given adequate time to rest and to recuperate, serious health problems may develop or existing problems may worsen or aggravate. Even a mobile phone, an essential gadget of one's life needs to be charged routinely for smooth functioning, the same also goes for the human mind and body.

Does Stress Affect Everyone in the Same Way?

Response to any external stimuli providing stress differs from person to person. Each person reacts differently to the same stimulus. For example, a marriage procession on the street may be enjoyable for those who are participating in it, but stressful and a nuisance for others due to the inconvenience caused. One of the most common transient stressful condition for students is the public use of loud speakers during examination time. Stress can cause anger, fear, guilt or anxiety in many individuals, and it may be difficult to keep calm. An attitude of *'chalta hai'* or *'koi baat nahin'* can save many but very few have it and may just crack with the situation getting out of control and sometimes they may take extreme steps such as commit suicide. Not able to repay the loan of private or government lenders is also a cause of concern and has increased the suicidal episodes and tendencies.

What Causes Stress?

Financial constraints, frequent change of workplace, high headedness of seniors, nagging neighbours, domestic problems and ill health are some of the common factors which can cause stress in our life. A few common ones include:

1. Unemployment and all the stigma that it carries.

2. Daughter's marriage.
3. Children living separately or studying outside.
4. Problem in personal relationship.
5. Work overload or fighting for free time.
6. Retirement – not having adequate preparations for it.
7. Legal problems – a time and money consuming process in India.
8. Property dispute – a never ending problem.
9. Perfectionism – an impossible proposition.
10. Failure or poor performance in exams.
11. Financial loss especially in the share market, business or ditched by a partner.
12. Costly treatment and drugs.
13. Incompatibility in marriage and ego.

Is Living Alone a stressful Condition?

Yes. All stress conditions are not bad. Marriage is a joyful bonding and emotional stress *(jo kare wo pachtaye jo naa kare wo bhi pachataye)*. Several studies have clearly documented that people without a spouse or life companion die earlier than married people. Thus, having a spouse is a joyful, emotional stress and it actually provides desired and significant emotional support and stability in life. The social taboo in India is such that a single person is not welcome in various social gatherings. Moreover, raising a family and enjoying life with your spouse and children is the best way of distressing yourself daily.

How should one Curb Stress?

When stress becomes prolonged, frequent and excessive it can cause physical, mental, emotional and behavioural problems that can damage health and mental performance. If you are under stress you are at risk of heart attack, angina, high blood pressure and stroke. Further over-reaction to any situation or an emotional outburst due to stress can cause awkward situations, unpleasant atmospheres and even social isolation. Frequently people start ignoring or overlooking you. This can increase the stress further. Stress disturbs all family members and adversely affects performance and relations. So, it is all the more important to curb stress – a positive approach towards life can dispel distress and many difficult situations. The best approach is not to be concerned about worries. A few tips for curbing stress are, never feel rushed, under pressure, and try to be cool under demanding or difficult situations. Don't avoid these situations, try to face the situation and find a possible solution by yourself. Sharing things with loved ones and someone you trust is also an excellent way of distressing yourself. Today, time management is a big problem for every urban dweller. Do not become a slave of time or compete with time. You should learn to manage time and take things one at a time and with priority. Try to satisfy yourself honestly and not others, and reward yourself whenever and wherever possible. If you think you can satisfy every individual who comes across then you have to make a lot of compromises and it can also compromise your health. As all individuals cannot be pleased, it is very important to learn to say NO. A simple NO helps in the longer run.

What are the Different Types of Personalities?

There are two common types of behavioural responses or personalities. These types are type A, the strict, rigid and the perfectionist type and type B, the relaxed individuals. Recently type C and D behaviour has also been described as those who are depressed all the time.

What is Type A Behaviour Pattern?

Type A personality, also known as the type A behaviour are frequently prompt, impatient, excessively time-conscious, insecure, highly competitive, ambitious, agitated, irritable, quick to anger, suspicious, hostile and aggressive, preoccupied with deadlines and impulsive. They frequently try to seek the attention of others and often interrupt others. These people may be highly successful but are often dissatisfied with their achievements. Few studies suggested that type A people are prone to hypertension, heart disease and stroke. However, an equal number of studies failed to support this association.

What is Type B and C Behaviour Patterns?

Type B personality is relaxed. They enjoy their work and have a positive approach towards life. They are less prone to heart disease. However, type C personality is concealed, compulsive and non-communicative. They are often introverts and prone to high blood pressure, obesity and diabetes due to their negative personality. They are also prone to heart disease.

What is Type D Personality?

In this group, the personality type is anxious, depressed and has a tendency of social inhibition and isolation. It has been observed that if a type D personality persists for a longer period, it can damage the cardiovascular system and make them prone to heart disease.

Can Management of Stress Reduce or Prevent Heart Disease?

To a large extent, maybe yes. Managing stress makes sense for your overall health. However, current data doesn't support stress reduction as a proven therapy for cardiovascular disease. After a heart attack or stroke, people who feel depressed, anxious or overwhelmed by stress should talk to their doctor or other healthcare professional. The most common feeling is that I am a patient and will remain a patient lifelong. I will not be able to enjoy life as before. People after a heart attack must be assured that they are not incapacitated by the disease; that there is a total cure and they will return to their normal activities with some lifestyle changes.

Ways to Reduce Stress

1. Identify the cause of stress and assess whether stress is related to, family, work or finances.
2. Share your feelings and thoughts with your loved ones.
3. Discuss the cause of stress openly with those around you.
4. Honestly assess yourself and simplify your life.
5. Realize that there are others like you, who feel stressed. Therefore, you are not alone so do not surrender.
6. Take time outs for hobbies, recreational and social activities which divert your mind away from stress.
7. An active outdoor life, games, regular exercise, walking alone or with children or pets, and indoor activities such as meditation, yoga and music help to reduce stress. The motto is to stay healthy.
8. Professional advice should be sought if stress gets out of control, but the help of alcohol, drugs and smoking should be avoided at all cost.

9. Sharing stress with someone in whom you confide helps to reduce it. An effort can be made by your confidant to give you sensible and sagacious advice. He/she may have a practical approach towards your problem.
10. Lay to rest your bloated ego.

Stress at a Glance

1. *Some degree of stress is normal and promotes performance.*
2. *Life without stimulus is incredibly dull, boring and unpleasant.*
3. *Stress in itself is not bad. The most important thing is how you handle it.*
4. *Prolonged and excessive stress can seriously interfere with your ability to perform effectively and may affect your mental and physical faculties.*
5. *The art of stress management is to keep yourself at a level of stimulation that is healthy and enjoyable.*
6. *Manage time and learn to say 'NO'.*
7. *Believe in yourself. Remember, you have the ability to handle whatever happens.*
8. *Do not try to change the world; try to change yourself accordingly but don't surrender.*
9. *Keep yourself calm and peaceful at home; read something spiritual, listen to music and create new hobbies. Humour and laughter are a must. Do not bring your office stress, problems home.*
10. *Recharge your energy by taking vacations at least twice a year with your family or friends.*
11. *Exercise regularly, practice body-mind techniques such as qi gong, yoga and meditation.*

Chapter 20
Complementary and Alternative Therapy

'Doctors give prescriptions to cure ailments, but you as doctor with a heart give remedies for life. Thanks for giving back my precious life and showing me the true meaning of it. Always be beside me and make a difference to others lives too.' Belief in the benefit of treatment is known as faith and it can improve the outcome even if the treatment is a placebo.

The American National Centre for Complementary and Alternative Medicine (NCCAM) defines complementary and alternative medicine (CAM) as covering 'a broad range of healing philosophies (schools of thought), approaches and therapies that mainstream western (conventional) medicine does not commonly use, accept, study, understand or make available'. More simply, it can be defined as traditional methods of therapy that have been accepted and practiced by other populations (outside its native culture). Alternative medicine and complementary medicine treatments differ slightly as the former is used as replacement and latter along with evidence based conventional standard medical treatments. However, CAM has originated from various civilizations and has been in practice before the advent of modern medicine which has a history of two centuries only. These treatment modalities include dietary supplements, use of vitamins, minerals, herbal preparations, relaxation techniques, massage therapy, magnet therapy and spiritual healing. Since many CAM therapies cannot be patented, it is difficult for these therapies to undergo case control trials. They also have different philosophies such as bio-energy and spirituality whose basis is still unclear. Since the basis of these therapies is not known or clear and they have not been proved by large randomized trials, they are not recognized and endorsed by western medical community. These therapies fail to prove beneficial in acute, life threatening conditions and are not recognized as standard therapy. Despite all this, CAM is popular in both developed and developing countries and almost one third of the world's population uses them for chronic medical conditions, especially to get rid of pain of any origin.

Complementary and alternative medicine (CAM) therapies as defined by NCCAM fall into five major categories or domains:

1. **Whole Medical Systems:** Alternative medical systems are built upon systems of theory and practice. It includes traditional Chinese medicine (TCM) and Ayurveda which were developed in China and India respectively. Homoeopathy and naturopathy originated from the western world.

2. **Mind-body Medicine:** It takes a holistic approach to health and explores the mind, body and spirit. It uses various techniques which increase the capacity of mind to influence bodily functions and symptoms. It includes meditation, prayer, mental healing and therapies that involve creative art such as folk dance, laughter and music.

3. **Biological Based Practices:** It uses substances present in nature such as herbs, spices, foods, vitamins, animals and other natural substances. Herbal therapy is the most common and often used both as dietary supplements and as drugs.

4. **Manipulative and Body-based Practices:** It includes movement and manipulation of one or more parts of the body. This type of therapy includes chiropractice, osteopathic manipulation and massage.
5. **Energy Medicine:** It involves the use of energy fields. There are two types of energy therapies – one is Bio-field based (Reiki, qi gong, healing, therapeutic touch) and the other is Bio-electromagnetic based (magnetic fields, alternating or direct current and pulsed fields).

The use of complementary and alternative medical (CAM) practices in the developed nations is growing rapidly. In developing nations, the access to essential medicine is restricted because of poverty and availability driving people to rely on traditional methods of treatment. In a majority of developing nations, it is used extensively as it is close to their culture, civilization, faith and regarded as safe and free from side effects. In some Asian and African countries, it is well accepted in the mainstream of medical care and almost 30-80 % of the population depends on traditional medicine for primary health care. In China and most of the East Asian countries traditional Chinese medicine and in India Ayurveda, yoga, unani, siddha, homoeopathy (AYUSH) are a part of primary health care delivery system and are widely practiced alone or with allopathic medicines. The most common CAM therapies practiced are prayer, use of herbs and spices, acupuncture, breathing techniques, yoga, meditation (Qi gong, Zen, Reiki, Vipasana), homoeopathy and chiropractice.

CAM is most frequently used for musculoskeletal complaints and is used to treat or prevent chronic or recurrent pain. It is also used to combat anxiety, depression, emotional health and stress. Women are more likely to use CAM than men. Use of CAM specifically to treat cardiovascular diseases is not popular and is not practiced widely. However, acceptance of herbal preparations and mind-body techniques are seen quite often.

Traditional Chinese Medicine (TCM)

Traditional Chinese Medicine (TCM) includes a range of traditional medicine practices that originated in China. TCM claims to be thousands of years old and is rooted in meticulous observation of how nature, the cosmos and the human body are interacting. It is widely practiced for the prevention and treatment of various diseases, either alone or along with the western medical therapies in China and other countries in East Asia.

Herbs and Chinese herbal medicines find a special role and are extensively used in TCM. Chinese herbs have been used for centuries and many of the modern day drugs have been developed from Chinese herbs such as those for treatment of asthma and hay fever, from Chinese ephedra. Ginseng, wolfberry, astragalus, cinnamon, ginger, licorice, peony, rhubarb, ma-huang are some herbs which are used extensively for the prevention and treatment of various diseases. Ginseng, a Chinese herb is the most common constituent of various preparations prescribed to increase stamina and reduce stress across the world.

Chinese traditional medicine also includes acupuncture, an important treatment technique where needles are used to prevent and treat diseases. Tui na, acupressure and shiatsu are the traditional hands-on therapy which include deep breathing, rotating, stretching as well as manipulating pressure points with fingers or thumb. These techniques are routinely taught and practiced in China, Japan and Korea for treatment and management of injury and pain.

Qi gong and Taijiquan are also closely associated with TCM. In Chinese, the word Qi gong has two characters, 'qi' (chi) means life energy and 'gong' means daily effort. Qi gong describe systems and methods of 'energy cultivation' and the manipulation of intrinsic energy within living organisms. It relaxes the body response to stress and increases the flow of blood and oxygen to the brain. This has proven effective for a range of conditions and diseases and is practiced extensively for self-healing and prevention of diseases.

Acupuncture

Acupuncture has been used for thousands of years in Chinese traditional medicine system to treat a variety of illnesses. The underlying basis of this modality of TCM is that the human body has a bio-energy circulation system similar to the blood circulation system which Chinese call qi. The bio-energy or qi, like blood, flows to each cell via a network of pathways called meridians or channels. There are 12 such main channels which are symmetrical on each side of the body. Each pair is related to a specific organ including the heart. According to this theory, when an imbalance develops in the normal energy flow pattern, qi gets stuck or congested at certain points in the body resulting in a block in the flow of chi which manifests as discomfort or even disease. Acupuncture points are those points or spots where qi or energy has the greatest tendency to get stuck. Traditional Chinese medicine, has identified more than 300 acupoints along the meridians. Stimulating these points with sharp and fine needles helps to release the congestion of qi and restore normal flow of energy via meridians which connect the acupuncture points to each other as well as to internal organs. Stimulation restores the normal qi circulation in the cells and helps the body organs to return to their normal healthy state.

In short, **acupuncture** is the art of assessing and then releasing the blocked or congested energy by stimulating specific points with sharp special needles. It helps in normalizing the impaired flow of energy and health.

Acupressure, a non-invasive method of applying pressure of varying intensity and duration, is a simple variation of this theme. It has the advantage that it can be practised easily without the use of needles or expensive acupuncture sessions.

The Japanese practice of **Shiatsu**, which literally means 'finger pressure,' is similar to acupressure. In acupressure and shiatsu, thumbs and fingers are most commonly used to apply pressure, although knuckles, palms and elbows; even feet can be used in some therapies. The degree of pressure that is applied varies, as does the duration. Anything from moderate to penetrating pressure is employed for several seconds to several minutes, and the treatment can be performed once or repeatedly.

The mechanism of action of acupuncture or acupressure is through the stimulation of peripheral points which trigger the brain through the nervous system to release certain chemicals which act as natural painkillers. The substances released from the brain are endorphins, endomorphins, or enkephalins which act as neuromodulators and inhibit the sympathetic outflow. High blood pressure, heart rhythm, blood circulation and heart function are all influenced by sympathetic activity. All can be taken care of by acupuncture. The magnitude of blood pressure reduction is not great but one can achieve single digit reduction which is comparable to salt restriction. Reduction of 5-10 mmHg is noted in several small studies. Acupuncture can also inhibit ventricular extra systoles or irregular heartbeats which can aggravate disease or precipitate sudden death. Blood flow to the working heart is increased more by reducing the demand rather than by increasing the flow of blood. Not only are clinical events reduced due to its ability to reduce heightened sympathetic activity in patients of heart disease, the benefits are also attributed to rebalancing the body's functions achieved by easing and curbing stress and tension.

Acupuncture or acupressure is not a substitute for standard medical care. It may be regarded as an appropriate complement to the standard medical treatment. It can sometimes aid a heart patient by alleviating some of the associated anxiety and pain of the disease. Acupressure and acupuncture, though largely accepted to be safe are not free from adverse effects. The adverse effects resulting from acupuncture are generally below 10 %. However, the risk of a serious adverse event such as pneumothorax (air in chest cavity), spinal cord injuries, infections such as liver (hepatitis) and HIV infections, heart (endocarditis), joints (arthritis), and bone (osteomyelitis) have been reported. Pneumothorax is the most common and severest of them. Though these serious events are relatively rare, yet they have a cognizable risk value. The frequency of an adverse event is inversely related to the skill and training of the acupuncturists.

Ayurveda

Ayurveda is an ancient medicine system of India that has been in use since 5000 years. Ayurveda is derived from two Sanskrit words, namely, 'ayur' and 'veda', meaning 'life' and 'knowledge', respectively. The literal meaning of Ayurveda is 'science of life'. Unlike other traditional medicinal systems, Ayurveda is more focused on simple and logical therapies and has developed its own tried, tested and unique approach to health and disease. It has in fact a set of practical and simple guidelines for long life and good health. The basic feature of this medicinal therapy is the internal harmony of various body parts as well as body's harmony with the surrounding nature and environment.

The knowledge of Ayurveda is believed to be of divine origin, its wisdom being communicated to the saints and sages of India through deep meditation. Ayurvedic knowledge was thereafter passed down orally through the generations and then written down in the Vedas, Atharva Veda in particular. Later on, Ayurveda emerged as a science of life and Ayurvedic methods of health promotion and treatment were compiled in Sushruta Samhita and Charak Samhita, the two famous books written by Sushruta and Vaidya Charak respectively. Ayurvedic medicinal therapy was mainly the result of careful observations of practitioners of ancient system of Indian medicine. It was one of the most advanced medicinal therapy of its time with the prescribed treatment for complex ailments like angina pectoris, diabetes, hypertension, stones and surgeries like plastic surgery, cataract surgery and anal fistulas. The Ayurvedic system of medicine lost its glory during British rule and later on after independence, it regained its ground and new schools began to establish. Today AYUSH (Ayurveda, Yoga, Unani, Siddha, Homoeopathy), a department in the Ministry of Health and Family Welfare of Government of India monitors Ayurveda and its practice in India.

Ayurveda is a vast and ancient medical science. Unlike other medical sciences, instead of focusing on treatment of any particular disease, Ayurveda promotes healthy lifestyle. It stresses more on healthy living and well-being. According

to Ayurveda, the three basic principles of a healthy and long life are:
1. *Ahar*, that is, prudent diet.
2. *Vihar*, that is, proper activities and behaviour.
3. *Brahmacharya*, that is, control of sexuality.

Ayurveda stresses on moderation in food intake, activities, sleep, sexual life and the intake of medicine. Thus, Ayurveda can address cardiovascular disease prevention through this approach to lifestyle.

Ayurveda mainly focus on the use of herbal drugs. However, use of metals such as arsenic, gold, lead, copper, sulphur and animal products like milk and bones are not prohibited. Herbs and herbal preparations are one part of treatment in Ayurveda. Diet, exercise, yoga, meditation, massage and other practices are equally important. In the western world, herbal preparations, yoga and massage are gaining popularity, being promoted and practiced as part of complementary and alternative medicine for various diseases.

Guggul, garlic, turmeric, ginger, arjuna are some herbs used in Ayurvedic medicine that hold great promise for the development and use as novel strategies in the prevention and treatment of atherosclerosis and coronary heart disease. The available evidences are yet not convincing enough to prove Ayurvedic herbal treatment as effective treatment of heart disease or hypertension. However, the use of certain spices such as garlic, ginger and turmeric in an overall healthy diet is appropriate and can be promoted as food supplement. Herbs such as guggul and arjunarisht used by Ayurvedic practitioners need to be considered as candidates for larger randomized trials. These modalities need to be scientifically evaluated using currently available research techniques.

Yoga

Yoga is an integral part of Ayurveda. Yoga techniques have been known for centuries to improve mental relaxation, physical well-being and overall quality of life. The more we cherish materialistic values, struggle for ambitions, desire for more and more, we force our body and mind towards restiveness. The pattern of life we choose to follow leaves no place for relaxation, spirituality and to think about our inner subconscious selves. The result is an overstrained body and mind. Development of disharmony between the mind and body invites passion, emotions, anxiety, stress, strain and disease. It is known that stress, especially mental stress has adverse effects on metabolism of lipid and glucose. It can also lead to abnormalities in platelet function and clotting mechanism, increase in the sympathetic activity and production of stress hormones. All these can be attributed to genesis and aggravation of coronary heart disease. All problems instigate from a state of imbalance between physical, mental and spiritual levels. Yoga teaches us how to attain and maintain a perfect balance and harmony among the body, mind and soul. Yoga reduces anxiety, promotes well-being and improves the quality of life. It encourages us to lead a healthier physical, mental and spiritual life. All this implies a total change in habit, behaviour and outlook towards life.

The holistic science of yoga may be one of the methods for prevention as well as management of chronic diseases including cardiovascular diseases. Stress is responsible for many diseases and the psycho physiological responses to yoga can be utilized to tackle these diseases. Stretching exercises along with progressive relaxation *(shavasan)*, *yogindra*, meditation *(dhyan)* and slow rhythmic breathing *(pranayam)* are very effective in calming and taming the mind. All promote physical and mental health. Heart patients are usually sensitive, emotional and anxious. Yoga techniques calm their minds and make them emotionally balanced. Consequently, minor disturbances do not cause emotional and physical upsets. It also helps in building a positive attitude towards life and health.

Various movements, positions and breathing exercises in yoga reduce both mental and physical stress. It provides mental and physical relaxation and improves the working of the heart. Yoga can improve physical fitness and alter breathing patterns with an increase in absolute and relative maximal oxygen uptake. There can be a decrease in the sympathetic response and changes in baro-reflex sensitivity. It results in lowering of blood pressure, decrease in resting heart rate and reduction in oxygen demand by the beating heart. It is also associated with a reduction of noradrenaline production in the brain and other tissues. Yoga also has an indirect beneficial effect on glucose and lipid metabolism. The therapeutic effects of yoga which are due to the management of stress, improvement in overall cardio-respiratory function and modulation in the sympathetic nervous system can be utilized for prevention as well as cure of coronary heart disease. Early results on patients of heart disease suggest that yoga along with other lifestyle management changes can influence the progression and regression of atherosclerosis by altering the lipid profile. The observation is substantiated by few small studies, however data from large trials about the effectiveness of yoga are lacking. Yoga, which is a part of Ayurveda, a traditional Indian medicine system has an excellent safety profile and can address cardiovascular disease prevention through changes in an individual's lifestyle. Its practice as a complementary therapeutic regimen under medical supervision is appropriate, has a promising role and is the need of the hour. It is worth considering in all cases of heart disease.

Mind-body Techniques and Body Energy

The face of exercise is changing in the world. Instead of relentlessly pursuing six pack abs and perfect physique, people are chasing longevity, stress reduction and improved health through mind-body practices. People are realizing that the inner health of body is just as important as the outer health. These relaxation techniques can reduce stress, promote blood circulation and lead to an improvement in several functions of the body. These practices have the potential to improve health and the capacity to reverse some of the effects of aging.

Modern medicine recognizes stress as a contributory factor for CHD. Stress results into elevated levels of *norepinephrine, epinephrine, cortisol* and growth hormone. Chronic stress may lead to hypertension; repeated blood pressure elevations can lead to diabetes and excess of cholesterol in blood. White cell count decreases during chronic stress leading to inflammation. All are important risk factors which accelerate atherosclerosis and the development of CVD. Individuals with mental stress have twice the risk of development of adverse cardiac events and depressed patients of heart attack die early.

Mind-body techniques believe that there is a link between our state of mind and physical health and the majority of time physical ailments are symptoms of inner turmoil. It works under the assertion that the mind can affect 'bodily functions and symptoms'. The various techniques practiced are zen meditation or sitting *dhyana* which are more 'insight' oriented and transcendental meditation, *yoganidra* and *vipassana* which are largely 'concentration' oriented. Numerous studies have shown that relaxation techniques have definite health benefits. Many of these benefits are related to the decrease in stress that is attained through these techniques and thus have a synergistic role in reducing the probability of heart disease significantly.

Energy medicine is a domain that deals with presumed and verifiable energy fields. The therapies are intended to influence energy fields that ostensibly surround and penetrate the body. The unique concept behind energy medicine is that cosmic energy has the capacity to reach physical, emotional, mental and/or spiritual levels and heal. No empirical evidence has been found to support the existence of the putative energy fields on which these therapies are predicated. Adjusting bioenergy fields through acupuncture, therapeutic touch, qi gong, johrei, a and/or Reiki (a Reiki healer channelizes the cosmic energy into the chakras of the patient and healing takes place by the power of universal energy).

Though, both the practices claim that they are superior, effective and beneficial. The extent of benefits and mechanisms responsible for it are not clearly known and are difficult to quantify. Some of the benefits can be summarized as:

1. Respiratory rate and oxygen requirement is reduced.
2. The blood flow to various organs including brain is increased.
3. It leads to a reduction in the heart rate and improvement in exercise tolerance in heart patients.
4. It helps in lowering the blood pressure and in controlling diabetes.
5. It reduces anxiety and improves relaxation.
6. Decreases muscle tension and headache.
7. It elevates mood and builds self-confidence.
8. It relieves depression and improves sleep.

Mind-body techniques and energy based therapies lack widespread acceptance by western medical practitioners.

There are many reasons for the reluctance in adopting these therapies, including a lack of understanding of their benefits and how they work, a scarcity of clinical trial results and an undefined scientific foundation.

Chelation Therapy

Chelation therapy involves administration of certain chelating agents to remove anxious agents from the body. This therapy is the treatment of choice for heavy metal poisoning such as lead, iron, arsenic, uranium or mercury. Chelating agents help in removing toxic metal ions from the blood. All chelating agents form chemical bonds with the metal ions and make them chemically inert resulting in formation of an inactive water soluble complex that can enter into the blood circulation to be safely excreted from the body. The therapy is administered orally, intravenously or intramuscularly.

Chelation therapy is another form of alternative medicine utilized in the treatment of cardiovascular disease. Some alternative medicine practitioners administer disodium — ethylene diamine tetraacetic acid (EDTA) by intravenous route along with some vitamins in patients of CHD and advocate that it dissolves the atherosclerotic plaques and restores the blood flow in the coronary arteries. According to them, this method of treatment is offered as a substitute to conventional therapies such as balloon angioplasty or coronary artery bypass graft surgery. They claim it to be a safe, effective, less traumatic and relatively inexpensive therapy for CHD. How it works is not clearly understood. One explanation is that it removes calcium from atherosclerotic plaques by an unidentified mechanism and can lead to regression of the lesion.

The use of EDTA chelation therapy as treatment for CHD has not shown to be effective over conventional therapies.

Chelation therapy has proven role and is approved in heavy metal poisoning and in removing toxic metals from blood. Till date, various scientific bodies including Food and drug administration of USA (FDA) have not approved EDTA chelation therapy for cardiovascular disease. Had the therapy been so effective, as claimed by its practitioners, it would have challenged the role of existing beneficial therapies becoming the therapeutic choice for CHD. The manufacturers of EDTA would also have left no stone unturned to promote it as the treatment of choice. Till date, barring few small uncontrolled studies and reports, claims for effectiveness of chelation therapy in heart disease have not been substantiated by any large clinical trial and is considered no better than a placebo.

Chelation therapy is not free of side effects. It has its own hazards and may be fatal occasionally. It can lead to irritation at the site of infusion, fever, nausea, headache, abdominal discomfort in the form of pain, cramps, burning sensation, nausea and vomiting, convulsions, partial or total kidney failure, hypotension or fall in blood pressure, sometimes leading to serious cardiac heart rhythm disturbances and respiratory failure. Multiple blood transfusions in a failing heart can aggravate or worsen the heart failure and can sometimes lead to hypocalcaemia or lowering of calcium levels in blood which can cause cardiac arrest.

Considering the recommendations of various scientific bodies, chelation therapy should not be promoted, practiced or advocated against the established modalities of treatment for CHD. At best, EDTA chelation therapy for atherosclerosis should be undertaken today only as an investigation protocol to ascertain safety of EDTA chelation and to study its effectiveness in improving the quality of life or survival.

Many cardiovascular symptoms are not treated easily and completely with the present medical therapy. Modern medical approaches of matching specific drugs to symptoms are used to eliminate or mask complaints and do not really cure and heal. They are life-saving. Modern medical therapeutic approaches are the treatment of choice and save lives in the majority of acute and chronic conditions of heart disease. Drugs to control angina, cholesterol, diabetes or high blood pressure are highly effective. However, in the majority, risk factors and symptoms promptly return if the medication is discontinued. Physical complaints such as chest pain, palpitations, short of breath, fatigue and weakness persist in a few despite all the medical treatment. Fear of next heart attack, feeling of life long debility, a sense of deprivation from quality foods and physical activity and a constant fear of death are some conditions which are related to the mind. These worries cannot be ignored or measured. They must be understood, discussed and tackled partly with modern therapeutic approach. This is common among the majority of patients who cannot afford definitive western therapies because of poor accessibility and poverty. It is clear that there is a pressing need for promoting complementary systems and techniques to augment modern medical care. They are natural allies and an ultimate merger shall greatly improve public health as well as health care delivery system, especially in third world countries. It may be promoted as complementary therapeutic regimen in selected cases under medical supervision and not as a replacement.

Chapter 21

Diet in Heart Disease

'Let the food be your medicine lest, the medicine will replace your food'.

— *Hippocrates*

Three basic requirements of a human being are food, clothes and shelter. A person can live without clothes and shelter but cannot survive without food. Food is not only responsible for living and survival but is also responsible for health and longevity. Food helps in building each and every cell in the body. Our body cells are responsible for the proper functioning of the whole body. Without adequate nutrition and proper food, we cannot expect ourselves to be healthy. Nutrition comes from what we eat and drink. It is important, therefore, to know what is good for our body and what is not. A healthy diet along with a proper lifestyle is the best weapon one has to fight against any disease, including that of the heart.

Today diet is an essential aspect of a healthy life. It plays an important role in health as well as in curing any disease. Healthy diet habits increase the ability of an individual to live longer and improve his well-being. It has a positive impact on the overall personality of the person.

What is a Healthy Diet?

A healthy diet should provide sufficient energy and nutrition which is the fundamental need of the human body. It should help in maintaining the normal functions of the body. It should also be such that it repairs and replaces body tissues from time to time and promotes growth. A healthy diet should also protect against disease and disability. Therefore, a diet which provides the desired amount of calories, minerals, vitamins, fats, carbohydrates and proteins is considered to be a healthy diet. Food items which are consumed raw, baked or grilled are considered best for health and may constitute a healthy diet.

What is an Unhealthy Diet?

Some food items, when consumed can increase the risk of development of disease. These are considered to be unhealthy diet. All food components are required for the proper health of the body and consumption of food items beyond what is required badly affects the normal functioning of the body inviting chronic diseases, as excess of anything is harmful. Excess and frequent use of refined food items such as refined flour, meat with fat, saturated oils, butter, whole milk and its products, sugar and sweets are few common food items which constitute an unhealthy diet. Overcooked, fried and highly processed foods are also unhealthy food items. These unhealthy food items increase the risk of heart disease, diabetes mellitus, hypertension, stroke, cancer, kidney and other problems.

Diet and Heart Disease

Various risk factors which are responsible for the development of heart disease can be directly or indirectly influenced by the diet. Some of the major risk factors for heart disease such as, cholesterol or fat content in the blood, diabetes mellitus, high blood pressure and obesity are directly influenced by what we eat. Even other risk factors such as, homocysteine level in blood, antioxidants and alcohol are also influenced by dietary factors. Sensible dietary and eating habits can modify these risk factors and make a quantum change in the disease pattern and outcome. Numerous epidemiological studies have identified dietary patterns and food categories associated with reduced risk of cardiovascular diseases especially heart disease. It is also observed that adherence to dietary recommendations is associated with reductions in cardiovascular disease risk by upto 30 % or more.

What is a Mediterranean Diet?

Increasing evidence suggests that a Mediterranean style diet emphasizing upon the consumption of fruits, vegetables, more of plant proteins and fish with little meat, tree nuts and seeds such as almonds, walnuts, pistachios, sesame and oil rich in unsaturated fat such as olive and canola oil with whole grains were associated with a marked reduction in future heart related adverse effects in patients of heart attack. It also helps in reducing cancer of the gut, especially that of the colon (large intestine). It has also been observed that a Mediterranean diet also protects one from the development of wrinkles. Olive oil, an integral part of Mediterranean diet is considered to be the healthiest of all edible oils and Homer called it 'Liquid Gold'.

What is an Indian Diet?

India is an agro based country hence the Indian diet is close to the Mediterranean diet as a majority of Indians consume vegetables and cereals. However, the pattern of cooking and the amount differs. Consumption of olive oil and nuts, an important ingredient of the Mediterranean diet is negligible as it is expensive and beyond the reach of common Indians. In India, food choices are governed by the cost of the food, availability and seasonal variations. It is also influenced by family traditions, religion and culture.

Diet and Heart Disease in India

In India, diet as well as the pattern of preparing food plays an important role in influencing the health of heart and body. Dietary factors such as a low intake of fruits, vegetables and nuts which are rich sources of vitamins, minerals, antioxidants and fibre, excess use of whole milk and its products, butter, high intake of *vanaspati* oil, an hydrogenated vegetable oil rich in trans-fats, high intake of sugar and sweets, less use of fish and more use of fatty meats with whole egg increases the chance of heart disease. The cooking pattern also influences the health of the heart, deep frying, reuse of oils, overcooking and garnishing the food with excess of butter or clarified butter (*ghee*) are few practices which not only destroy the important minerals and vitamins but also increase the saturated fat content of the food. All this may contribute to a high CHD risk in India. Mustard oil with low content of erucic acid, which is a popular cooking oil amongst North Indians is rich in omega fatty acids along with refined oils made from sunflower, rice bran, ground-nut and sesame-all are considered to be heart healthy oils. Coconut oil is a common cooking medium among South Indians. It is rich in saturated fats and is a cause of concern as it can increase the risk of coronary heart disease. We cannot blame the rapid surge of heart disease among Indians to the food items alone but extensive use of tobacco and sedentary lifestyles are also factors which enhance the likelihood of development of heart disease. To address the relation between diet and IHD, we should know the various food groups consumed.

In general, the food items which are commonly consumed can be placed under five separate groups (Table 21.1). The five groups are:

1. Cereals and grains.
2. Pulses or legumes.
3. Milk, eggs and flesh foods.
4. Fruits and vegetables.
5. Fats, oils and sugar.

Fats and carbohydrates are the primary source of energy in the body. Vitamins, minerals and trace elements in food are helpful in enzymatic and metabolic activities. Most of them are required in small quantities and contrary to carbohydrate, protein and fat, do not provide energy to the body.

Table 21.1: Common Food Groups and Respective Energy and Contents

Food Group	Amount (gm)	Protein (gm)	Fat (gm)	Carbo-hydrate (gm)	Energy (kcal)
Cereal	100 gm	12	Nil	80	350
Legumes and pulses	100 gm	24	Nil	60	350
Milk (cow)	100 ml	3.5	4	4	65
Milk (buffalo)	100 ml	4.5	8	5	110
Oil	10 ml	Nil	10	Nil	80
Meat	100 gm	10	8	Nil	125
Sugar	10 gm	Nil	Nil	10	40
Fruits	75 gm small	Nil	Nil	10	40-60
Vegetables-green leafy	100 gm	Nil	Nil	6	30-40
Vegetables-others (tuberous)	100 gm	Nil	Nil	6-10	50-60

Source: Gopalan G, Rama Shastri BV, Balasubramanian SC, 2007, Nutritive Value of Indian Foods, National Institute of Nutrition, ICMR, Hyderabad.

Proteins

Protein is present in every cell of our body. The heart muscle in itself is a muscular organ and contains protein termed as myoglobin. Protein is essential for body's functions and is an important constituent of diet. In the human diet, protein can be obtained both from plant and animal sources. Pulses are the main source of protein in the primarily vegetarian Indian diet. In India, other plant sources of protein are nuts and oil seeds. Milk and cereals and their products are the other options for protein. In the Indian diet, animal source of protein includes egg, poultry, meat and fish. It should be emphasized that the plant source of protein is the main source of protein in the Indian diet because the majority of Indians are life long, strict vegetarians. The remaining who are non-vegetarian consume animal food products occasionally and only a few consume it regularly. The other reason may be that pulses and legumes are cheaper options as compared to animal food products. Common pulses consumed in India are pigeon pea (*arhar* or *tur*), chik pea or Bengal gram (*chana*), lentil (*masur*), green gram (*moong* or *mung*), green pea (*matar*), kidney bean (*rajma*), black gram (*urad*) and cow pea (*lobia*).

Pulses are dry seeds. When their seed coat is removed, it is called as '*dal*'. It is used as the staple diet in India. The most common pulse used in a major part of India is *arhar* or *tur* or yellow dal. The other commonly used dals are *chana, urad, masur, and moong*. Dal in the Indian diet provides 17-25 gms of protein consumed per 100 gms of dal or pulses and the energy content is similar to cereals which is approximately

350 kcal of 100 gm dal or pulses consumed. Every Indian daily consumes dal with rice or rice with *sambar* or *chapatti* with *dal*. Dal is also an essential ingredient of *khichari, pongal* or *dhokla*. Dal or pulses are very low in fat and are a rich source of iron, calcium and vitamin B.

Nuts and Oil Seeds

Nuts and oil seeds are another source of plant protein. Some of the commonly consumed nuts in India are groundnut, coconut, dry cashew nuts (*kaaju*) gingelly seeds (*til*), mustard seeds (used as oil) almonds, walnuts (*akhrot*) and pistachios (*pista*). Groundnut, coconut, gingelly and mustard seeds are cheap and are used by most people. Groundnut, gingelly seeds (til), and niger seeds (*kala til*) are frequently used with jaggery during winters, especially during *lohri* or *Khichari* or *Makarsankranti* festival.

Milk and Milk Based Products

Milk has a very special place in the Indian diet. The morning starts with a cup of tea or coffee with milk. Owning cows, buffalos, goats or camels is a sign of prosperity in India. Milk obtained from different animals is used as food. In India, milk obtained from cow and buffalo is the most important sources of food. Milk is an important source of protein, especially for infants and children, postmenopausal women, people who are strictly vegetarian and during pregnancy.

Milk and milk products are the main dietary source of calcium which is mandatory for strong bones and teeth. It also plays an important role in nerves and muscle function and clotting of blood. Calcium plays a positive role in controlling high blood pressure and stroke. Whole milk and its products are a rich source of saturated fat and may increase the cholesterol level in blood thereby increasing the risk of heart disease. Considering this, the best strategy is to consume more of skimmed or low fat milk in place of whole milk or its products. Skimmed milk contains only 0.3 % fat as compared to whole milk which has fat as high as 3.25 %. The benefit of skimmed milk is not only to cut down your fat intake but also calorie intake while retaining the benefit of calcium.

A common practice is to boil milk before it is consumed. Curd is the second most common milk product consumed in India. *Paneer*, cheese, buttermilk *(mathaa), lassi, rabari* and *khoya* are other forms popular all over India. Milk is an important ingredient of many household desserts such as pudding, *kheer* and *halwas* which are consumed routinely in India. Milk and milk products are also used to make delicious sweets. Some of the Indian desserts such as *halwa* are very high in calories, even more than ice cream or cakes.

Eggs

The diet of low and middle income countries is deficient in protein and protein deficiency is common. This can be met by the consumption of eggs. Eggs are cheaper than meat, poultry, fish or even pulses. Eggs have excellent nutritive value and contain 10-12 % of protein. The yolk or yellow portion of an egg is rich in fat and contributes to the calories supplied by eggs. Yolk is not always bad as it is a good source of iron and vitamin A and D. It also contains calcium, sulphur and phosphorus. With these properties, eggs may be considered more useful than milk; besides, affording milk may not be easy for poor and low income groups, and more so during summer season when its production goes down and demand increases. Today, egg is no more considered non-vegetarian. It is now considered as an important food item in breakfast by a majority of Indians. Various preparations of egg along with bread are popular breakfasts all over India. Hens remain the most common source of egg on the breakfast table. The whole egg contains 65 % water, 10-12 % protein and 10-12 % fat. The yolk of an egg contains approximately 250 mgs of cholesterol. This makes the egg an unfavourable diet for heart patients. An average Indian hen's egg provides 70 kcal. It is advisable to restrict the intake of egg yolk or yellow portion, to reduce the calories and cholesterol in diet. However, if one wants to consume 2-3 eggs per week you can continue with the whole egg and if you want to consume it daily, it is better to avoid the egg yolk or yellow portion of egg. Various popular egg preparations include-boiled egg, fried egg, poached egg, scrambled egg, omelette, custard, pudding, pies, foam cakes and egg curry.

Meat and its Products

Meat is the third most common food item which is rich in proteins. Meat contains 15-20 % protein which is less than that present in pulses. However, meat proteins are a good source of essential amino acids. Common items consumed are fish, chicken and red meat. Consumption of pork and beef is popular amongst poorer communities as it is cheap. Lamb, turkey, duck, goose, camel and sea foods are less commonly consumed except along the coastal regions. Globally, pork and beef are consumed quite frequently. However, its consumption is strongly influenced by religion in various countries including the Indian subcontinent.

Red meat is high in both fat and cholesterol. Studies have shown that a diet rich in red meat increases the risk of heart disease and also the risk of colon, rectal and prostate cancers. The irony is that the content of fat is further increased while cooking meat by adding more saturated fat. Considering the nutritive value of meat, it is advisable to use fish and skinless poultry products more frequently as compared to red meats with fat. Secondly, roasting or baking these products reduces the fat content. Avoid frequent consumption of burgers with meat as these are prepared in vegetables oils, fried and contain trans-fats which are as harmful as saturated fat.

Role of Fish and Fish Oil in Diet

Both freshwater and sea fish are good for the heart. Fish oil and fish are a rich source of omega 3 fatty acids, which have been shown to protect you against CHD. The use of fish and fish oil has shown to reduce the episodes of chest pain in patients with CHD. Fish are of two types - one is lean while the other is a fatty fish. Both are excellent for the heart. Consuming 100-200 gm of fish twice a week is recommended. Fish oils are marketed in capsules. However, its consumption can increase the calorie intake as some of the capsules are high in calories. Hence, it is advisable that one should get fish oil from the natural source that is, by regularly eating fish. Mackerel, herring, sardines, lake trout, salmon, tuna along with the Indian variety of fishes such as *hilsa, purava, seer, pomphret, murrel, katla, rohu, mackerel, bam, bombay duck* and *bhekti* are good sources of omega 3 polyunsaturated fatty acids and helps in preventing coronary heart disease. It is best to avoid fish fingers, fried fish or fish roe. However, shrimps, prawns, lobsters, squids, mussels and cockles can also be eaten in moderation as they are rich in cholesterol and low in saturated fats.

Fish Intake at a Glance

1. *It was observed that Greenland Eskimos and Japanese fishermen have low prevalence and death rate associated with heart disease.*

2. It was suggested that this beneficial effect was due to their high intake of fish.
3. Fish oils are rich in polyunsaturated fatty acids such as omega 3 fatty acids which are associated with a reduction in the occurrence of heart disease.
4. The mechanism by which fish oil or fish can protect are multiple. Some of the mechanisms have clot bursting property (antithrombotic), maintain the rhythm of the heart (antiarrhythmic), decreases triglyceride cholesterol, improves the intactness of the inner lining of vessels (improves endothelial function) and makes plaque stable.
5. It is proved that habitual intake of oily fish appears to offer protection against heart disease.
6. Intake of two portions of oily fish once a week is associated with a reduction in the prevalence of heart disease.

Fish oils are rich in omega 3 fatty acids which have anti-inflammatory, clot busting properties. It also has the property to boost the immune system. It also helps in lowering blood pressure, reduce triglycerides and prevent heart rhythm abnormalities, making fish oil a perfect cardio-protective substance. Some physicians recommend fish oil capsules. The usual dose is 3000 mg per day and that too after meals. People with diabetes should take 2000 mg per day as it may worsen blood sugar control in some. Side effects of fish oil capsule include a fishy after taste or smell. Sometimes it can cause abdominal upsets such as belching, bloating, indigestion and pain. However, high doses of fish oil that is, 8000 mg or above may result in internal bleeding and weight gain. Cod liver oil should not be substituted for fish oil capsules as it contains high doses of vitamin A and D. Always stick to the natural thing as eating fish twice or thrice a week is better than taking fish oil supplements.

Choose Low-fat Protein Sources

Although meat, poultry and fish along with dairy products and eggs are some of the best sources of protein, they are high in total fat, saturated fat and cholesterol. Skimmed milk rather than whole milk or skinless turkey or chicken breast rather than fried chicken patties are lower fat options and may be substituted for the above. Fish is another good alternative to high fat meats. Soybeans may be especially beneficial to the heart and may be regularly substituted for animal protein. Legumes and pulses can be cheap and a good source of protein. They may be considered as the best source of low fat high protein diet in the vegetarian dominated Indian culture or in a majority of low and middle income countries. The intake of the white portion of egg can increase the protein in the diet and is pocket friendly for both, the poor and rich alike. Table 21.2 depicts various protein contents in common food items.

Table 21.2: Protein Content of Common Foods

Food Item	Protein %
Legumes and pulses	18-24
Milk	3-4
Groundnuts	26
Gingelly seeds	18
Paneer	18
Cheese	26
Egg	10-12
Red meat	15-20
Fish	6-9
Vegetables	2-6
Fruits	< 1

Oils and Fats

Fats and oils are an essential ingredient of diet and an important source of energy. Fat in itself is not harmful as it is used to make body cells, absorb fat soluble vitamins, help in the production of hormones and of course makes the food tasty. Since a major part of fat is synthesized in the liver, a very small quantity of fat is required in the diet. Fat is the only food item which people try to avoid completely and its relationship with health is more misunderstood than any other aspect. It should be emphasized that a small quantity of fat is an essential component of our diet and is necessary for health. Though consumption of fat is mandatory, foods rich in oil and fats, if consumed in excess can lead to serious health problems such as obesity, cancer and heart disease.

Fat is obtained from either animal sources such as red meat, butter or vegetable source as it is present in various vegetable oils especially coconut and palm oil. Egg yolk, lard, almonds, avocados, chocolate, cheese, cream, puddings and fatty meat cuts are other important sources of fat. A majority of people in developing countries depend mainly on oil seeds to meet its oil or fat consumption. Butter is not cheap and its consumption is limited to the middle and higher income group. Other animal fats such as lard and tallow are not consumed because of religious reasons and sentiments. Nowadays, poor in developed countries and rich in developing countries consume the highest amount of saturated fat.

Mustard Oil and Erucic Acid

Mustard oil is composed of fatty acids such as oleic, linoleic and erucic acid. It is widely used in North India. Mustard oil is considered unsuitable for human consumption due to its high concentration of erucic acid (20-50 %). Erucic acid has been found to be carcinogenic for rats. However, consumption of routine amounts of mustard oil has not shown any carcinogenic property in human beings. United States and Europe regard the use of mustard oil as unsafe due to its high erucic acid content and is sold for external use only. Now mustard oil has been genetically modified by scientists in India and the new product is healthier. In India, mustard oil has been in use since ages and is generally heated almost to boiling point before being used for cooking. This may be an attempt to reduce the noxious substances such as erucic acid. It may also be used with other oils to avoid its odour.

Choice of Cooking Oils

Cooking oil contains fat which is essential for daily use not only for taste but also for its nutritive value. It is wise to use more of unsaturated rich oils than saturated rich oils. There should be a good balance of omega 3 (alpha-linolenic acid) and omega 6 (linoleic acid) fatty acids (1:3). One should choose a variety of vegetable oils available as opposed to sticking to one single source. Mixture of two or more oils of different sources may be more beneficial. It is wise to mix MUFA rich groundnut or mustard oil with PUFA rich corn, safflower or sunflower oil. One can also try rice bran or corn oil with sunflower or canola with sesame oil. Considering the eurcic acid content, mustard oil used as the only cooking oil may not be a good choice unless it is obtained from genetically engineered mustard seeds with low erucic acid (less than 2 %). If one can afford, then olive or canola oil can be the best choice. However, it may not be pocket friendly for a majority of people. Various fatty acid composition of common edible oils are summarized in Table 21.3.

Table 21.3: Fatty Acid Composition of Common Cooking Oils and Fats

Cooking oil	Unsaturated (%)	Saturated (%)	Predominant Fatty Acid (%)	Remarks
Olive oil or jaitoon	86	14	Monounsaturated (75)	Excellent
Almond or badam Oil	87	13	Monounsaturated (70)	Excellent
Canola or rapeseed oil	91	09	Monounsaturated (59)	Excellent
Mustard oil	88	12	Monounsaturated (56%)	Excellent (euricic acid < 2%)
Peanut oil	82	18	Monounsaturated (49)	Good
Cod liver oil	74	23	Polyunsaturated (47%)	Good
Sunflower oil (Linoleic)	89	11	Polyunsaturated (70%)	Excellent
Safflower oil	77	23	Polyunsaturated (70%)	Excellent
Rice bran	76	22	Polyunsaturated (41%)	Good
Sesame or gingelly or til	82	14	Polyunsaturated (42%)	Good
Corn oil	87	13	Polyunsaturated (57%)	Good
Soya bean	85	15	Polyunsaturated (57%)	Good
Walnut or akhrot	87	10	Polyunsaturated (63%)	Good
Cotton seed oil	74	26	Polyunsaturated (51%)	Fair
Palm oil	50	50	Saturated (50%)	Bad
Butter	31	69	Saturated (69%)	Bad

Margarine (hard)	20	80	Saturated (80%)	Bad
Margarine (soft)	80	20	Monounsaturated (47%)	Good
Palm kernel oil	14	86	Saturated (86%)	Bad
Coconut oil	08	92	Saturated (92%)	Bad
Ghee	04	96	Saturated (96%)	Bad

Source: Gopalan G, Rama Shastri BV, Balasubramanian SC, 2007, Nutritive Value of Indian Foods, National Institute of Nutrition, ICMR, Hyderabad.

Should one Practice a Total Fat-free Diet?

The concept of prescribing or suggesting a fat-free diet to heart patients is not only wrong but is detrimental to health also. Even then many physicians advocate extremely low fat or fat-free diets for treatment of established coronary heart disease. It not only makes the food tasteless but increases more stress as one cannot enjoy good quality food. Fat-free diet is not only ineffective and harmful but cannot be continued for long periods. A fat-free or a very low fat diet causes deficiency of fat soluble vitamins such as vitamins A, D, E and K. It can also make the person devoid of essential fatty acids which are not synthesized in the body. It can increase the total small dense LDL and triglycerides in blood. Total reduction of fat in diet can also reduce HDL cholesterol in blood which actually protects the heart. It also increases insulin resistance. Therefore, one should reduce the fat content in diet but should not practice a fat-free or extremely low fat diet.

What are the Food Items which may Increase Cholesterol in Blood?

Food items rich in animal fat such as fatty meat and its products, egg yolk, organ meats (heart, liver, brain, kidney, etc.), poultry meat such as goose, duck, chicken and turkey with skin, whole milk, cream, ice cream, chocolates, fudge, whole milk cheese, *paneer* and butter, are rich in total fat. They increase the cholesterol content in the blood (Table 21.4). Food items prepared in butter, hard margarine, ghee, coconut oil are rich in saturated fats and *vanaspati* oil (partially hydrogenated vegetable oil, rich in trans-fatty acids) can also increase cholesterol levels. Food items commonly used as snacks before meals such as sausages, salami, ham or hog burger, bacon, fried steak, meat pies, pastries, cookies, crackers, cakes, French fries, pizza full of cheese or deep fried Indian food items such as *chole bhature, samosa, puri kachori, tikki* and *chat* or *sweets*, puddings are not only a rich source of saturated and trans-fats but also add up an excess number of calories in your diet. Similarly, cream soups, salad cream, creamy dressings, chocolate spread and full fat drinks should be reduced to the minimum to reduce cholesterol levels in blood.

Table 21.4: Cholesterol Content in Common Food Items

Food Item	Cholesterol mg/100 gm	Remarks
Skimmed milk	2	Ideal
Whole milk	14-16	Occasionally
Fish	25-50	Ideal
Chicken without skin	60	Ideal
Red meat or Mutton	65	Occasionally
Beef	70	Occasionally
Pork	90	Occasionally
Chicken with skin	100	Occasionally
Cheese	100	Occasionally
Prawns	150	Occasionally
Butter	250	Occasionally (rich in fat also)

Ghee	300	Occasionally (rich in fat also)
Whole egg	400	Occasionally
Cooked egg (omelette, poached, scrambled, boiled or fried)	450-550	Occasionally
Liver	500	Avoid
Kidney	550	Avoid
Cod liver oil	570	Avoid
Egg yolk	1120	Avoid
Brain	1350	Avoid

What are the Food Items which will Lower the Cholesterol in Blood?

Food items prepared in oils rich in poly and monounsaturated fats will reduce the cholesterol level. Consumption of olive, canola, mustard, sesame, soya, corn, safflower, sunflower seed oils are good for health. Frequent consumption of skimmed milk and its products, especially yoghurt are good for health. Nuts are a good source of healthy fat. Soft margarines and spreads made from vegetable oils are also low in cholesterol and saturated fats. Fish and fish oil also reduce the bad cholesterol and increase the good cholesterol. One should keep in mind that all fats are rich in calories and should be consumed in moderation.

What are Tropical Oils?

This term refers to coconut, palm kernel and palm oils. Like all fats and oils, these three oils contain various types of fatty acids. But unlike other plant oils, they contain a lot of saturated fatty acids. Coconut oil contains 92 %, palm kernel oil has 82 % and palm oil has 50 % of saturated fats.

What is Refined Oil?

It is a popular and highly advertised cooking oil in India. It is commonly used to make bakery products. Refinement means purifying fats and oils. This process helps in removing, toxic substances, suspended materials and fatty acids. The colour and odour is also removed during this process. Though the process makes the oil tasteless, it becomes more stable. Refined oils have a longer shelf life than unrefined oils of the same kind. Fortification with vitamins can also be done during the process. In urban areas, refined oils have been popular, while in rural areas mustard, sesame and coconut oils are preferred because of their purity, availability and aroma.

What is Hydrogenated or *vanaspati* Oil?

Vanaspati or vegetable oils or hydrogenated oils are popular oils in India. They are produced in bulk by the process of hydrogenation of vegetable oils. During the process of hydrogenation, the unsaturated fatty acids are converted into trans and saturated fat. Since these oils are the cheapest of all oils, and stable therefore their use is popular all over India. Foods cooked in *vanaspati ghee* have a long half-life with little taste and flavour. Clarified butter or *ghee* has been popular because of its aroma, however it is costly. In India, *vanaspati* is used as a substitute for ghee and often fortified with vitamin A. Its physical appearance and texture often resembles ghee. Hydrogenated fats or *vanaspati* ghee are used to make commercial snacks.

What is Invisible Fat?

Fat in the diet is in two forms – visible and invisible. Everyone is conscious and aware of visible fat such as oils, butter and ghee and try to curtail them. People know very little about the invisible fat present in food which is also important for health. A small quantity of invisible fat is present in cereals and pulses. Bengal gram and soya bean are a fairly good source of invisible fat in diet. Spices used daily in the Indian kitchen, especially dry chilly, cumin seeds, coriander seeds, and fenugreek seeds are a good source of invisible fat. Nuts and oil seeds such are groundnut, sesame, coconut, mustard seeds along with dry fruits are a good source of invisible fat. A non-vegetarian diet consisting of meat with fat, organ meat such as brain, liver, kidney, egg yolk, fatty fish especially shrimp or prawn can provide a good quantity of invisible fat. An adult Indian diet which is cereal based gets 20 gm of invisible fat. An average adult with sedentary work habits needs only 40-50 gms of fat daily. Therefore, it is wise to consume not more than 4-6 teaspoonful of visible fat daily. If you are suffering from heart disease it should be reduced to 2 teaspoonful (10 ml) daily but never try and consume a fat-free or a zero fat diet.

How to Determine what Oil is Rich in which Type of Fatty Acid?

Oils rich in saturated fats and trans-fats are harmful and are solid at room temperature. Oils rich in monounsaturated fats are liquid at room temperature but solidify during refrigeration. However, oils rich in polyunsaturated fats are liquid at room temperature and remain so even if refrigerated.

Some Practical Tips for Cooking Oils

1. Oil provides fat and is a high calorie food. Each gram of fat gives 9 calories, merely double the number of calories in carbohydrate and protein.
2. Vegetable oils such as olive oil or canola are best for use but sunflower, mustard, safflower, sesame, soya bean and peanut oils are also good substitutes.

3. Restrict the use of oils rich in saturated fats such as butter, hard margarine, lard, ghee, coconut and palm oil.
4. Avoid hydrogenated or vanaspati oil as they are rich in trans-fatty acids.
5. Avoid heating oil to a high temperature.
6. Do not use leftover oil again or add fresh oil to the fried oil.
7. Store oil in an airtight container.
8. 4 tablespoonful or 60 ml of vegetable oil is sufficient for a healthy adult per day and will provide approximately 500 calories and 60 gm of fat.

Nuts

Nuts are a good source of monounsaturated fatty acids, fibre, flavonoids, magnesium and copper. Walnut is particularly rich in polyunsaturated fatty acids such as linoleic and alpha-linolenic acids. It is a vegetarian source of omega 3 fatty acids. Almond is also a good source of unsaturated fats. Groundnut is the cheapest source of protein. Various studies revealed that people who consumed a small quantity of nuts (50-70 gm) twice a week had 47 % reduction in the risk for heart attack and related diseases compared with those who rarely or never consumed nuts. Nuts are very rich in calories, so one should consume them in a small quantity (Table 21.4). A hundred grams of edible nuts contain calories which are almost equal to a major meal. It is often used as a concentrated source of energy by trekkers and mountaineers.

Table 21.4 : Common Dry Fruits and Nuts and Their Nutritive Value:

Food Item (per 100gms) Edible Portion	Common Name	Protein (gm)	Fat (gm)	Carbohydrate (gm)	Energy (kcal)
Raisin	Kishmish	1.8	0.3	75	308
Currant	Munakka	2.7	0.5	75	316
Dates	Khajur	2.5	0.4	76	317
Groundnut	Moongphali	25	40	26	567
Cashew	Kaju	21	47	22	596
Pistachio	Pista	20	53	16	626
Almond	Badam	21	59	11	655
Coconut (dry)	Nariyal	16	65	11	662
Walnut	Akhrot	16	53	162	687

Source: Gopalan G, Rama Shastri BV, Balasubramanian SC, 2007, Nutritive Value of Indian Foods, National Institute of Nutrition, ICMR, Hyderabad.

Carbohydrates

Carbohydrates are the cheapest and most abundant source of energy. They are synthesized by the process of photosynthesis. The process of photosynthesis in plants involves sunlight which converts carbon dioxide and water into carbohydrates. Since animals cannot synthesize carbohydrates, they obtain their carbohydrate from plant sources. Carbohydrates in the human diet are supplied by simple sugars, fruits, cereals, vegetables and milk.

Cereals

Cereals supply the bulk of food consumed because it is the cheapest source of energy. India is basically an agriculture based economy and cereals are grown in India in large quantities. The main cereal crops are paddy (rice), wheat, maize (corn), sorghum *(jawar)*, millet, barley, oats and rye. Carbohydrates are the major constituents of cereals and comprise 80 % of dry weight. Maize consumption as staple diet is common in a large part of the world. It provides the maximum amount of carbohydrates followed by rice, sorghum and wheat. In the majority of low and middle income countries, paddy or rice production is the highest followed by wheat, barley, maize, sorghum and the rest.

Rice

Rice is the staple diet for the Indian subcontinent. It is the most common source of carbohydrate in diet. Asia produces almost 90 % of the total world production of rice. The cooking method mainly involves boiling it with water and it is consumed with pulses *(dal)*, *vegetables*, sambar, fish or meat or milk and sugar. The other rice products are *dosa* and *idli* which are consumed mainly in the southern states of India. *Dhokla*, a delicious preparation of rice is not only common to Gujaratis but also popular all over the country. Rice bran is used to prepare edible oil. Rice flakes *(chiwra)* or rice puffs *(murmura or muri)* are commonly used to prepare various homemade and commercial snacks and *namkeens*. *Biryani*, whether vegetable, mutton or chicken is another delicacy made from rice. The city of Hyderabad is famous for its biryani throughout the world.

Wheat

Wheat is consumed in the form of flour which is obtained by milling the grain. It is the major staple diet of Punjab and other northern parts of the country. It is also consumed with rice, almost all over the country. In India, it is commonly used to make *chappati or roti*, and is prepared in almost all household kitchens and restaurants in India. *Chapati* is the staple diet of

North India. It is a type of unleavened bread that is cheap, quick to cook and very delicious to eat. *Tandoori roti, naan, parantha, bhaturas* and *poori* are other forms of wheat preparation. Bread, commonly used in breakfast is made with white flour by mixing water, yeast and salt. Breads available in India are fine breads. Breads made from whole flour, corn bread and garlic bread are less popular. *Paranthas* and *poori* are fried by using oils or ghee; if stuffed, especially *paranthas* with various ingredients such as *paneer* (Indian cottage cheese), meat or vegetables, it makes them highly nutritious and rich in fat and calories. Biscuits, cakes, cookies, pastries and muffins are other baked products usually used as desserts or in breakfast.

Maize

Commercially available cornflakes are commonly used with milk. It is a popular breakfast among urban children. Shorgum (*jowar*), barley and millets (*bajra* and *ragi*) are other cereals consumed in India, especially in rural India because they can be cultivated with less water and manures, making them cheap options to eat.

Sugar and Sugar Based Products

Sugar and sweets are a quick source of energy. Refined white sugar, molasses and honey are commonly consumed daily. Jams, jellies, candy, syrup or sherbet and sweets are other concentrated sources of sugar. Fruits, cane, beet sugar are the natural sources of sugar. Sugar is a major source of carbohydrate but it lacks proteins, vitamins and minerals. Hence, they have a poor nutritive value. Fruits are an exception. They are not only rich in sugar but have adequate amounts of vitamins and minerals. Excess of sugar can lead to obesity, increase in cholesterol level, tooth decay and pyorrhoea.

Indian sweets and sugar based products occupy a privileged place in our life and are associated with happy occasions such as birthdays, marriages and success celebrations. Indian sweets are manufactured locally and differ from region to region depending upon the prevailing culinary taste and preferences. The shelf life of Indian sweets is short. Indian sweets are prepared from milk products such as *khoya* (used for preparing *burfi, gulab jamun* or *pedas*), *chhena* (used for preparing *rasogulla, sandesh, chhena kheer, chamcham*) and mixed with sugar. Major ingredients used in sweet preparations are *khoya* or *chhena*, sugar, *vanaspati ghee* (a rich source of transfat), edible oil, *maida* (refined flour) and dry fruits. *Khoya* and *chhena* are obtained from whole milk. Indian sweets contain a high sugar content that is between 30-50 %. The fat content is also high as whole milk is used. Thus, Indian sweets provide high fat and calories. Since they are consumed as desserts or as snacks, they cause obesity and increase the cholesterol content of the body.

Fruits and Vegetables

India, because of its favourable climatic conditions produces a wide variety of seasonal fruits and vegetables. A majority of fruits contain a lot of water and a small quantity of protein and fat. Vegetables are low in fat and proteins (except peas and beans). Vegetables are low in calories except starch containing vegetables such as potato, sweet potato and tapioca. Fruits and vegetables are low in calories, a good source of vitamins and minerals, and rich in dietary fibre, making them the healthiest of all foods. Citrus fruits along with Indian gooseberry, strawberry, melons and guava are a good source of vitamin C. A 100 gm of orange juice provides 50 mg of vitamin C which is almost equal to the daily requirement of an adult. Green leafy vegetables, tomatoes and green pepper are also rich in vitamin C. Yellow fruits and vegetables along with dark green leafy vegetables are rich in vitamin A and contain carotene. Vitamin B is relatively low in fruits. Green leafy vegetables and legumes contain a fairly good amount of calcium and iron. Fruits and vegetables also provide other essential minerals in diet. Green leafy vegetables and cruciferous vegetables such as broccoli, cabbage and cauliflower provide the maximum benefit to health.

The key component of the Mediterranean diet was 4-6 (350-500 gm) servings of vegetables and fruits which showed a 30 % reduction in risk of CVD. A majority of Indians are vegetarians and vegetables constitute as an essential food item for both the poor and rich. Even though we are vegetarians, the intake of vegetables is lower than recommended and we depend more on cereals. Vegetables and fruits are consumed less in comparison to cereals, the main reason being the cost. We also underestimate the vast potential benefits of vegetables and fruits. Vegetables are served as part of the main meal, and apart from their nutritive value they add colour and flavour to the food. Vegetables can be served raw or cooked. They also contain phytochemicals substances, found in plants that may help to prevent cardiovascular disease. Vegetables and fruits are a good source of fibre in the diet. Eating more fruits and vegetables helps us indirectly also by satisfying our hunger and thereby reducing the intake of high fat foods. Consumption of whole fruits and not the fruit juices should be practiced. A majority of us live in the false belief that red colour fruit juices, especially pomegranate juice increase the blood content or haemoglobin or orange juice will give instant energy. However, in order to take out the juice of a fruit, we discard the pulp which is rich in fibre. Whether it is mere convenience or myth, the practice should be discouraged. Don't smother fruits and vegetables in butter dressings, creamy sauces or other high fat garnishes. Serve it as fruit salad or vegetable salad with a little salt, pepper or lemon. The rule should be to serve it in its most natural form, fresh and not with cream or heavy sauces. Table 21.5 depicts the nutritive value and energy content of common fruits in the ascending order.

Table 21.5: Various Contents and Energy Provided by Common Fruits

Fruits (100 gm)	Indian Name	Carbohydrate (gm)	Protein (gm)	Fat (gm)	Energy (kcal)
Watermelon	Tarbuj	3.3	0.2	0.2	16
Papaya	Papita	7.2	0.6	0.1	32
Sweet lime	Musambi	9.3	0.8	0.3	43
Strawberry	Kash or istabari	9.8	0.7	0.2	44
Pineapple	Ananas	10.8	0.4	0.1	46
Orange	Santra	10.9	0.7	0.2	48
Guava	Amrud	11.2	0.9	0.3	51
Pear	Nashpati	11.2	0.6	0.2	52
Apricot	Khumani	11.6	1.0	0.3	53
Apple	Seb	13.4	0.2	0.5	59
Litchi	Litchi	13.6	1.1	0.2	61
Jamun	Kalajamun	14.0	0.7	0.3	62
Pomegranate	Anar	14.5	1.6	0.1	65
Grapes	Angoor	16.5	0.5	0.3	71
Mango	Aam	16.9	0.6	0.4	74
Jack fruit	Katahal	19.8	1.9	0.1	88
Sapodilla or sapota	Chiku	21.4	0.7	1.1	98
Custard apple	Sharifa	23.5	1.6	0.4	104
Banana	Kela	27.2	1.2	0.3	116

Source: Gopalan G, Rama Shastri BV, Balasubramanian SC, 2007, Nutritive Value of Indian Foods, National Institute of Nutrition, ICMR, Hyderabad.

Fibre is Another Form of Diet

Dietary fibre is the term used for food items which the body cannot digest or digests partially. Fibre is also known as roughage. Increased consumption of foods rich in fibre are associated with positive health benefits. It relieves constipation, a common bowel problem, by making the diet bulky. It reduces the risk of cardiovascular disease by delaying the absorption of fat and carbohydrates. It also reduces serum fibrinogen which lowers the chances of blood clot formation in the blood thereby reducing the chances of heart attack. High dietary fibre also reduces the blood pressure, obesity and insulin resistance as all are independent risk factors for CHD. Dietary fibre may make you feel full which may help you to decrease the total amount of calories you eat. Soluble fibre reduces the cholesterol in blood. Oats, contain the highest amount of soluble fibre than any other grain. Apart from oats, psyllium, pectin and guar gum are also rich sources of soluble fibre in diet. Studies have shown that a diet enriched with soluble fibre is effective in lowering total cholesterol and LDL cholesterol (the bad cholesterol) levels. However, the levels of triglycerides and HDL cholesterol (the good cholesterol) were not significantly influenced. Psyllium seed husks (*isabgol*) have been used in herbal remedies. It can alleviate constipation and is commonly used as a gentle bulk forming laxative. Other foods which are rich in fibre include beans, peas, rice bran, citrus fruits, apple pulp and strawberries.

There is enough scientific data to support that fibre when included as a part of the diet low in saturated fat may reduce the risk of heart disease. Daily requirement of fibre in the diet is approximately 50 gm per day. Diet which is based on grains, pulses and vegetables provides 50-100 gm of fibre per day. It contains enough fibre to meet the daily requirements and usually no fibre supplementation is necessary. Western diets or diets rich in processed foods are low in fibre and require fibre supplementation. Those who are fond of consuming large amounts of milk and milk based products, processed and refined foods are advised to consume enough vegetables, grains and fruits to meet a desired dietary requirement of fibre. To increase the dietary fibre content in diet, one should consume oats and its preparations, dried beans and peas. Among all pulses, Bengal gram is the richest source of fibre in the Indian diet. Choose green vegetables and salad every day. Fruits with or without skin such as apple, pears, sapota, Indian gooseberry, guava, dates and figs are all excellent sources of fibre in the diet and should be consumed routinely. Choose whole grain cereals and pulses, and brown rice instead of white rice. Whole wheat flour should be used for preparing *roti or chappati*. Use of *naan, roomali roti* and common bread should be limited. Refined and processed food items along with sugar, milk, all types of meat, oils and fats are poor sources of fibre in the diet and should be consumed in moderation.

Tips for Adding Fibre into Diet

1. Use whole grain cereals and pulses.
2. Baked goods or breakfast cereals containing oat or oat bran and psyllium husk are preferable.
3. Use fresh fruits and not juices.
4. Try to consume enough green salad and vegetables every day.
5. Use germinated pulses, dried beans and peas frequently.
6. Use fenugreek seed, flax seed, sesame and coconut.
7. Use brown rice and not polished or white rice.
8. Try to consume foods in their most natural form.

Minerals and Vitamins

Sodium

Most of us know that too much salt is bad for health, but few are aware of the fact regarding how much is needed and how much they are consuming. Salt is essential for health as well as taste. On an average, the body needs 2-5 gm of salt each day depending upon the climate you are living in. An Indian adult requires 5-8 gm of common salt or one or one and half teaspoonful of salt per day. Enough salt is added during cooking of daily foods and Indians get 90 % of their salt quota from the meals they consume. We fail to realize that there are certain food items which are rich sources of hidden salt and are consumed daily. Such items are, *papad*, chutney, wafers, chips, ketchup, cornflakes, bread, salted biscuits, *namkeen*, packaged soups, canned vegetables, salted nuts, dried salted fish, etc. They contain a good amount of salt (Table 21.6). Some western processed foods like bacon, baked beans, corned beef, cured ham, pepperoni, pork pie, sausages, spaghetti hoops, pasta sauce, salted nuts or crisps, frozen or canned fish, canned foods, packet soups, pies, onion rings, cheese and some salad dressings are very rich in salt content. Baking soda and *ajinomoto* are high in salt content. Most spices used during cooking also contain a small amount of sodium. It is the sodium in the common salt which is the culprit and a teaspoonful of common salt contains approximately 2.4 gm of sodium. Considering the climatic condition of tropical countries including India, consuming one or one and half teaspoonful will be sufficient to keep us healthy. However, people with high blood pressure and heart failure, require less of salt and should avoid all sources of invisible sodium in the diet apart from curtailing the daily intake of common salt or sodium chloride. 3-5 gm of common salt per day is the recommended amount, if you are suffering from high blood pressure or heart disease. Practicing or consuming a salt-free diet in tropical climate may cause electrolyte imbalance (sodium and potassium deficiency in the body), sometimes leading to serious complications. It should be discouraged unless you are suffering from a severe degree of heart failure and have been advised by your physician to do so.

Table 21.6: Some of the Common Indian Foods rich in Salt Content

Food Item	Amount (gm)	Salt Content (gm)
Wafers	100	2-2.5
Bread-sliced	100	1
Pappad	100	10-12
Salted biscuits	100	2-3
Pickles and chutney	100	3-4
Cornflakes	100	1-2
Bhajjias	100	2
Cheese	100	2.5
Sauce and ketchup	5 ml or 1 tsf	0.1-0.2
Packaged soup	100	10

How can I Reduce the Sodium in my Diet?

Limiting salt intake is very important to keep an individual well. It is a known fact that too much salt can make high blood pressure worse. A majority of Indians consume homemade food; canned or preserved foods are not a routine habit. However, the following steps will help in reducing the salt in the diet:

1. Limit salt while cooking.
2. Do not use table or extra salt.
3. Select fresh foods instead of canned and processed foods.

4. Know the hidden source of sodium in your diet and avoid it.
5. Consume plenty of fresh fruits and vegetables.
6. Encourage the use of lemon juice, vinegar, curd, unripe mango (*amchur*) and spices like *ajwain* and pepper to curtail salt intake and to maintain the taste.
7. Restaurant, *dhaba* and chat corner foods are a rich source of salt. Try to avoid them and if necessary ask them to use less salt for your dishes.
8. Use less of salt with nuts or choose their unsalted version.

Potassium

Foods high in potassium include banana, mango, Indian gooseberry, sapota, lemon, sweet lime, peaches, plums, guava, grapefruit, oranges, tomato, prune juice, honeydew melons, prunes, molasses, coconut water and potatoes. Some foods rich in potassium are also high in calories. When weight control is important, eat more low calorie foods. Foods high in potassium help in preventing or lowering high blood pressure and may also decrease the risk of heart disease and stroke.

Vitamin E

Because of its antioxidant and cell membrane protection properties, it offers safety against heart disease, cancer and other chronic illnesses. Vitamin E is a fat soluble vitamin containing four major forms of tocopherols. Alpha-tocopherol is the most common and most effective of all. Observational data suggests that it can prevent cardiovascular disease by reducing the harmful effects of LDL cholesterol, reducing the process of inflammation and clot formation. Initially, vitamin E supplementation was found to be beneficial in reducing the overall adverse outcome in patients of heart disease. Later on, larger clinical trials failed to show similar beneficial results. Considering the current scientific knowledge, Vitamin E supplementation for the prevention of heart disease cannot be recommended. However, dietary supplementation should be encouraged. The usual dose of vitamin E is 400-800 units per day. It should be taken along with meals and vitamin C as both increase the effective absorption in the gut. Whole grains, germinated pulses, green leafy vegetables, vegetable oils and seeds of almonds and sunflower are rich sources of vitamin E in the diet.

Vitamin C (Ascorbic Acid)

It is a water soluble vitamin and is necessary for the growth and repair of cells. Its deficiency is known to produce scurvy (bleeding and swollen gums), particularly in long distance sailors whose diets are deficient in fresh fruits, especially citrus fruits which is a rich, source of vitamin C. It is also, known as ascorbic acid which is derived from – 'a' (meaning none) and 'scorbutus' (meaning scurvy). Sufficient amounts of vitamin C in diet not only protects the gums but can also protect you against cardiovascular diseases, cancers, cataracts and joint problems. The common belief that it may protect you from colds is purely a myth. It acts as an antioxidant and can slow down the progression of atherosclerosis. Till date, scientific studies have not proved that taking vitamin C supplements will prevent heart disease or stroke. The best strategy is to get enough vitamin C through your diet. For an adult, the daily requirement is 500 mgs which should be obtained from dietary sources as it is neither manufactured nor stored in the body. A glass of 200 ml freshly squeezed orange juice can provide 100 mgs of vitamin C. Foods rich in vitamin C are citrus fruits, berries, kiwi fruit, green leafy vegetables, capsicum, tomatoes and wheat germs. These should be consumed in their natural form as heating destroys the vitamin C content.

Folic Acid

Folic acid or folate is a water soluble vitamin worth mentioning as it can prevent heart attack and stroke by reducing the levels of homocysteine in blood. Homocysteine is an amino acid like substance which at high levels can damage the inner lining of blood vessels. Folic acid is critical in the prevention of formation of atheromatous plaques and clots inside the blood vessels, maintaining smooth and uninterrupted blood flow. It regulates the production of homocysteine as high level of homocysteine is an emerging risk factor for stroke and heart disease. However, insufficient scientific data is available to support folate supplementation to reduce or prevent the risk of heart attack or stroke. But still, intake of folic acid should be encouraged in the diet. It is present in abundance in green leafy vegetables, beans and whole grains. The name folic acid is from the Latin word 'foliage' or 'leaf' as it was first isolated from the spinach leaves. In developing countries, to encourage the intake of folic acid, some refined food products are fortified with folic acid. For good health and prevention of heart diseases, it is advisable to take 400-800 mcg of folic acid per day combined with other vitamin preparations.

Beverages

These are liquid food items which are consumed with or without food. Water, an absolute ingredient of any beverage is essential, especially in tropical countries. Water is free from calories. The myth with drinking water is that one should drink only when he/she is thirsty. It should be emphasised that water is not only meant to quench thirst but it is essential for the movement of food in the gut and body. Considering the dry hot climate of tropical countries, it is wise to consume fluids, preferably water, liberally; 10 to 12 glasses per day is recommended. Beverages have been in the food culture of various religions and they are served to guests and fellow colleagues as a warm gesture of welcome and hospitality. Beverages can be served hot or cold. Hot tea and coffee are the essential morning beverages for adults. However, hot milk with or without flavouring agents is common for children. Hot soups as starters are an excellent stimulant or appetizer before meals. Fruit juices, *lassi*, sherbet, milk shakes, cold coffee, buttermilk and soft drinks are served cold. Fruits and vegetables based on beverages are a rich source of minerals and vitamins and are low in calories. Milk based beverages such as *lassi* and buttermilk are not only nourishing but are good for the bones and teeth, and for the growth of young ones. Beverages which are rich in sugar should be consumed less or occasionally. Calorie contents of various beverages are summarized in Table 21.7.

Table – 21.7: Calorie chart for common beverages

Beverage	Serving Size	Amount	Energy (kcal)
Water	One glass	200 ml	00
Fresh lime juice or nimbu pani without sugar	One glass	200 ml	10
Jal jeera	One glass	200 ml	20
Clear vegetable soup	One cup	150 ml	20
Tomato soup	One cup	150 ml	40
Tomato juice	One cup	150 ml	45
Coconut water	One glass	200 ml	50
Tea with sugar 10 gm	One cup	150 ml	80
Tea without sugar	One cup	150 ml	22

Buttermilk	One glass	200 ml	60
Orange juice	One glass	200 ml	70
Sugarcane juice	One glass	200 ml	80
Coffee with sugar 2 tsp (10 gm)	One cup	100 ml	110
Coffee without sugar	One cup	100 ml	25
Milk (cow) no sugar	One glass	200 ml	100
Pineapple juice	One glass	200 ml	140
Pomegranate juice	One glass	200 ml	150
Non-vegetarian soup	One cup	150 ml	100-150
Soft or cold drinks	One can	200 ml	150
Milk (buffalo) no sugar	One glass	200 ml	175
Milk shake	One glass	200 ml	200
Syrups (Sherbat)	One glass	200 ml	200
Bournvita	One cup	150 ml	200
Mango juice	One glass	200 ml	200
Cold coffee	One glass	200 ml	250
Lassi	One glass	200 ml	250
Beer	One glass	650 ml	400
Wine	One glass	100 ml	100
Whisky	One small peg	30 ml	90
Rum	One small peg	30 ml	110
Gin	One small peg	30 ml	110

Coffee and Tea

Morning tea is popular in North, East, West and Central parts of India. Darjeeling tea is world famous and exported to various countries. Coffee is a basic beverage in South India. Caffeine and tannin are present in tea and coffee. Coffee contains thrice the amount of caffeine as compared to tea. Chocolate and cocoa are also rich in caffeine. A moderate amount of tea or coffee is not bad and calorie content of coffee or tea comes from the addition to sugar and milk. Excess of calorie, which is contributed by addition of milk and sugar can increase obesity and bad cholesterol in the blood that is, LDL cholesterol. A cup of tea or coffee with two teaspoonful of sugar, consumed five times a day provides the maximum permissible sugar and this is an invisible source of calories. Caffeine has a stimulating effect on the brain. Thus, a morning cup of coffee and tea sharpens our mental edge and performance. It also helps fight muscle fatigue or relieves one from migraine or headache. Excessive use of caffeine can cause palpitation (racing of heart beats), irregular heartbeats, excessive urination and disturbances in sleep. It can even cause heartburn or hyperacidity and restlessness. Whether excess use of caffeine results in causing heart disease is uncertain. However, in patients of heart disease, it should be restricted to two to three cups per day as it may precipitate life threatening arrhythmias (irregularity in the heart beat).

What is the Role of Green Tea?

Green tea *(Camellia sinensis)* to a large extent and black tea to a certain extent may protect your heart. If one consumes it in moderation then it may prevent stroke, heart attack or cancer. Green tea contains an anti-oxidant compound known as polyphenols which is present in a lesser quantity in black tea. This antioxidant is destroyed while preparing black tea leaves which are prepared by drying and crushing followed by fermentation later on for several hours. This process of fermentation destroys polyphenols. The antioxidant content of green tea is preserved, its process of preparation involves steaming and drying the tea leaves and fermentation is not done.

Carbonated Drinks

These are commercially manufactured beverages made by adding sugar, water, citric acid and various colours and flavours. It is charged with carbon dioxide and bottled under pressure to produce effervescence. These drinks have little or no nutritive value and only add calories which are provided by the sugar present in it. Their habitual consumption is associated with obesity.

Junk or Fast Food

What is Junk or Fast Food?

The food items which are only rich in calories and have little or no nutritional value are classified as junk foods. Junk foods are rich in refined sugars and fats. It lack necessary vitamins and minerals and are loaded with extra calories and hidden salt. These foods when consumed in abundance can cause heart disease, obesity, high blood pressure, diabetes and cancer. Therefore, these food items are considered unhealthy. Due to urbanization, a variety of junk foods are available. Since these items are cheap, served quickly, come in attractive packages, they are popular and acceptable to all ages, especially children and young ones. The fast developing mall culture has more fast food joints than the shops meant for other items. Today, youngsters of developing nations have more money to spend than their parents. These food items are consumed as snacks followed by regular meals. And these eating habits are making them obese. You will be surprised to know that almost a quarter of the children living in metro cities are obese and consume junk food daily before meals. We live in the false belief that fast food includes only western foods. Thus we try to blame and prohibit burgers, French fries, pizzas, steaks, sausages, pies, cookies, colas, chips, hot dogs, sugar donuts, puddings, muffins, etc. Indian food items which are commonly consumed as snacks such as *poori, parantha, bhatura, naan, samosa, tikki, pakoda, kachori,* potato or banana chips, *vada, stuffed dosa, sweets,* and *halwa* are all categorized as junk food as they are also rich in calories and contain excess of sugar or salt. Other than *idli* and *dhokla,* remaining Indian snacks are very rich in calories and fat. These food items are prepared by deep frying in oils which are either saturated or trans-fats raising the level of bad cholesterol in blood. Excess of sugar in the food is converted to fat and salt is detrimental for blood pressure. Some Indian snacks are served faster than some western snacks and should be included in the fast food items.

Should we Ban these Fast or Junk Foods?

For a heart healthy diet, one should definitely know which foods to eat and how much to consume. It is the food habit and not the food item which should be blamed. One should count how often and how much you consume junk food. Consuming once in a fortnight may not be harmful but making it a routine or consuming twice a week can definitely prove to be a health hazard. Today, a majority of parents pamper their children by taking them out and giving them food which is easily available. Advertisements and attractive packaging makes a child pick up these foods but it is the duty of the parents to give them healthy choices and homemade snacks frequently rather than unhealthy snacks which may be given occasionally. Nuts can replace chips. However, they are not cheap except for groundnuts. The best approach is not to avoid these food items or ban them. Therefore, they should be used in moderation and with caution.

It may Dig Less to Pocket but may Rig Deep in the Heart

Snacks which are rich in calories are more dangerous, though they may cost less. These snacks are usually consumed in between meals. Some of these snacks contain approximately 500 calories or more. Examples of such snacks are a packet of potato chips (100 gms), large cheese or chicken burger, large piece of cake or ice cream, French fries, two egg omelette with bread, a medium size pizza, two large *samosas*, 10-12 pieces of *pakoras*, two bread rolls, a plate of *chole bhatura*, *four pooris* with vegetable, two big stuffed *paranthas* with curd, *pao bhaji*, *jalebi* with four *kachoris*, or 100 gms of *halwa*. All may not cost much, but their frequent consumption can lead to obesity, high blood pressure and heart disease. These portions of meal can easily distort your body and health and it is not easy to burn off these 500 calories. Burning 500 calories is no joke. It requires one hour of brisk walking at a speed of 6 kms/hour, one and half hour of cycling at a speed of 10-15 kms/hour, 45 minutes of swimming or playing outdoor games for an hour. In the process of maintaining ideal weight, this knowledge is crucial. To lose 1 kg weight, one needs to burn 7700 calories. It means for reducing 1 kg weight we have to reduce our daily intake of calories by 500 kcal for a fortnight, or a month for 2 kgs. Things do look difficult but not discouraging, and nothing is impossible when it concerns health.

What is Meant by Serving Size?

For excellent health, it is mandatory to know which food to eat and how much to consume. Introspect yourself and keep a track of how much and how many times you eat. Excess can lead to overloading and overloading can lead to consumption of extra calories, excess of sugar or carbohydrate, excess of fat and cholesterol, which all can cause problems for your heart by increasing the risk factors such as obesity, diabetes and hypertension. The caloric value of various cooked and uncooked food are calculated as per the amount of food served, which is commonly referred to as the serving size. A serving size is defined as specific amount of food measured and, in India, it is measured as cups, *katori* or bowl, glass, plate, pieces, teaspoonful or tablespoonful. In USA, the food guide pyramid measures one serving as a size of an ice cream scoop or half cup of pasta. A meat serving is equivalent to 60 to 90 gms in weight. It is not a common practice in India to measure serving size in grams or litre, in fact it is a skill which can be acquired over several years and with experience. A majority of Indians are comfortable with their own skill and judgment. Whatever the diet schedule is, one should always be aware of the number of servings and the proper serving size to know how much to eat and how much is good or bad for health. The following measurement or serving is practiced in India:

One teaspoon	5 ml or 5 gms
One tablespoon	15 ml or 15 gms
One *katori* or bowl	150 ml
One glass	200-250 ml
One cup	125 ml
One serving of fruit or vegetable	75-80 gms
One *chappati*	20 gms
One serving of rice	50 gms

Tips For a Healthy Diet

1. Enjoy foods of all colours and taste.
2. Eat a variety of locally available foods.

3. Eat in a balanced quantity; every food item that is necessary.
4. Eat plenty of seasonal fruits and vegetables.
5. Curtail both visible and invisible fat in the diet.
6. Use less of sugar and sweets.
7. Take plenty of fluids, especially water.
8. Avoid alcohol; green tea is good.

'The key message is to consume a variety of food items and that too in a balanced quantity'. The various food groups which are good for the heart are grouped in Table 21.8.

Table 21.8: Food Groups and Their Role in Heart Health

Diet Component	Choose	Restrict	Avoid
Oils	Olive, canola, flax seed, sunflower, safflower, mustard	Rice bran, corn, peanut or soyabean with omega fatty acids	Coconut, palm, ghee, vanaspati, butter
Eat omega rich foods, 2-3 times a week	Fresh water fish, flax seed, spinach, walnuts	Shrimps, prawns, lobsters, crabs, oysters	Deep fried fish, fish sticks or fingers, fish cutlets
Add nuts and beans	Soybean, green beans, kidney beans, lentils and nuts of all kinds like almonds, walnuts, cashewnuts etc.	Heavily salted nuts and groundnuts	Stale or rancid nuts

Fats-saturated	Fish, lean meat with trimmed fat, chicken with no skin, dairy products made with skimmed milk, yoghurt, egg white	Processed low fat meat, cottage cheese, soft margarine, paneer	Desi ghee, butter, cream, hard margarine, lard, organ meats such as liver and brain, whole milk and its products, ice cream, egg yolk, high fat snacks
Carbohydrate	Cereals, wheat, rice, bajra, ragi, jowar and maize	Maida or refined flour and its products, naan, roomali roti, jaggery	Poori, parantha, kachori, samosa, bhatura, all sweets and simple sugars, doughnuts, biscuits, buttered popcorn
Proteins	Pulses, sprouted legumes, fish, meat with no or little fat, skinless chicken or turkey, egg white, skimmed milk, tuna	Bhajiya, vada, lean cuts of red meat, real crab meat	Organ meats such as brain, liver, chicken nuggets, imitation crab meat, sausages, salami, meat pies and visible fat on meats or fatty meats
Fibre	Whole grain breads and cereals, brown bread, brown rice, vegetables, fruits with skin, dates and figs	Mashed potatoes, egg noodles, noodles	White bread, milk and its products, simple sugars, sweets
Miscellaneous foods	Salad, pepper, mustard, raw vegetables, herbs, spices	Salad cream, mayonnaise, honey, jam, marmalade, low fat cottage cheese	Creamy dressings, toffees, fudge, chocolate, crisps, chips, pies

Water and fluids	Drink 12-15 glasses of water or 3-4 litres per day, skimmed milk 250-500 ml, pure fruit juices 200 ml, tea or green tea upto 3 cups, lassi made with non-fat curd with little or no sugar or butter-milk	Coffee, artificially sweetened fruit juices, squash, rhooafja (rose box), sports drink, low fat and malted drinks	Soft drinks with sugar, milk shakes, excessive alcohol, cream based drinks
Fruits and vegetables	Use seasonal or all variety of fruits-2 servings of fruit preferable per day, apple, watermelon, papaya, pears, guava, etc.; 4 servings of vegetables, all green leafy vegetables, raw steamed vegetables are better than overcooked vegetables, salad made of cucumber, onion, garlic, lettuce, carrot, radish, etc.	Fruit juices less than 200 ml, dried fruits, canned fruits and juices, excess of banana, mango, potatoes, fruit salads, fruit punch	Overcooked vegetables, vegetable pakodas, fruit custards, vegetables prepared in heavy cream or rich with gravy containing butter or ghee

| Salt | Indian diet gives enough salt, can replace need of salt by lemon, unripe mango or vinegar | Salt dressed salads and fruits, bread, cheese, cornflakes | Pickles, sauces, papads, namkeens, ketchup, wafers, packet or canned foods, bacon, baked beans, corned beef, cured ham, pepperoni, pork pie, sausages, spaghetti hoops, pasta sauce, salted nuts or crisps, frozen or canned fish, onion rings |

To minimize the risk of CHD amongst the population, dietary and nutritional improvements are of great importance and cannot be ignored. To achieve this goal, the American Heart Association has outlined certain guidelines and practical means for making therapeutic lifestyle changes in the diet which may be applicable globally (Table 21.9).

Table 21.9: The American Heart Association Recommends the Following Therapeutic Lifestyle Changes (TLC) in Diet

Food Compositions	Recommendations
Total fat	25-30% of total calories
Saturated fat	< 7% of total calories
Polyunsaturated fat	Upto 10% of total calories
Monounsaturated fat	Upto 15% of total calories
Carbohydrate	50-60% of total calories
Protein	15% of total calories
Fibre	20-30 gms/day
Cholesterol	< 200 mg/day
Total calories	Sufficient to maintain desirable body weight

Heart Healthy Diet Recommendations at a Glance

1. *The aim should be to include a variety of seasonal fruits, vegetables, grains, pulses, legumes and to consume them in their most natural form.*
2. *Include fish, skinless poultry and lean meat in the daily diet. Avoid organ meats and fried meat contents.*
3. *Low fat dairy products or skimmed milk and its products, cow milk instead of buffalo milk, should be a part of the daily diet and consumption of whole milk, butter, cheese and ghee should be restricted.*
4. *Avoid simple sugars and sweets in diet, replace them with fruit salads and desserts.*
5. *Use a combination of oils. Use mustard (with low erucic acid) or refined oils such as sunflower, safflower, peanut, corn oils rich in unsaturated fat. Avoid saturated and trans-fat. Exchange a variety of cooking oils as no oil is ideal for heart health, and use no more than 2 litres per month in a family of four.*
6. *One tablespoonful (15 ml) of vegetable oil gives approximately 130 calories.*
7. *Fried and fast food should be avoided or consumed once in a fortnight. Food should preferably be grilled, steamed, boiled or micro-waved.*
8. *Limit salt and alcohol intake and maintain a healthy body weight. Watch salt intake to prevent and control blood pressure.*
9. *Base your dietary habits as per your liking, interest, culture, family tradition, availability and cost.*
10. *Extreme dietary modifications are injurious to health. They cannot be followed long term and should never be practiced.*

Chapter 22
Alcohol

Alcohol is the only substance which has global popularity and acceptance. It is the most common chemical for intoxication used by humans during the present age as well as in the past. You will be surprised to know that in ancient times alcohol was consumed in powder form and not liquid. Its use has been mentioned as for medicinal, social, religious and recreational purposes across different cultures of the world. It affects all walks of human life and causes hazards to health and welfare. Heavy alcohol intake reduces life expectancy by 10-12 years and it also badly affects the financial status of both the individual and the family.

Alcohol consumption in the Indian culture can be traced as far back as 2000 BC. The Hindu mythological descriptions mention *somras* and *sura*. *Somras*, believed to be an alcoholic beverage was common amongst the upper and rich class of people including kings and Gods like *Indra* and *Shiva*. *Sura* was meant for lower classes, to relieve them of their physical and mental hardships. History is full of stories of *sura* and *sundari* (alcohol and damsel) which have been responsible for the downfall of many a kingdom in the past. Though there is a long tradition of alcohol intake, today alcohol consumption in the Indian subcontinent has been influenced by European and American culture. Alcohol consumption is common in both the rich and poor class of Indians. However, religions like Islam, Jainism and Buddhism preach strict prohibition of alcohol. Alcoholism is a complex psychosocial habit. It should be emphasized that everyone who drinks is not alcoholic, however, those who drink are definitely at risk of becoming alcoholics. It can lead to impairment of judgment and affect the way one thinks and perceives the world. Alcoholism can cause diseases and contribute to automobile related accidents and deaths. In India, on an average 270 people are killed and 5000 are injured every day due to drunken drivers. A majority of them are poor and innocent pedestrians. It is a major cause of domestic violence and broken families. There is always a risk that alcohol intake may lead to irresponsible behaviour which can be mild to violent and is unacceptable in society. In India, alcohol use is believed to be a social taboo and its sale is banned in some states like Gujarat.

How Drinking Helps the Heart?

Alcohol protects the heart by raising the level of HDL cholesterol that is, good cholesterol. Two small drinks a day increase the level of HDL cholesterol by 17 %. Most heart attacks or strokes are caused by formation of blood clots and blocking of already narrowed arteries. Alcohol inhibits clot formation and increases the body's ability to break up the clots soon after they form. Alcohol drinking reduces the clotting by reducing the stickiness of platelets in blood thereby decreasing the short term risk of heart attacks. When it comes to alcohol and the heart, it seems that what matters is not what you drink but how much and how often. The ultimate outcome also depends upon the age and gender of the person.

What are the Adverse Effects of Alcohol on the Heart?

Adverse effects of alcohol include, damage to the liver (cirrhosis), development of gastric irritation, garlic ulcer and social problems. Excessive (more than 2 pegs per day) alcohol consumption can weaken the heart muscles and dilate the heart resulting in poor cardiac function and finally cardiac failure, a condition known as alcoholic dilated cardiomyopathy. Alcohol consumption causes awareness of your increased heartbeat (palpitation) or irregularity in heartbeat. The most common irregularity is atrial fibrillation. Excessive alcohol intake can result in high blood pressure. It also increases the level of triglyceride cholesterol in blood.

Alcohol and Women

Alcohol protects a woman's heart just as well as it protects a man's, but this benefit is most significant after menopause. Although alcohol intake in India by women is uncommon as compared to men, it still poses as a more health risk to women as it leads to the development of a large liver, fatty liver and cirrhosis of liver. Alcohol during pregnancy or during child bearing age should be strictly avoided. The body mass of women is less than men and the enzyme that breaks alcohol in the body is also secreted in lower concentration, so the consumption of alcohol in women should be half than what is recommended for men. In India, the pub and club culture and use of alcohol during social gatherings is increasing fast amongst urban women. This is a cause for concern, especially for young women of child bearing age.

Is Wine Safe?

Research on wine, especially red wine has shown that it contains flavonoid by the name resveratrol which acts as an antioxidant which helps in relaxing arteries and reducing the clot burden. Red wine, in particular, has been thought as healthy for the heart. Various studies on the heart health benefits have reported mixed results and other studies show that red wine is not healthier than other alcohols. However, their effect on cardiovascular health have not been fully explored and there is no concrete evidence suggesting that red wine in particular may provide any benefit to the heart. The benefit of moderate drinking comes from the ethanol component of alcohol and not the type of alcohol consumed. Wine drinking, still uncommon in India, has been shown to be associated with the affluent class of society which has better education, healthier lifestyle and better accessibility to health services as compared to spirit and beer drinkers, falsely perceived as more beneficial than other forms of alcohol.

What is a Safe Quantity?

If you know your limit and remain restricted to it, then drinking alcohol is a pleasure and joy; otherwise it will be the pain and sorrow of your life. Alcohol content is highest in whisky where it may be up to 42 % followed by 10-12 % in wine and 4-10 % in beer. A safe or moderate drinking is considered when one consumes 50-60 ml (2 small pegs) of spirit, 250 ml of beer and 125 ml of wine daily with meals. However, it should be emphasized that no amount of alcohol is safe as it is highly addictive, and as tolerance level increases with consumption, the control decreases resulting in excessive alcohol intake which may invite all the ill-effects of alcohol intake and abuse.

Sensible drinking of a moderate amount may be considered safe but is not true for all as there is always a chance that too much alcohol will make you inebriated.

What is 'holiday heart'?

Consuming a large amount of alcohol or binge drinking on Friday and Saturday is associated with an acute rise of alcohol in the body resulting in racing of heartbeat (palpitation). Sometimes irregular heartbeats called arrhythmia and a steep rise in blood pressure results. This can lead to breathlessness, change in blood pressure, syncope or even sudden death.

Alcohol Intake and Stroke

Heavy drinking is a risk factor for high blood pressure as well as both types of strokes (ischaemic or blood clot and haemorrhagic or brain haemorrhage). Moderate drinking reduces the risk of ischaemic stroke but the risk of haemorrhagic stroke increases.

What about Binge Drinking?

Drinking alcohol with meals every day is a healthier pattern as compared to consuming 3-5 pegs on Friday or Saturday or occasionally. Food slows the absorption of alcohol in the blood and prevents an abrupt rise of alcohol in blood stream as seen with binge drinking. A Finnish study found that middle-aged men who typically drank 6-7 bottles of beer at one sitting were more likely to have fatal heart attacks. They were also seven times more prone to violent death related with traffic accidents.

Facts of Alcohol Consumption in India

Widespread alcohol consumption is not popular and is regarded as a social taboo in India and the amount of alcohol consumed per person per year is very low when compared to Europe or America. Alcohol use is permitted for magical rituals in the Hindu religion and is offered as *prasad* or offering in a few temples of God *bhairavji*. Alcohol intake is associated with fun and gaiety in parties and social gathering, the so-called page 3 culture. Its use is also said to get rid of pain, failure and miseries of life. These facts are often depicted in Indian cinema by actors, who are the icons of the masses and have a vast influence over the alcohol consumption in India.

Some facts related to alcohol consumption are as follows:

1. Hard liquor such as whisky, rum, vodka, gin, feni, etc. are consumed more.
2. Wine is not a popular alcoholic drink among Indians.
3. Beer consumption is linked with adolescents and young adults.
4. Binge drinking is the most common form of drinking habit in India and is harmful.
5. Alcohol intake in women is common either in the affluent society or in the poor and rural set up. In the middle income group, women rarely consume alcohol.
6. It is believed to give warmth and is common during winters, more so in hilly regions.
7. Country made alcohol and adulterated alcohol (*tharra, daru,* etc.) is common among the poor socio-economic strata and in rural areas. It is prepared locally, either in villages or in the home by fermenting grains, fruits (*mahua*) and sugarcane and its products. It is also obtained from palm trees (*tadi*). These country made liquors are not stable and get spoiled readily. As it is easily available and cheap,

it is popular in the rural set up among men and women alike. These alcoholic beverages have caused deaths and blindness from time to time in various parts of India due to the combined effects of methanol, high alcohol content or deliberate adulteration.
8. Alcohol consumption is associated with consumption of fried unhealthy foods.
9. It is a social taboo and is associated with other social problems such as smoking and consumption of tobacco, drugs and prostitution. All these go hand in hand.

Should Alcohol be Recommended for Prevention of Heart Diseases?

Today, there is strong evidence that regular intake of relatively small amounts of alcohol may protect the heart after middle age and considering this, one can argue about its use. Pub culture is spreading in India as part of globalization and young people argue that anything done with a sense of responsibility is fine. The sense of responsibility may vary from person to person and it is our duty in society to impose the strictest penalties on those who cross the limit. The relationship between alcohol and heart is complex and there is a thin line between moderate to heavy drinking and between reported benefits and risks. Today, the relation between alcohol and heart disease is like a double edged sword. The risks and benefits of alcohol consumption should be understood clearly and before taking any action the physician should be consulted. The risks and benefits should be reviewed as part of the medical care and should be discussed in length. In my opinion, considering the pattern, type, amount and education, heart protection benefits of alcohol are nullified by the risks of alcohol consumption in India, and I would personally be hesitant to recommend it as a routine measure. Teetotaller's should not be advised to start consuming alcohol for heart protection. Instead, a healthy diet and exercise will pass all the benefits. That is why doctors will tell you 'If you don't drink, don't start'. People with a family history of alcoholism, high triglyceride levels, heart failure, irregular heartbeats, uncontrolled high blood pressure, pregnant women and abdominal problems such as hyperacidity, liver disease, pancreatitis (infection of pancreas), should abstain from consuming alcohol.

Alcohol and Heart at a Glance

1. Alcohol intake is a globally accepted habit and is a part of culture in many societies.
2. Moderate alcohol intake is beneficial for the heart as it raises the good HDL cholesterol and has clot buster properties.
3. Red wine may not be beneficial over other forms of alcohol.
4. Alcohol with meals delays its absorption.
5. Consumption of fried and unhealthy snacks and food along with it is detrimental to health.
6. Binge drinking and consumption of large amounts of alcohol is harmful to health.
7. Women should consume half the recommended alcohol quantity as compared to men. It should be avoided completely during pregnancy and breast feeding.
8. If you do not take alcohol do not start it for protecting your heart. Exercise and a healthy diet will be more beneficial for your health.
9. Physicians should encourage heavy drinkers to drink less, rather than recommend alcohol. As the overall health benefit is uncertain, the gap between sensible and safe drinking is unknown and the risk of addiction is unpredictable.

Chapter 23

Antioxidants, Heart Healthy Foods and Herbs

Antioxidants are natural substances which are present as vitamins, minerals and other substances. Antioxidants are believed to fight against free radicals to prevent disease and keep the body healthy. Free radicals are formed in the body, either naturally or by various external stimuli such as smoking, diabetes, hypertension, etc. Free radicals travel throughout the body and if left unchecked, can damage cells.

What are Free Radicals?

Free radicals are the molecules which are produced normally in the body as a part of cell function and quickly react with other molecules to achieve stable configuration. Under normal circumstances, these molecules are continuously cleared from the body with the help of various enzymes produced in the body. Free radicals can also be cleared by certain vitamins such as vitamin C (ascorbic acid) and E (alpha-tocopherol).

Free Radicals and Heart

When excess of free radicals are produced in the body, they can damage the inner lining of blood vessels by enhancing the process of atherosclerosis. Oxidation, meaning addition of a molecule of oxygen is the key step in the formation of free radicals. Cholesterol molecules, especially LDL cholesterol, to become toxic need to be oxidized and once oxidized they are taken up by the artery wall much more easily thus commencing the process of atherosclerosis. This oxidative stress in the coronary arteries which supply blood to the heart plays an important role in the development of coronary heart disease.

Antioxidants

Antioxidants are the substances which reverse the process of oxidation. Their major function is to stop the free radicals from attacking and damaging healthy cells of the body. Antioxidants include various vitamins namely vitamin E, vitamin C, beta-carotene and flavonoids. All these antioxidants have the property to reduce the risk of heart attack and stroke as well.

How to Increase Antioxidants in Body?

Antioxidants are natural substances that are present in abundance in plant and plant based foods. So to get enough antioxidants, one should consume more plant based foods.

Which Food is Rich in Antioxidants?

To enjoy healthy eating and to get enough antioxidants one should enjoy different colours and all tastes of natural food. The pigments present in some fruits and vegetables give them different colours such as red, orange, green or yellow. These pigments are called carotenoids and these natural pigments are potent disease fighters. Spinach, broccoli, cabbage and capsicum are dark green in colour and are rich in antioxidants. Yellow and orange fruits and vegetables such as oranges, lemons, grapes, papayas, mangoes, guavas, pineapples, carrots, and tomatoes are all excellent sources of antioxidants. Apple, apricot, berries, potatoes and pumpkins can also provide abundant antioxidants. Whole grains, cereals, especially pulses contain tocopherols, flavonoids and isoflavonoids all of which act as antioxidants. Germination increases the antioxidant content by two to three times. The immature green pulses and germinated pulses along with dry pulses are a fairly good source of antioxidants in the cereal-pulse-based diet. To get significant amount of antioxidants, it is advised to take fruits and vegetables along with cereals and pulses. Tea, especially green tea, and dark chocolate are also good sources of antioxidants. Various antioxidant groups and common dietary sources are enumerated in Table 23.1.

Table 23.1: Antioxidant Groups and their Dietary Sources

Antioxidant Group	Dietary Sources
Flavonoids	Fruits: Apple, berries, citrus fruits, grapes, pears, pomegranate Vegetables: Beetroot, broccoli, lettuce, onion, pepper, spinach, tomatoes Legumes: Horsegram, greengram, beans. Spices: Cardamom, cinnamon, cloves, coriander, cumin Beverages: Coca Cola, tea, wine (red and white wine, sherry) Oils: Olive oil Dark chocolates
Carotenoids	Fruits: Apples, apricots, bananas, berries, cherries, grapes, lemons, mangoes, melons, oranges, papayas, peaches, pears, plums Vegetables: Amaranths, asparagus, brinjal, broccoli, cabbage, cauliflower, cucumber, carrots, lettuce, mushroom, onion, pepper, potato, pumpkin, spinach, tomato Legumes: Bean and bean sprouts, pears Spices: Chillies, saffron Oil: Red palm oil Dairy products: Butter, cheese, margarine, milk, yoghurt

Vitamin C	Indian gooseberry (amla), citrus fruits and juices (oranges, lemons), broccoli, red capsicum, dark green vegetables, strawberries, papayas, kale, kiwi fruits, guavas, mangoes, pineapples, tomatoes
Vitamin E	Germinated pulses, green leafy vegetables, whole grains, nuts and seeds, vegetable oils (almonds, palm, cotton seed, corn, soybean, sunflower)

What about Antioxidant Pills?

When the concept of antioxidants and disease protection became popular, plenty of antioxidants and vitamin supplements were made available in the market. However, at this stage there is enough scientific data and evidence supporting that these supplements do not provide extra advantage in treating or preventing heart disease. The best strategy is to consume plenty of fruits, vegetables, cereals and pulses to ensure that you get enough antioxidants and it is better to avoid artificial supplements.

Heart Healthy Foods and Herbs

Lyon heart study revealed that people who ate four to five servings of fruits and vegetables, three servings of low fat dairy products along with grains and fish could reduce their risk of heart disease and cancer significantly. The diet had a beneficial effect in lowering of blood pressure also.

Fruits

Most of the fruits provide fibre which not only relieves constipation, a common problem but also lowers blood cholesterol and risk of heart disease. Fruits are also low in sodium and high in potassium - a novel combination which lowers the risk of high blood pressure. Fruits are rich in plant chemicals such as flavonoids which may protect against cancers especially breast cancer. Enough scientific data is available regarding the role of flavonoids which act as antioxidants and help in lowering the risk of heart disease by preventing the oxidation of bad cholesterol. Apples, berries, citrus fruits, grapes, papayas and mangoes are excellent sources of flavonoids.

Garlic (*Allium sativum*)

In many countries including India and China, garlic has been used both as a food and medicine for many centuries. Regular consumption of one or two cloves of garlic or 500 to 1000 mg garlic supplement each day may reduce the risk of several diseases including heart problems. It also lowers blood cholesterol, especially triglycerides and thins the blood by reducing the tendency of blood to clot. In heart diseases, garlic is used to lower blood pressure, causes thinning of blood and lower cholesterol levels prevent heart attack and angina. It can take care of minor infections as it also has antioxidant, antifungal and antibacterial properties.

Ginger

Ginger is an important herb for a healthy heart. Ayurvedic physicians suggest that eating a little bit of ginger every day will help to prevent heart attack. It reduces cholesterol and improves blood circulation. It also reduces blood pressure and prevents blood clots. This helps to prevent clots that can lodge in narrow coronary arteries and set off a heart attack. It is widely used to treat coughs, common colds and nausea. Ginger is frequently used in making tea.

Turmeric

Turmeric lowers blood cholesterol levels by stimulating the production of bile. It may also prevent the formation of dangerous blood clots that can lead to a heart attack.

Onions

Onions contain adenosine and other 'blood thinners' that help to prevent the formation of blood clots. In addition to thinning the blood, onions can help keep the coronary arteries open and clear by increasing HDL.

Green Tea (*Camellia sinensis*)

Tea alone is good, it is the sugar and milk that provide extra calories and fat in tea. Tea consumption has been linked with a reduction in strokes, heart attacks or cancers. It also helps against infection and promotes longevity. This benefit is well established for green tea but black tea also protects you to a certain extent. People who are sensitive to caffeine should limit the intake to not more than 2-3 cups per day as each cup contains about 40 mgs of caffeine.

Yoghurt

Yoghurt made up of skimmed milk is a good source of calcium and can help in reducing blood pressure.

Olive oil

Olive oil is the best balanced oil as far as the health of heart is concerned, and probably the finest. However, its high cost is a cause of concern in developing nations. It contains omega fatty acids which reduce the cholesterol level and help in thinning the blood.

Flax Seed

Flax seed, also known as linseed is native to Europe and are used for therapeutic purposes. Flax seeds are rich in essential fatty acids which the body cannot manufacture. Apart from fish, flax seeds are the vegetarian source of omega 3 fatty acids which protect against heart disease. It is also a rich source of fibre in diet.

Green Leafy Vegetables

Green leafy vegetables are excellent natural sources of fibre, vitamins and antioxidants. They help in correcting the various risk factors associated with heart disease such as obesity, diabetes, high cholesterol and high blood pressure.

Fish

Eskimos and other fish eating communities in various parts of the world enjoy almost complete freedom from cardiovascular diseases. It is attributed to the beneficial fatty acids present in oily fishes which help in increasing the level of good HDL cholesterol, help in lowering bad cholesterol LDL and triglycerides. They also reduce the risk of development of clots which can block blood vessels. Fresh water fish is good for the heart. Flesh of the fish is rich in vitamin B, selenium and fluoride which are present in marine fishes.

Nuts

Nuts are regarded as bad for heart's health as they contain plenty of oil and fat. However, this conception is a myth and nuts are one among the good sources of omega fatty acids and are a substitute for fish in vegetarians. Walnuts and apricots are a rich source of omega 3 fatty acids. Consuming 50-60 gm of nuts twice a week is good for the heart. Nuts also reduce the risk for the development of blood clots that can cause a heart attack. Nuts are a concentrated source of energy and contain excess fat. Hence, their consumption should be limited to avoid obesity. Nuts are also rich in proteins excluding chestnut.

Germinated Pulses

It is a common, popular and cheap alternative for both breakfast and salad. It not only provides adequate fibre but is rich in antioxidants.

Fenugreek Seeds or *Methi*

A common Indian spice, which is also rich in fibre and reduces cholesterol. It also increases the excretion of bile acids and helps in deleting cholesterol stores from the liver. It is believed to be helpful in preventing diabetes mellitus.

Indian Gooseberry or *Amla*

This fruit is a rich source of pectin and vitamin C. The content of vitamin C in *amla* is 20 times higher than in an orange. It has excellent antioxidant properties and *amla* finds a number of medicinal uses in indigenous medicine also.

'An apple a day keeps the doctor away' is an old saying. It has always been linked with good health and quercetin, an antioxidant, present in the apple may be the magic ingredient.

Food consumption and practices are specific to different populations and vary widely. Today, the very concept of food habits is changing from mere health maintenance to the use of foods to promote health and to prevent chronic diseases. Food items which are rich in antioxidants, essential vitamins and nutrients are classified as 'functional foods' as they provide something more than the simple basic nutritional needs. They contribute additional physiological benefits to the consumer. Considering this, the healing power of fresh fruits, grains, vegetables and spices should be known to every individual who is interested in enhancing their vigour, vitality and over all well-being especially the health of their heart.

Herbal Treatment for Heart Disease

Herbs and their extracts have been known for thousands of years as medicinal agents. Their use has been mentioned in various ancient treatment philosophies. The use and practice is still popular and well accepted in traditional Chinese medicine and Ayurveda. Herbs and herbal preparations as medicine are not admired by the western world. Even then they are immensely popular and widely promoted in a large part of the world as they help to attain or maintain good health, prevent diseases and treat chronic or mild health problems. Herbs and herbal medicines are rarely recommended and promoted for acute or severe, life threatening diseases.

The various parts of herbs such as leaves, stems, buds, flowers, bark or roots are used alone or in combination. They can be used in their natural form or can be extracted and refined into oils, tablets, capsules, powder, tinctures or other formulations. One such example is of garlic which can be used raw or as garlic pearls. In modern medicine, many physicians and patients use herbal medicine frequently for common health problems. However, its use in cardiovascular disease is not accepted in the western world, but a majority of patients in Asia and other continents frequently use them with or without the consent or knowledge of their treating physician. In Asia and Africa, it is a part of their traditional medical therapy and some of the herbs and its products are used in main stream therapy. In developed countries, herbs and its preparations are used by almost one third of the population and are sold as dietary supplement and not for diagnosis, prevention or treatment for any particular disease.

Almost 80 % of the people living in developing countries still rely on traditional medicine, largely based on various species of plants. Modern medicine cannot deny the role of herbs in preventing and curing various diseases and many of the modern day drugs have been developed from herbs. Some of the commercially available, time tested cardiovascular medicines such as digitalis, atropine or amiodarone were also first obtained from herbs. The most abundant herb in use is digoxin or digitalis which has an interesting history. As early as the eighteenth century, an English lady in Shropshire use to treat patients of dropsy or congestive heart failure with extracts of 20 herbs including foxglove. After meeting this 'wise lady', Dr William Withering discovered that the leaves of foxglove contained the natural form of digoxin and described in detail the medicinal value and side effects of digitalis. Since then, digoxin or digitalis is widely used in modern medicine for the treatment of congestive heart failure as it helps the heart muscles to pump more powerfully. It is particularly of great use if heart failure is associated with irregular heartbeats caused by atrial fibrillation. There is a long list of herbs and its products that claim to be effective in the treatment of cardiovascular diseases but because of lack of evidence, their use in clinical practice needs further evaluation. Some of the herbs and their preparations have an important place and role in heart diseases which is worth considering. Both in traditional

Chinese medicine and in Ayurveda, herbs are still used extensively. Some of these herbs are:

Hawthorn *(Crataegus Species)*

It is also known as mayflower. It is a popular herb both in Europe and China and is used as a potent heart tonic. It contains a combination of flavonoids (especially procyannidolic oligomers) which are powerful antioxidants and are responsible for heart protection effect. Hawthorn improves the working of the heart by dilating the blood vessels, increasing the energy supply to the heart and reducing the load on the heart by increasing urine discharge (diuretic effect). It improves heart failure, relieves chest pain by dilating coronary blood vessels, corrects irregular heartbeats and may help in reducing blood pressure to a certain extent. In various human trials hawthorn treated patients showed significant improvement in their clinical symptoms like, chest pain, exercise tolerance, fatigue, palpitations, breathlessness, etc. Also, their quality of life improved significantly as compared to placebo. In some countries, it is widely prescribed for 'mild cardiac insufficiency'. The property of diuresis was used extensively during the Ancient Greek period for the treatment of kidney and bladder stones. The recommended dose of hawthorn extract is 300-450 mg per day. Leaf extracts of hawthorn are safe, however, it should not be prescribed with digitalis as it potentiates the effects of the latter.

Ginkgo Leaf Extracts *(Ginkgo biloba)*

Ginkgo leaf extracts improve the flow of blood throughout the body. It is also an antioxidant and therefore can benefit the cardiovascular system by preventing the formation of free radicals. It is used to prevent claudication or leg pain arising due to peripheral arterial disease and is supposed to act by increasing the capillary blood flow. It significantly improves attention and memory and may be beneficial in cases of dementia. However, recent controlled trials with Ginkgo biloba failed to show any positive benefits in patients of dementia. Ginkgo should not be used in patients who are taking anticoagulant (blood thinning) or antidepressant drugs.

Ginseng *(Panax ginseng)*

It is the most popular herb all over the world. It has been used historically in traditional Chinese medicine for thousands of years. The, name ginseng is derived from the Ancient Chinese word 'jen shen' meaning 'man root'. The root is mainly used to enhance vitality, longevity, potency, as well as general well-being. In today's context, it is the most widely consumed herb and ginseng finds its place from fruit juices to vitamin supplements. In China, it is used to treat various heart problems such as angina, heart attack and heart failure. Its dose is 100-250 mgs, once or twice a day. It should be avoided with excess caffeine as it potentiates the effect of caffeine. It is a fairly safe herb, however, in a few cases it may cause stomach upset, headache, breast congestion and an increase in menstrual bleeding at higher doses.

Arjuna *(Terminalia arjuna)*

Arjuna, an Indian medicinal plant, has been reported to have beneficial effects in patients with heart disease. It protects the heart, strengthens circulation of blood, and helps to maintain the tone and health of the heart muscle. It is also useful in promoting healing after a heart attack. It is a perennial plant found in the Indian subcontinent and in Mauritius. Its bark powder is used as medicine and is the most widely prescribed Ayurvedic preparation for heart patients in India. The bark stem powder contains arjunine, arjunoside, bioflavonoids (natural antioxidants) and minerals such as magnesium, calcium and zinc. Inside the body it also enhances prostaglandin E2 like activity. Some, Indian studies have shown that bark powder is very effective in patients with coronary heart disease, high blood pressure, heart failure and some other heart problems. It relieves symptoms, improves exercise tolerance and the quality of life. It was also observed that arjuna significantly reduced the elevated cholesterol and increased the levels of HDL cholesterol. Considering the improvement in overall symptoms and its cardioprotective effect, the drug has a promising role in overall management of coronary heart patients, however, larger and longer follow up results are still warranted. Arjuna bark powder is regarded a safe drug and is recommended in the Indian Materia Medica for various heart diseases as well as a heart tonic in doses of 1.5 to 2.0 gms per day, with or without toned milk.

Guggul or Gugulipid *(Commiphora mukul)*

The medicinal property of this herb has been known for thousands of years and is used for lowering blood cholesterol since 600 BC by ayurvedic physicians in India. It is derived from the dark, gummy resin of thorny mukul myrrh tree, native to India. The extract of guggul resin is known as gugulipid. The active ingredients in gugulipid are known as guggulsterones. It has a mild to moderate cholesterol and triglyceride lowering effect and may raise levels of HDL cholesterol. Gugulipid has been approved for clinical use in India.

Horse Chestnut *(Aesculus hippocastanum)*

Horse chestnut seed extract (HCSE) contains escin, and is used to treat venous insufficiency. Horse chestnut is known as kanor or pankor in India and is commonly found in the Himalayan forests. It is often used to treat piles. In some countries, it is extensively used to treat chronic venous insufficiency and can take care of leg pain, itching, redness and tenderness. Side effects with horse chestnut are uncommon but gastrointestinal irritation and toxic nephropathy may occur and should not be used in cases with kidney or liver impairment. Drug interactions are rare but it may sometime interfere with the anticoagulant coumarin and may increase the risk of bleeding.

White Willow Bark

It contains salicin, an aspirin-like compound. The salicin in the body is metabolized to active compound salicyclic acid, which helps in reducing pain, fever and inflammation. It has been used for centuries, much as aspirin is today. Aspirin is routinely recommended for prevention of cardiovascular diseases including heart attack. This herb is often referred to as 'herbal aspirin' and may provide the same protection without stomach upsets associated with aspirin. It is a very safe herb in therapeutic doses. However, in large doses it may cause nausea, vomiting, heartburn or a ringing sensation in the ears. It should not be used by people who are sensitive to aspirin.

Soy or Soya

Soy bean products have long been popular in Asia. Apart from their beneficial use around menopause, soy also protects against heart disease by lowering LDL cholesterol and increasing HDL cholesterol. It acts as an antioxidant and helps to prevent blood clots from forming inside the blood vessels. Its effect is best seen in people with high cholesterol levels than in normal cholesterol levels.

Plant Sterols and Stanols

These have important cardiovascular benefits. The beneficial effect is due to the fact that it is absorbed in the intestine in place of dietary cholesterol and/or slows the absorption of cholesterol, ultimately helping in lowering blood cholesterol levels. It has been shown that 2 gm of plant sterols taken per day can reduce the LDL cholesterol by 10-20 %. However, it has no or little effect on triglycerides or HDL cholesterol levels. All whole grains (rice bran, brown rice, oat bran, whole wheat), legumes (peas, beans and lentils) and vegetables are not only rich in plant sterols but also provide sufficient fibre and can be regarded as heart healthy food.

Coenzyme Q10

Coenzyme Q10 or co Q10 is a natural substance produced by the body. It is also known as ubiquinone. It is present in abundance in nuts and oils but is also present in many other foods. It acts with enzymes responsible for speedy metabolism. It plays an essential role in energy production and also acts as an antioxidant. It is a popular dietary supplement in many countries, more so in Japan where its consumption is trendy to prevent heart attacks and cancers. Its usual dose is 50-100 mg per day in two divided doses.

Efficacy, Safety and Side Effects of Herbs

Herbs and herbal therapies have their own philosophies and backgrounds. Claims regarding their efficacy and safety are high. Even in general public it is believed to be a safe option. A vast majority of herbs are considered safe, however, certain herbs may not be safe and can cause minor problems such as stomach upset or skin reactions. Some of the herbs may be toxic or poisonous; in certain doses they may even cause liver or kidney damage. Scientific evidences are sparse as tests done to evaluate the safety and effectiveness of herbal medicines are limited, costly and complex. Not only it is difficult to study finished herbal products but large pharmaceutical companies find little motivation and are reluctant to fund larger trials as a majority of the herbs cannot be patented.

Use of various heavy metals and toxic herbs is common in traditional ayurvedic treatment and is a major concern. Various minerals, metals (lead, gold, mercury, arsenic), gems and saturated fats are often added to various herbal preparations which may cause toxicity or can aggravate heart disease. A whole list of toxicities are mentioned in ayurvedic textbooks but practitioners as well as patients are often reluctant to accept or are ignorant of the fact that herbs and its preparations could be toxic. The claim that there is no need to worry about safety as these preparations have been in practice for many years may be misleading. Many a times it is difficult to obtain reliable toxicity and side effects of finished Ayurvedic herbal preparations. Majority of manufacturers and suppliers often fail to mention properly the list of all the ingredients and side effects on product labels.

The safety, effectiveness and quality of finished herbal medicine products depends on proper recognition of herbs, prudent selection of parts to be processed and how ingredients are handled during production. Each step should be executed meticulously observing stringent quality control otherwise the finished product may cause unsatisfactory response and unwarranted adverse effects. To avoid all this and to get maximum benefit it is sensible to shop with due care and choose brands with a reputation of quality. Always read and follow the product monograph, take the recommended dose, avoid self-medication and choose a qualified practitioner.

Herbs and Safety in Heart Disease

Herbal medicines are used by many patients with hypertension and cardiovascular diseases. Scientific knowledge about their efficacy and safety is lacking. People prefer herbal medicines because they perceive that plant based remedies are safe and free from undesirable side effects. Physicians are frequently unaware that their patients are using these non-traditional forms of medical care. Patients usually do not take their physician's into confidence as they anticipate the physician's disapproval of their use and fail to realize that some of the preparations may counter with modern medicines.

For heart patients, modern medicine frequently uses blood thinning agents such as aspirin and heparin, diuretics which increase the urine output, angiotensin converting enzyme inhibitors for remodelling of heart, anti-cholesterol agents which lower cholesterol in blood, anti-angina agents to relieve angina or heart pain and anti-depressants, either alone or in combination. Adverse drug interaction with herbs and these medicines are known and should be considered before practicing herbal therapy. Some important herbs such as ginseng, ginger, licorice, yohimbine and ephedra (ma-huang) can increase blood pressure; garlic and gingko can interfere with the blood thinning agents, and hawthorn can potentiate the effect of digitalis.

The safety profile of many herbal medicines looks great and this has led to a steep rise in the use of herbal medicines all over the world. However, heart patients should take due care as accumulated data shows evidence of significant interactions with cardiovascular medications. This can sometimes place individual patients at enormous risk. Practitioners in cardiovascular medicine should be competent and patients should be vigilant about the current scientific knowledge for benefits and adverse effects of herbal supplements. Physicians should be taken in confidence so that they can provide reasonable suggestions to the patients.

Recommendation

Herbs and its products are commonly used for treatment of minor illnesses and some chronic conditions such as common cold, depression, painful body conditions and skin diseases. Use of herbs and its preparations specifically to treat cardiovascular conditions is comparatively less common. Based on the review of available studies, the evidence is not convincing that any herbal treatment is effective in the treatment or prevention of heart disease or hypertension. Therefore, it appears prudent to consult your doctor about the use of herbs and herbal products as a treatment for high cholesterol, high triglycerides, heart disease, heart attack and heart health. However, the use of garlic, green tea, ginger, ginseng, olive oil and turmeric in an overall healthy diet is appropriate and worth considering. Many herbs used by traditional Chinese and ayurvedic practitioners show promise and could be appropriate for larger randomized clinical trials. Patients interested in the use of herbal medicines should observe the following precautions:

1. Herbal therapies should not be perceived as the sole approach for prevention, cure or to treat a heart disease.
2. It cannot be used in emergency situations such as heart attack, heart failure or stroke.
3. It cannot be replaced or substituted for the existing treatment modalities and should not be practiced alone in established heart disease patients. So, never stop the prescribed medicines.

4. Take only one herbal preparation at a time and avoid herbs with the same effect as you are already taking medicine for the illness.
5. It should be perceived and enjoyed as diet therapy and not as drug therapy.
6. Herbal therapy acts slowly but has a definite role in medical self-care. It should be encouraged as healthy food supplements and not as an alternative to cure heart disease.
7. Food supplements cannot replace the essential nutrients must for body or it cannot counter the poor dietary habit such as a high intake of saturated fat.
8. Food supplements cannot compensate for bad habits such as smoking and physical inactivity which are known to contribute to heart disease.
9. If any side effects are experienced or observed, consumption of herbs should be stopped immediately.
10. Avoid herbal remedies if you are pregnant or nursing.
11. Avoid new, unproven, sure shot or wonder remedies.

Chapter 24

Cardiovascular Diseases– Prevention and Practice

Improving public awareness regarding cardiovascular health should be the mission to combat this deadly disease all across the world. It should be perceived as a public health problem and individuals, community workers, teachers, policy makers, politicians, academicians, professionals, clinicians, health service providers, NGOs and pharmaceutical industries, all should be involved in tackling the CVD epidemic in the world, especially in the developing world. Setting up a 'defeat the heart disease' campaign should be multilevel, multimedia project based on total risk care and management of CVD. We have been successful in almost eradicating polio by a multipronged approach and there is no reason why we won't be successful in 'defeat the heart disease' mission. The mission should be aimed at identifying the risk factors and reverse them through awareness. Action must be directed towards both the healthy individual and the patient of established heart disease.

Changes in the prevalence of risk factors may be an important factor for the declining trend in this disease. Therefore, all efforts should be directed to identify the risk factors prevalent among all developing nations and preventive measures should be initiated right from childhood. Researchers should be encouraged to find new risk factors, trend of existing risk factors and to develop a novel way of reducing its impact on individuals as well as on the community.

The western world has witnessed a declining trend as well as a decrease in heart related deaths by a population-wide improvement in the major risk factors. The decline in death rate of heart patients is also attributed to the awareness towards the disease and advancement in the treatment which includes thrombolysis, statins, angiotensin converting enzyme inhibitors, blood thinning agents such as aspirin and clopidogrel, and revascularization procedures such as coronary angioplasty (PCI) and coronary artery bypass graft surgery (CABG). Advancement in treatment has a positive role but the power of prevention is of utmost importance as a vast majority of patients of heart attack have little time for treatment and may not reach the hospital alive. Considering the cost of therapy and uneven distribution of health services, prevention remains the best way out for low and middle income countries including India to counter heart diseases.

Is CVD preventable?

The fact that CVD is one of the biggest public health problems, both in developed and developing countries is well known. The INTERHEART study is a large international study of myocardial infarction (MI) or heart attack risk factors with 15,152 cases (patients) and 14,820 controls that were followed for 4 years. It was conducted in 52 countries and included every inhabited continent. The objective of the study was to determine the relation of smoking, history of hypertension or diabetes, waist/hip ratio, dietary patterns, physical activity, consumption of alcohol, blood apolipoproteins, and psychosocial factors to heart attack or myocardial infarction.

The number of centres involved in this trial made the results applicable to global risk including India. As *demonstrated in INTERHEART, these 9 risk factors account for 90 % of the risk for a first myocardial infarction or heart attack in both sexes and at all ages throughout the world.* The most encouraging part in this trial was that all important risk factors were modifiable and could be prevented or controlled through implementation of lifestyle changes and medication or both.

The WHO European Health Report, 2005 also points out that the burden of death and disability adjusted life years (DALYs) for the 7 leading conditions – coronary heart disease, depressive disorders, stroke, alcohol abuse, chronic lung disease, lung cancer and road-traffic injury which can be attributed to just 7 leading risk factors like tobacco use, alcohol, high blood pressure, high cholesterol, being overweight, low fruit and vegetable intake and physical inactivity. WHO also estimates that by modest population-wide approach and a reduction of these factors would reduce the CVD burden by more than half.

Aim of Prevention

The aim of prevention should be to address the population at large and a person in particular to reduce the burden of the disease. Its aim should be to reduce the incidence, to postpone and prevent CVD, to reduce disability, increase quality of life and longevity. Therefore, prevention should be an integral part of every health care interaction.

What are the Common Hurdles Against Prevention?

Awareness about any disease is the key to success. Even after advancement in communication, very few individuals are aware about the heart disease or the risk factors which make them prone to it. Staggering cost to the health system is another important reason. Majority of individuals are unaware of the benefits of medical insurance. General practitioners are usually the first people who attend the heart attack or related disease and often fail to recognize the early symptoms of the disease. Failure to accept the disease and relating it with common problems such as abdominal discomfort is common. This often delays the diagnosis. Gender bias against women also prevents them to get early attention and treatment. Sure shot cure by various medicines and dietary habits also delays and worsens the disease. Asymptomatic status, illiteracy, ignorance, poverty, cost, fear and confusion regarding allopathic medicines reduce the adherence to treatment. These factors are more prevalent and important in the developing countries.

World Heart Day

It is being observed on the last Sunday of September ever since 2000. Its main aim is to arouse awareness regarding the importance of CVD as the world's major killer and that its preventability measures should be taken at the right time. It is getting an increasing response from all countries around the world-both developed and developing countries. On this particular day, organization of media campaigns for raising awareness about CVD, walkathons, cycling, other athletic events are a feature along with face to face question and answer sessions between laymen and the physicians. In India, the participation of common man in the event has gained momentum in recent years and it is a heartening feature indeed.

The Blame Game

Government and government officials are often blamed for not providing adequate measures. Government is held responsible for uneven distribution of health facilities, lesser number of specialized centres, more urban than rural doctors and health providers, staggering population burden and apathy of the government health delivery system. Physicians are often criticized for not taking the disease seriously, for devoting less time to patients and prescribing costly medicines. Patients are often blamed for not adhering to the treatment protocol-they either modify the dose or reduce or stop the drug therapy by themselves. Physician's apathy is either because of lack of knowledge or is driven by pharmaceutical industries, while the patient's negligence is because of many type of pathies prevalent and non-professional advice which results more in confusion than cure. Deteriorating faith and communication gap among patients and physicians is a cause of concern today. The blame game is not going to solve the problem, it only worsens it. Considering this, a person with high CV risk should be encouraged from all quarters whether it is government or health providers to take an active interest in his or her well-being and should view his or her diet, exercise and make other lifestyle changes with medicines which are an integral part of a healthy life.

Role of Government and the Limitations

Health care facility in India like other developing countries is not available to all though the constitution supports a view that the right to health is an aspect of our fundamental rights. Provision of a health and a healthy atmosphere is the duty of state agencies. However, in practice its provision is unequal among different states. It is often said that the government is unable to provide health services for all because the government does not have enough money and facilities. It is true that in India to provide huge budgets only for treatment of heart disease is something next to impossible. In a democratic set up, people expect the government to work for their welfare. This could be achieved through the provision of education, employment, housing, health, provision of safe drinking water and a pollution free atmosphere. However, all of the government's efforts are nullified by the exponential growth of population in India.

Is the Government Sitting Idle?

Safe drinking water, provision for proper disposal of wastes, open sewage system, and air pollution need to be tackled efficiently and effectively, as all these affect health directly or indirectly. Provision for curbing the growing population is not effective. Even then, the government is trying in its limited resources and is allocating more money for the health sector.

In India, curative medicine has progressed a lot more than preventive medicine. We have very few world class hospitals which can only cater to a fraction of wealthy Indians who can afford it. We pat our back for medical tourism but simultaneously forget that the majority of Indians cannot afford drugs. Preventive medicine is the fundamental need of any health care delivery system, as it not only cuts the health care related financial burden in the long run but simultaneously reduces the pressure over the already burdened health care delivery system. Today we are facing the disease profile of both developing (infectious diseases and malnutrition) and developed (lifestyle diseases or chronic diseases) nations. We are still fighting these diseases and have failed miserably. Today almost half the children are malnourished and we witness sporadic cases of starvation. Almost two million cases of malaria are reported annually and half a million people die from tuberculosis every year. The irony is, these figures are not changing despite all our efforts.

Communicable diseases such as diarrhoea, cholera, hepatitis or jaundice and worm infestation are water borne diseases and still, we cannot provide safe drinking water to almost 20 % of the population. We should introspect the reasons, fund allocation and intentions are not the problem of policy makers, it is the failure in implementation, lack of will power and determination. We are in the habit of talking mission and vision but we never accept the failure of not achieving the target. After all it is the tax payer's money and they have every right to know the reasons so that the measures for rectification may be incorporated in the future. We all know that the government is not sitting idle. It has its own limitations and financial crunch. Today, almost 40 % or 400 million people in India live below the poverty line or are classified as poor. They are more in need than the rest of the population. Let us not politicize the matter. In fact, we should evolve means for better health understanding, awareness and implementation by making involvement both at the public and the private level.

What should we do?

Let us focus more on preventive measures and change our strategies for treating the heart disease from intervention to prevention. It may sound ridiculous with such a large number of existing heart patients but a reduced disease burden in the future should be our mission. Today, the biggest hurdle is how do we achieve it? This is not only the government's responsibility or a personal choice; it should be a collective approach. Let us agree on a minimum common agenda and allow the government to have the main thrust on communicable diseases which are rampant in rural areas where almost two third of India resides. Let them have the major chunk of fund expenditure for them because they need it more than the urban dwellers. The government can boost the health of rural India by making a provision for safe drinking water, linking the roads, preventing the dumping of garbage in nearby rural locations and making provisions for safe disposal and treatment of waste. Strict measures must be taken to reduce the burden of the growing population otherwise all efforts will be nullified. A slogan 'one child only' for a nation like India may sound crazy and the majority may not agree to it, but it may be the only choice in the near future and will dilute all efforts if not implemented urgently.

The second aspect is the reduction of chronic or lifestyle diseases which as the name suggest, is the choice of an individual and the government cannot force upon anyone. So for curbing these diseases, the approach should be from the individual; the government can only help by imposing certain rules and regulations to encourage healthy lifestyles among people. Policy makers have already initiated it by discouraging people against tobacco or alcohol abuse by imposing various legislations. Probably, much more is needed as law enforcement is not effective as far as the sale of tobacco products to minors is concerned. Cost of *gutaka* or chewing tobacco is another reason. It is fast replacing cigarette smoking in urban areas among young people and it needs more heavy taxation than those present right now. Ban of smoking at public places should be implemented strictly and simultaneously surrogate advertisements should be penalized heavily. The government should restrict the shrinking green space by maintaining the present space and expanding the cities properly to provide more green spaces for recreation and physical activities. Use of tobacco and physical inactivity are the two most important risk factors as far as the heart of Indians is concerned. Choosing unhealthy food and making yourself obese is your choice. One can again argue and shift the responsibility to the government stating, why don't they ban this? It is the duty of the government to enforce various food compositions to be mentioned on food items marketed and foods rich in trans-fat should be made costly. Remember it is not the food item which is harmful, it is the amount and choice which is wrong. It is a wrong plea and notion as we are to be blamed for the sale of junk food. The government does not force us to purchase these junk food, it is our own inherent weakness. Now it is your turn to take the responsibility to avoid or restrict this habit. Obesity can make you prone to diabetes which, coupled with physical inactivity can invite high blood pressure, abnormal cholesterol levels and heart disease. India is a tropical country. A variety of fruits and vegetables are grown here, but even then their consumption is not adequate. Of course, cost is a major barrier but the use of seasonal and locally available items may solve the problem to a certain extent.

Some may need drug therapy to reduce heart disease, especially high blood pressure and diabetes. In this matter, the help of the pharmaceutical industry may be sought and with them one can formulate cheaper drugs and options. Concept of a single pill, a cheap alternative that is, using aspirin-a blood thinning agent, statin-a cholesterol lowering agent and ramipril - an angiotensin inhibitor agent with or without a beta blocker is fast gaining acceptability for primary and secondary prevention against heart disease. All these medicines have proved their role in reducing disability and death. They also enhance the patient's compliance and acceptability.

The government can play a vital role in spreading the preventive measures and enforcing all hospitals and clinics to display health educative materials mandatory, either in the form of posters or audio-visual displays of their respective discipline. One can call it the health gallery and the help of local doctors, chief medical officers, Indian Medical Association, computer professionals, NGOs and the pharmaceutical industries can be sought to prepare the relevant materials. The average waiting time in an outdoor clinic is almost an hour. During this time, the patients and their relatives can be easily educated by adopting this simple approach.

Print and electronic media is the most powerful and accessible medium to approach the majority of people. Their help will be vital in spreading this message. Some national and local newspapers are already spreading the message by devoting one column or one page, once a week to health. Magazines need more initiative in this matter. Electronic media can advertise the messages for the sake of fellow citizens and the nation. Seminars can be organized for an hour, once a week by inviting both experts and health providers. One example can be to deliver a 10-15 minute lecture on the prevention of the disease through slides by a local expert keeping in mind that the viewers are common people. Then questions can be invited from the audience and viewers for the next 45 minutes or so. This will be of importance in spreading the message to the masses. Now the problem may be - who will sponsor the programme? Corporate hospitals, companies that manufacture health instruments or food products and/or drugs would be of immense help and use in this regard. Short messages pertaining to health can also be displayed frequently.

Health education can play a major role in the modern era. It can spread the messages on prevention of non-communicable diseases. Health education should start early during childhood, as many personal habits and lifestyle choices are formed early in life. Schools and home are the best places to initiate health education. Health education in schools can help young people make sensible choices. Apart from providing ample opportunities to be physically active, their cafeteria should serve healthy snacks and meals. Today, children are much more high tech, are ready to accept the things and their habits can be changed easily as compared to adults. An annual check-up of height and weight will help in fighting childhood obesity and selected obese children should get counselling along with parents for lifestyle and eating habits. Schools should follow strict tobacco-free policies and impose heavy penalties both on the parents as well as the pupil in case of policy violation. Schools should allot periods once a week or fortnight for health interaction and invite doctors or take the help of local health authorities, Indian Medical Association or a chief medical officer or an NGO interested in the matter of health. The formulation should be such that it focuses more on behaviour and lifestyle changes rather than on statistical data. The junior wing can learn more about hygienic conditions and eating habits, while the senior wing can have lifestyle incorporation lectures and interactions. Schools can also display health preventive messages once a week as thought for the day. Health festivals can be organized once a year on a holiday with the help of local physicians, authorities and NGOs. Healthy lifestyle measures which should emphasize upon hygiene, physical activity, dietary practices, saying no to tobacco, should be displayed in school premises as well as at the back of every school diary or almanac.

Various bodies, especially national and regional bodies of cardiologists and physicians should devote various lectures, articles and books on prevention of heart disease. Also, the theme and thrust of some conferences had been mainly the prevention of this disease. The conference deliberations always lay emphasis on their delegates to make prevention an element of every health care interaction. Physicians are encouraged to promote preventive strategies locally and to distribute materials in local dialect among patients and general people. But still preventive advices lack in routine prescriptions considering that distribution of preventive strategies and display of preventive methods in their clinics should be the part of daily patient care.

The time tested role of relaxation exercises such as qi gong, yoga, meditation, spirituality, music therapy, etc., can be added to modern medicine which can definitely add a new dimension in controlling the CHD epidemic. However, these practices alone should not be promoted as panacea. All the relaxation exercises demand punctuality, regularity and devotion, only then can one benefit with emotional, physical, mental and spiritual well-being. Enough scientific data is available today which supports that it not only controls risk factors for coronary heart disease but can retard or reverse the disease process in a few cases.

Yoga, nowadays, is very popular in India but it should not be perceived as treatment of all diseases and one should not live in the false sense of well-being that merely practicing it will guarantee a disease-free life or will cure the chronic diseases. Yoga should not be practiced as just a few postures or *'assans'*. The first two steps in yoga are *yama* and *niyama*, that means don'ts and do's. Therefore, one should preach the yogic way of life which includes truthfulness, non-violence, self-control, non-greed, purity, contentment and surrender to the will of God. Along with *asanas* (different postures) and *pranayam* (control of bio-energy), one should also practice other rules of the yogic way of life that include a low fat vegetarian diet with plenty of fruits, physical exercise, meditation, alcohol and tobacco abstinence. The basic advantage of yoga is that it can be practiced at home with no financial obligation. However, it definitely needs self-discipline and determination. These methods along with modern medicine can make a sea of changes in the scenario of CHD epidemic, as the developing world requires a little effort to be convinced about the positive role played by the relaxation exercises. Proposed health interventions to reduce the burden of cardiovascular disease by various bodies at various levels in a society are summarized in Table 24.1.

Table 24.1: Possible Roles and Responsibilities For the Various Bodies Concerned For Facilitating the Movement to Defeat Cardiovascular Diseases

Bodies and individuals	Roles and responsibilities	Limitations
Policy makers and politicians	Framing of laws and legislations, health care facilities and provision for safe walking and cycling lanes (policy and funding)	Funds, population outburst, failure in effective implementation and other priorities
Physicians	Devote more time for lifestyle modifications and preventive strategies and prescription is a must for patients	Less time for patients, intervention in cardiology more lucrative than prevention
Presidents of various bodies	Organizing—Continued Medical Education program (CME) for prevention which includes identification of risk factors, their diagnosis and treatment, framing guidelines which are socially, financially and culturally beneficial	Few sponsors for preventive education and efforts

Patrons of NGOs and charitable organizations	Help in organizing and spreading the message of prevention, population screening and public education	Fund and lack of co-operation from both, the physicians and the public
Patients	Awareness, and responsibility for their illness	Asymptomatic status, health priority, health initiative is low and costly treatment
Public	Mass education for a healthy lifestyle	Do not know how to get all and lack of initiative due to other engagements
Print and television media	Can spread the message at a large scale and more effectively	Lack of sponsorship
Pharmaceutical industries	Can formulate cheaper drug formulations and help in sponsoring various public and physician interaction programmes, both at local and national levels	Preventive aspects yield little profit
Packaged food Industry	Provision of law for low sodium, high potassium foods, less use of saturated and no use of trans-fat in food preparations, labelling of calories and ingredients	May loose the market share to local manufacturers
Principals of schools	Can spread the message to children effectively for better habits about exercise and diet	Lack of green spaces, fierce competition among students and schools for better academic results
Parents and guardians	Inculcate and practice healthy diet habits, encourage use of fish, fruits, vegetables, skimmed milk and its products, consume less fried foods, spent time with children and encourage them for outdoor activities and games	Both parents working, less time to spent with family, more time devoted to social media, easy accessibility (just a phone call) and less expensive availability of fast foods

Today, CHD is the leading cause of death in a majority of countries including the Indian subcontinent. It is comparable to the industrialized and affluent countries. There is a definite evidence that coronary heart disease is preventable, because a majority of the risk factors can be controlled, avoided or treated. Therefore, it is necessary to develop strategies to prevent the rising incidence of coronary heart disease. There are well recognized approaches identified by international studies with proven role which can be modified and implemented, according to the regional population. Income growth, improvements in medical technology, public health programmes combined with the awareness and spread of knowledge about health are some of the major factors that can cause a dramatic and unprecedented decline in cardiovascular disease burden in all parts of world and will help in defeating the heart disease.

The aim of all these efforts is to reduce the disease burden and suffering, to increase the quality of life and to increase the healthy life expectancy for all irrespective of an individual's wealth. Whatever be the message and how it spreads, all efforts will be in vain if you don't take charge of your health. So your involvement, determination and action are of paramount importance as today we are in the middle of an epidemic of various chronic diseases and at this point, we cannot afford failure as an option.

Appendix and Tables

Approximate Calorie Value of Common Indian Food Items

Vegetarian Dishes

Food	Quantity	Calories
Phulka	One	80
Chappati	One	100
Tandoori roti	One	145
Missi roti	One	125
Makke ki roti	One	275
Poori	One	100
Parantha	One	125
Stuffed parantha	One	175
Naan	One	190
Butter naan	One	250
Boiled rice	One cup	100
Fried rice	One cup	170
Khichdi	One cup	200
Coconut rice	One cup	255
Vegetable pulao	One cup	200
Biryani-vegetarian	One cup	200
Biriyani-mutton	One cup	250
Dal-tur or arhar	One cup	50

Dal makhani	One cup	210
Dal fry	One cup	90
Kadi	One cup	40
Rasam	One cup	30
Sambhar	One cup	110
Vegetable curry	One cup	175
Potato curry	One cup	200
Bharta-brinjal	One cup	175
Malai kofta	One cup	320
Navratan korma	One cup	320
Palak paneer	One cup	240
Vegetables-dry	One cup	150

Non-vegetarian dishes

Egg curry	One cup	225
Mutton curry	One cup/2 pieces	260
Chicken curry	One cup/2 pieces	240
Fish curry	One cup/2 pieces	125
Prawn curry	One cup	270
Crab	One cup	70
Keema	One cup	240
Fish fry	2 big pieces	220
Fish fingers	3 pieces	160
Fish cutlet	2 pieces	190
Tandoori chicken	One piece	120
Seekh kebab	One piece	160

Approximate Calorie value of Common Indian Snacks

Snacks Popular All Over India

Bread	Two	120
Bread with butter	Two + 10 gms butter	200
Boiled egg	Two	160
Poached egg	Two	300
Omelette	Two	500
Cheese sandwich	One	250
Vegetable sandwich	One	150
Finger chips	100 gms	350
Chips	10 piece	150
Papad (grilled)	Two	50
Papad (fried)	Two	80
Patties	One piece	320
Vegetable burger	One	400
Chicken burger	One	500
Pizza	One slice	160-200
Spring rolls	Two	320
Popcorn	50 gms	200
Chowmein	One plate	200
Potato chips	100 gms	500
Bhajias and namkeen	100 gms	400

Snacks Popular in North and Central India

Poori	4 in number	400
Parantha plain	Two	250
Stuffed paratha	Two	350
Bhelpuri	One plate	200
Bhatura	Two	450
Chole	One cup	170

Dahi vada	Two	360
Pav bhaji	One serving	500
Kachori	Two	400
Kachori with jalebi	One serving of two	700
Poha	One serving	250
Samosa	Two	500
Dhokla	Six medium pieces	130
Chiwda-fried	100 gms	400
Aloo tikki	Two	150
Cutlet	Two	300
Mathri	100 gms (4 small)	400
Pakoras	Eight pieces	300
Bread roll	Two	500
Papari chat	One plate	300

Snacks Popular in South India

Plain dosa	One small	150
Masala dosa	One small	230
Idli	Two small	150
Rava idli	Two small	375
Vada	Two small	280
Chakli	500 gms	550
Upma	One cup	270
Sambhar	70 ml	75
Uttapam	One piece	170
Aloo bonda	One serving	125

Common Sweets or Sweet Meat and their Approximate Calorie Value

Sweet meat	Pieces	Cal
Burfi	One	110
Peda	One	55
Jalebi	Two/40 gms	200
Rasogulla	Two	250
Gulab jamun	Two	350
Balushahi	Two/80 gms	540
Laddoo	Two/80gms	500
Shrikhand	125 ml	340
Rasmalai	80 gms	500
Malpua	80 gms	520
Mysore pak	1 piece	357
Puran poli	Two	600
Custard	125 ml	160
Fruit salad	125 ml	100
Rabadi without sugar	125 ml	60
Kulfi	Two	640
Kulfi falooda	Two	750
Pastry	One	400
Ice cream	150 ml	160
Chocolate	One	200
Cake	One	140
Kheer	150 ml	260
Gajar ka halwa	125 ml	290
Moong ka halwa	125 ml	300
Chikki	One	135

Dietary guidelines for Indians, *National Institute of Nutrition.* ICMR, Hyderabad. 1998.

Common Complications of Diabetes from Head to Toe

Organ	Disease	Manifestation
Brain	Cerebral infarct or haemorrhage, transient ischaemic attack (TIA)	Stroke, coma, paralysis, loss of speech or memory
Eyes	Retinal haemorrhage, exudates, detachment, cataract, retinal vascular thrombosis, macular oedema, optic nerve atrophy	Gradual or sudden impairment in vision or blindness
Ear	Infection in ear (otitis).	Ear discharge and pain.
Teeth	Gingivitis, periodontitis, Pyorrhoea, dry mouth, oral thrush, dental decay	Mouth sore, gum swelling, pain, bleeding, cavities
Heart	Coronary heart disease, cardiomyopathy	Chest pain, breathlessness, heart attack, heart failure, sudden death
Lungs	Chronic infections such as tuberculosis, pneumonia	Fever, shortness of breath, prolonged cough
Gastrointestinal-system	Delayed emptying, reflux and candidiasis	Fullness, dyspepsia, nausea, vomiting, hiccoughs
Kidneys	Kidney or urinary infections, glomerulosclerosis, pyelonephritis, urinary tract infections (UTI), proteinuria	Swelling of body, painful and frequent urination, reduced urinary output
Sexual function	Impotence or loss of libido	Decreased performance or erectile dysfunction

Appendix and Tables | 427

Nervous system	Diabetic neuropathy	Numbness, tingling, constant pain or loss of sensation or feeling, postural hypotension
Skin, nails, limbs	Infections, boils, carbuncles, cellulitis, gangrene	Redness, pain and swelling with poor healing, occasionally gangrene leading to amputation
Limbs	Peripheral artery disease, infections, cellulitis	Pain on walking, ulcers, gangrene, painful joints

Common Complications of High Blood Pressure from Head to Toe

Organ	Disease	Manifestations
Brain	Cerebrovascular disease or stroke, transient ischaemic attack (TIA), Hypertensive encephalopathy, vascular dementia	Ischaemic or haemorrhagic stroke, coma, paralysis, loss of memory, problem in vision and speech or trouble with understanding
Eyes	Hypertensive retinopathy, conjunctival haemorrhage	Partial or total blindness or bleeding
Heart	Left ventricular hypertrophy or dysfunction, coronary heart disease	Myocardial infarction or heart attack, angina pectoris leading to chest pain or even sudden death, congestive heart failure leading to difficulty in breathing, weakness and easy fatigability
Kidneys	Chronic kidney disease, hypertensive nephropathy, albuminuria	Renal failure, body swelling, reduced urinary output, protein leak in urine
Limbs	Peripheral artery disease.	Intermittent claudication, leg pain or difficulty in walking.
Aorta	Dissecting aneurysm	Severe chest or back pain, can be life threatening

Your Health Care Goals and Responsibilities to Defeat Heart Disease

Blood pressure	<139/89 mmHg
	< 120/80 mmHg with diabetes
Blood sugar	Fasting < 100 mg or HbA1c < 7.0%
LIPIDS Total cholesterol LDL cholesterol Triglyceride HDL cholesterol	< 200 mg/dl < 100 mg/dl < 150 mg/dl > 40 mg/dl males > 50 mg/dl females
Waist circumference (Asians)	90 cms (36 inches) for male 80 cms (32 inches) for females
Basal metabolic rate (BMI)	18-22.9 kg/ m^2 for men and women
Total fats in diet should be restricted to	20-25% of total calories Saturated fat around 7-10%, prefer oils which are liquid at room temperature
Lipoprotein Lp(a)	< 20 mg/dl
Salt intake	5 gms or one teaspoonful daily
Physical activity	About 45 to 60 minutes daily apart from routine work
Tobacco	Total abstinence
Alcohol	Preferably NO to alcohol, 30-60 ml/day with meals on a regular basis
Fruits and vegetables	Three to four servings (300-400 gm) per day
Dry fruits	100 gm per week, prefer walnut, pistachio, apricot, almond
Fish	2 portions (200 gm), twice a week
Avoid whites in your diet	Sugar, flour, whole milk except white of egg
Medical check up	Annually after 30 years of age, irrespective of asymptomatic status

Glossary

Acute: Describing a disease and its events which occur in a short period of time.

Aneurysm: An abnormal balloon-like swelling or bulging in the wall of the artery or heart.

Angina: Pain in the centre of the chest, which is induced by exercise and relieved by rest; may spread to arms, back or jaws.

Angiography: Imaging of heart or blood vessels by injecting a specific dye or a contrast medium, which can be detected by X-ray or by other means of imaging.

Angioplasty: A method of repairing or fixing narrowed or completely blocked blood vessel. Today, in medical practice this term commonly refers to percutaneous trans-luminal angioplasty (PTA) or balloon angioplasty in which an inflatable balloon, mounted on the tip of a flexible catheter is placed within the lumen of the affected vessel at the site of the narrowing or blockage under X-ray control and then inflated and deflated several times to open the blocked site.

Antioxidants: Substances capable of neutralizing oxygen free radicals, the highly active and damaging atoms and chemical groups produced in the body. Antioxidants occur naturally in the body and in certain foods, especially plant based foods and beverages. They prevent the fat from becoming oxidized.

Aorta: The main artery of the body from which all others derive. It arises from the main and most robust chamber of the heart that is, the left ventricle.

Arrhythmia: A rhythm disturbance of heart or irregular heartbeat.

Artery: A blood vessel carrying blood away from the heart; it carries oxygen rich blood except the pulmonary arteries which carry deoxygenated blood from the heart to the lungs for oxygenation.

Aspirin: Commonly used drug to reduce stickiness and accumulation of platelets. It is used to dissolve clots.

Atherosclerosis: A disease of the arteries in which a fatty build up develops on the inner wall of the artery and eventually obstructs the lumen and blood flow.

Atrial fibrillation: Irregular heartbeats arising from the atria.

Atrium: Either of the two upper chambers of the heart; they are thinner than the lower chambers that is, the ventricles. The right atrium receives oxygen poor blood from the body via veins and the left atrium receives blood from the lungs which is rich in oxygen.

Bacon: The salted and dried or smoked back and sides of the hog.

Blood clot: A solid or semisolid mass of blood coagulation, either within the blood vessels and or in the heart. A blood clot consists of a meshwork of protein fibrin in which various blood cells are trapped.

Blood pressure: Pressure of blood in the arteries.

Blood vessels: Tubes or pipe-like structures through which blood flows (arteries and veins).

Body mass index (BMI): The weight of a person in kilograms divided by the square of the height measured in metres, used as an indicator of whether or not a person is over or underweight. A BMI of less than 18.5 is considered underweight, between 20-25 is normal, between 25-30 is overweight and above 30 is seen as obesity. BMI more than 40 is considered morbid obesity.

Bradycardia: Slow heart rate that is less than 60 beats per minute at rest.

Bronchogenic: Related with the lungs such as bronchogenic malignancy or lung cancer.

Calorie: A unit of heat equal to the amount of heat required to raise the temperature of 1 gram of water from 14.5 °C to 15.5 °C. This unit is used to indicate the energy value of foods.

Capillaries: Finest blood vessels joining arteries to veins.

Carbohydrates: It is one of the three main important food constituents and is manufactured by plants. Carbohydrates are an important source of energy and all ingested carbohydrates are broken down in the body to simple sugars that is, glucose which can take part in energy production. Sugar and starch are the main constituents of carbohydrates.

Cardiac cycle: The sequence of events between one heartbeat and the next, normally occupying less than a second.

Cardiac output: The amount of blood pushed out from the heart each minute. It usually ranges between 3-5 litres per minute in an adult at resting state.

Cardiac: Related to heart.

Cardiomyopathy: Disease of heart muscles which dilates and weakens the heart.

Cardiovascular: Related with heart and vessels of the body.

Carotid arteries: Arteries running up both sides of the neck. They supply blood to the brain.

Cerebral embolism: Blood clot which has travelled to the brain.

Cerebral haemorrhage: Commonly known as brain haemorrhage. It is defined as bleeding inside the brain due to leakage or rupture of a blood vessel.

Cerebro-vascular accident: Commonly termed as CVA or stroke. It is death of a part of the brain due to a clot or blood.

Cerebro-vascular: Any disorder of blood vessels of the brain or its covering.

Chagas disease: A disease caused by the protozoan parasite *Trypanosoma cruzi*. It affects the heart muscles and brain. The disease is limited to poor rural areas of central and South America.

Cholesterol: Fat-like material present in blood and most tissues of the body. It can be obtained from food and manufactured by the body in the liver.

Chronic: Occurring in a span of long periods - in months or years and describing the disease or process as gradual and involving a slow change. It has nothing to do with the severity of disease.

Claudication: Is a cramping pain, induced by exercise and relieved by rest. It is caused by an inadequate supply of blood to the affected muscles, often seen in calf and leg muscles.

Clopidogrel: A common drug which inhibits platelet accumulation and clot formation. It is used as clot buster.

Coarctation of the aorta: Narrowing of a short segment of the aorta present since birth. This results in high blood pressure in upper arms and body and low blood pressure in the legs.

Computed tomography (CT imaging): A form of X-ray examination in which the X-ray source and detector rotate around the object to be scanned and the information obtained can be used to produce cross-sectional images with the help of a computer.

Coronary arteries: The arteries supplying blood to the heart.

Coronary artery bypass surgery (CABG): It is a surgical process in which a segment of the coronary artery narrowed or blocked is bypassed by a healthy blood vessel obtained from the same person's body which can be leg veins or arteries from the chest or arm to restore the blood flow beyond the blocked area and improving the blood circulation through the grafted healthy vessels.

Coronary heart disease: Atherosclerosis of the coronary arteries which may cause various manifestations. The most common are angina pectoris or myocardial infarction, commonly known as a heart attack.

Cushing's syndrome: The condition resulting from excess amount of corticosteroid or *growth hormone*. It is associated with weight gain and excessive body growth.

Diabetes mellitus: A disorder of carbohydrate metabolism in which sugar in the body is not utilized to produce energy either due to reduced production of insulin or dysfunctional insulin from the pancreas, a hormone responsible for shifting sugar from the blood into the body cells for utilization. This results in an excess of sugar in blood and urine. The common complaints of diabetes are excessive production of urine, thirst, excessive eating and weight loss. Diabetes mellitus is commonly referred to as diabetes.

Diastole: The period of cardiac cycle during which the heart relaxes.

Diastolic blood pressure: The lower reading of blood pressure.

Dyspnoea: Breathing difficulty or shortness of breath.

Echocardiography: Ultrasound based technique to assess heart function and structure at rest or during exercise.

Ejection fraction: Amount of blood pumped out of the heart after each beat, normally more than 52 %.

Electrocardiography: A technique of recording the electrical activity of the heart with the help of a machine and surface electrodes. The record is called electrocardiogram or ECG.

Embolism: A condition in which an embolus (common is blood clot) becomes lodged in an artery and obstructs its blood flow.

Emphysema: The air sacs of the lungs are damaged and enlarged, which reduce the surface area for exchange of oxygen and carbon dioxide.

Endothelium: A single layer of cells that lines the blood vessels and heart from the inside.

Exercise or stress test: Synonym for TMT.

Fats: A substance that contains one or more forms of fatty acids and is the main source of energy which is stored in the body. Fat is one of the three main constituents of food (others are proteins and carbohydrates). It is essential for health.

Fatty acids: Fatty acids are the fundamental constituents of all lipids. A majority of them are synthesized in the body by the liver. However, some fatty acids must be obtained from the diet and are called essential fatty acids.

Fibrillation: Erratic and irregular contraction of either atria (atrial fibrillation) or ventricle (ventricular fibrillation). In ventricular fibrillation, blood is not ejected from the heart and it may stop in a few minutes.

Gangrene: Death or decay of a part of the body due to deficiency or cessation of blood supply.

Genetic disease: Inherited diseases or disorders from the parents sharing a common genetic structure.

Haemoglobin: A substance present within the red blood cells which is responsible for the colour of the blood. Haemoglobin contains a pigment 'haem' and a protein 'globin'. It has the unique property of combining reversibly with oxygen and is the medium by which oxygen is transported within the body.

Haemorrhage: Loss of blood, internally or externally.

Ham: The thigh of a hog, smoked or salted.

Heart attack: A common term for myocardial infarction in which one of the blood vessels supplying blood to the heart are completely blocked. The subsequent loss of blood supply causes death of a part of the heart muscle.

Heart block: When the heart beats less than 40 beats per minute due to failure of the normal function of natural pacemaker that is, sino-atrial node.

Hog: A pig, especially the fully grown pig.

Homocysteine: It is a sulphur containing amino acid. Its elevated level in blood is recognized as a risk factor for vascular disease such as a stroke or heart disease. Its level is also elevated in vitamin B12 deficiency.

Hyperlipidaemia: Presence of abnormally high level of lipids in blood.

Hypertension: Is high blood pressure or elevation of arterial blood pressure above the normal range.

Hypotension: Low blood pressure.

Hypothyroidism: Subnormal activity of thyroid gland; often associated with weight gain.

Incidence: A number of new patients arising in the population over a period of time.

Infarction: The death of a part or the whole organ that occurs when the artery carrying its blood supply is completely obstructed by a blood clot or thrombus. Example is myocardial infarction, affecting the muscles of the heart following coronary thrombosis.

Inflammation: The body's response to injury, a defence mechanism.

Ischaemia: The inadequate flow of blood to a part of the body caused by constriction or blockage of blood vessels supplying it. Ischaemia of heart muscles can produce various symptoms and is grouped as ischaemic heart disease.

Lipids: Lipids and fats are interchangeable and are an important dietary constituent.

Lipoproteins: These are protein molecules which are combined with lipids (which may be cholesterol, triglyceride) and are responsible for the transportation of lipids in blood.

Low density lipoprotein or LDL: Bad cholesterol in the blood which sticks to the inner lining of arteries.

Lumen: Inside of a tube or vessel through which blood flows.

Magnetic resonance imaging (MRI): A diagnostic imaging technique based on the emission of electromagnetic waves from the body when a person is placed in a strong magnetic field and exposed to strong radio--frequency radiations.

Malignancy: Medical term used for cancer.

Mediastinum: Midline portion of the chest cavity.

Metabolic syndrome: It is a combination of insulin resistance and Type 2 diabetes, central obesity, high blood pressure and lipid disorder. It is associated with the risk of early atherosclerosis.

Morbidity: The state of being ill or diseased.

Mortality: Related with death; the mortality rate signifies the rate of death in the population in a given period.

Myocardial infarction: Reduced blood supply to heart muscles; also known as heart attack in common terms.

Myocardium: It is a cardiac muscle and forms the greater part of the heart. It is thicker in the ventricles than in the atria.

Necrosis: Death of body tissue.

Nitroglycerine: A common drug used to treat angina pain.

Nutrients: A substance that must be consumed as part of the diet to provide a source of energy and material for growth. Nutrients include carbohydrates, fats, proteins, minerals and vitamins. When taken in a balanced amount, they sustain good health and well-being.

Obesity: Being overweight; it is defined as more than 20 % of your ideal height and weight.

Occluded: Total block.

Oils: A cooking medium which is a rich source of fat in diet. It is liquid at room temperature.

Omega fatty acids: A type of unsaturated fatty acid, out of which some are essential fatty acids whose moderate consumption promotes good health.

Open heart surgery: Surgical procedure on the heart after opening the chest. It is commonly referred to a bypass surgery or valve surgery.

Pacemaker: A structure or device used to produce and maintain the normal heart rate. The part of heart that regulates the heart rate at which it beats is known as 'sino-atrial node' or natural pacemaker. When an artificial device is used to regulate the heart rate, especially in heart block, then it is known as an artificial pacemaker and consists of a battery and circuit which stimulate the heart rate through an insulated electrode wire or lead inserted into the heart chambers.

Palpitation: An awareness of the heartbeat; it is normal with fear, emotions, exertion and anxiety.

Pancreas: A linear organ or gland in the abdomen, below the stomach. It produces the hormones-insulin and glucagon which regulate carbohydrate metabolism in the body.

Paralysis: Loss of function of a part or one half of the body because of muscle weakness. It varies in extent from total to partial loss and denotes disease of the nervous system.

Passive smoking: Breathing in or inhalation of other's tobacco smoke.

Pepperoni: It is a spicy Italian-American variety of salami (a dry sausage) usually made from cured pork and beef, but poultry may be added.

Pericardium: A membrane-like structure surrounding the heart.

Plaque: A deposit, consisting of a fatty core covered with a fibrous cap that develops on the inner wall of an artery in atherosclerosis.

Platelets: A disc-like cell present in blood. It has a role in arresting bleeding by formation of blood clot. It is also responsible for clot formation in the heart and brain.

Pleura: Covering of the lungs and of the inner surface of the chest wall.

Porphyria: One of a group of rare disorders due to inborn errors of metabolism in which there are deficiencies in enzymes involved in the biosynthesis of haem.

Postprandial: After meals, and it refers to blood sugar estimation.

Prevalence: A measure of current sickness or disease at a particular time or period.

Proteins: Are complex structures made up of amino acids – an essential ingredient of diet. It is necessary for muscle tissues, bones and various organs of the body. Excess of protein in diet is converted into glucose.

Pulmonary: Related with lungs.

Renal: Related with kidney.

Risk factors: Certain disorders, diseases or habits which make a person prone or at risk to the development of disease.

Saturated fat: Fats which are bad for health and solid at room temperature.

Sausage: Finely chopped and highly seasoned meat, commonly stuffed into a prepared animal intestine or other casing.

Sodium: Sodium chloride is the chemical name for common salt.

Sphygmomanometer: A device or instrument with which blood pressure is measured.

Steak: A slice of meat or fish, especially of beef, usually fried or boiled.

Stenosis: It means narrowing.

Stent: Metal mesh or cage inserted after balloon dilatation of blocked artery to prevent its re-closure. It holds the artery open. When it is coated with a drug, it is called drug eluting (DES) or coated stents.

Sternum: Breast bone.
Streptokinase: Clot dissolving drug which is used following heart attack; also known as thrombolytic drug.
Stroke: A sudden attack of weakness affecting one side of the body or part of the body due to interruption in the flow of blood to the brain.
Syncope: Sudden loss of consciousness.
Systole: The period of the cardiac cycle during which the heart contracts.
Systolic blood pressure: The upper reading of blood pressure.

Tablespoonful: A measurement which denotes approximately 15 ml or 15 gms.
Tachycardia: Heart rate more than 100 beats per minute or fast heart rate.
Teaspoonful: A measurement which denotes approximately 5 ml or 5 gms.
Thallium testing: A nuclear scan of heart using radioisotopes to assess the heart function and extent of damage to the heart muscle.
Thrombolysis: The process of breaking down blood clots.
Thrombolytics: Agents that break up blood clots.
Trans-fats: They are unsaturated fatty acids that adapt a saturated fatty acid-like configuration by the process of hydrogenation. By this process, the shelf-life of polyunsaturated fatty acids is increased.
Treadmill test (TMT): A type of stress test to evaluate chest pain and related disorders in which a person is asked to exercise on a treadmill machine with simultaneous monitoring of ECG, heart rate and blood pressure. It is also referred to as stress test.
Triglycerides: Fats that may be bad for health. Their high level increases the risk of heart diseases.

Unsaturated fats: Fats that are liquid at room temperature.

Vein: Blood vessels carry blood towards the heart and contain oxygen poor blood. The only exception is pulmonary veins, which carry oxygen rich blood from the lungs to the left side of the heart.

Ventricles: The lower chambers of the heart. They are more muscular than the upper chambers. The left ventricle is the ejecting chamber and most robust of all four chambers of the heart.

Vessels: A tube or conduit pipe-like structure which carries body fluids such as blood.

Vitamins: A group of substances that are required in a very small quantity and are mandatory for growth and development. They are an essential constituent of diet as they are not synthesized in the body. There are two groups of vitamins-water soluble vitamins such as vitamin B and C, and fat soluble vitamins such as vitamin A, D, E, and K.

Xanthelasma: Yellow plaques or deposits around the eyelids. In some cases, it may be a manifestation of a disorder of fat metabolism, but in a majority of elderly people it is quite common and of no more than cosmetic importance.

Xanthoma: Yellowish skin lesions of deposition associated with various lipid disorders.

X-ray: Electromagnetic radiation of extremely short wavelength used for diagnostic purposes, mainly for bones or to monitor and guide various procedures.

References and Suggested Readings

Chapter 1

Enas EA. Coronary Artery Disease Epidemic in Indians: A Cause of Alarm and Call for Action. *J Indian Med Assoc* 2000; 98: 697-702.

Miranda JJ, Kinra S, Casas JP, Smith GD, Ebrahim S. Noncommunicable Diseases in Low and Middle Income Countries: Context, Determinants and Health policy. *Trop Med Int Health* 2008; 13: 1225–1234.

Reddy KS, Yusuf S. Emerging Epidemic of Cardiovascular Disease in Developing Countries. *Circulation* 1998; 97: 596–601.

Padmavati S. Prevention of Heart Disease in India in the Twenty-first Century: Need for a Concerted Effort. *Indian Heart Journal* 2002; 54: 99–102.

Chapter 3

Gaziano JM. Global Burden of Cardiovascular Disease in: Braunwald's Heart Disease: A Textbook of Cardiovascular Medicine. Eighth Edition, page 1-22. Elseviers Saunders: 2008.

Gupta R, Joshi P, Mohan V, Reddy KS, Yusuf S. Epidemiology and Causation of Coronary Heart Disease and Stroke in India. *Heart* 2008; 94: 16-26.

Gupta R. Burden of Coronary Heart Disease in India. *Indian Heart Journal* 2005; 57: 632-638.

Jafar TH, Qadri Z, Chaturvedi N. Coronary Artery Disease Epidemic in Pakistan: More Electrocardiographic Evidence of Ischaemia in Women Than in Men. *Heart* 2008; 94: 408-413.

Leeder S, Raymond S, Greenberg H, Liu K. A Race Against Time: The Challenge of Cardiovascular Disease in Developing Economics. New York: Columbia University, 2004.

Lopez AD, Mathers CD, Ezzati M, Dean T Jamison, Murray L. Global and Regional Burden of Disease and Risk Factors, 2001: Systematic Analysis of Population Health Data. *Lancet* 2006; 367: 1747–57.

Mensah GA. Ischaemic Heart Disease in Africa. *Heart* 2008; 94: 847-852.

Reddy KS. Cardiovascular Disease in Non-western Countries. *N Engl J Med* 2004; 350: 2436-2440.

World Health Organization. Preventing Chronic Diseases: A Vital Investment. Geneva. World Health Organization, 2005.

Yusuf S, Reddy S, Ounpuu S, Anand S. Global Burden of Cardiovascular Disease: Part II: Variations in Cardiovascular Disease by Specific Ethnic Groups and Geographic Regions and Prevention Strategies. *Circulation* 2001; 104: 2855-2864.

Yusuf S, Reddy S, Ounpuu S, et al. Global Burden of Cardiovascular Disease: Part I: General Considerations, the Epidemiologic Transition, Risk factors and Impact of Urbanization. *Circulation* 2001; 104: 2746-2753.

Chapter 6

Deedwania P, Singh V. Coronary Artery Disease in South Asians: Evolving Strategies For Treatment and Prevention. *Indian Heart Journal* 2005; 57: 617-631.

Enas EA. How to Beat the Heart Disease Epidemic Among South Asians: A Prevention and Management Guide for Asian Indians and Their Doctors. Downers Grove. Advanced Heart Lipid Clinic USA. 2007.

Ghaffar A, Reddy KS, Singhi M. Burden of Non-communicable Diseases in South Asia. *British Medical Journal* 2004; 328: 807-810.

Gupta R. Recent Trends in Coronary Heart Disease Epidemiology in India. *Indian Heart Journal* 2008; suppl. B: B4-B18.

Reddy KS. Cardiovascular Diseases in the Developing Countries: Dimensions, Determinants, Dynamics and Directions for Public Health Action. *Public Health Nutrition* 2002; 5: 231-237.

Chapter 7

Chambers JC, Obeid OA, Refsum H et al. Plasma Homocysteine Concentrations and Risk of Coronary Heart Disease in UK Indian Asian and European Men. *Lancet* 2000; 355: 523-527.

Enas EA, Dhawan J, Petkar S. Coronary Artery Disease in Asians Indians : Lessons Learnt and the Role of Lipoprotein (a). *Indian Heart Journal* 1997; 49: 25-34.

Ezzati M, Lopez AD, Rodgers A, Vander HS, Murray CJ. Selected Major Risk Factors and Global and Regional Burden of Disease. *Lancet* 2002; 360: 1347-1360.

Gronbaek M, Deis A, Sorensen TI, Becker U, Schnohr P, Jensen G. Mortality Associated With Moderate Intake of Wine, Beer or Spirits. *British Medical Journal* 1995; 310: 1165-1169.

Gupta A, Gupta R, Lal B, Singh AK, Kothari K. Prevalence of Coronary Risk Factors Among Indian Physicians. *J Asso Physicians of India* 2001; 49: 1148-1152.

He J, Vuputuri, Allen K, Prerost MR, Hughes J, Whelton PK. Passive Smoking and the Risk of Coronary Heart Disease--A Meta Analysis of Epidemiological Studies. *New Eng J Med* 1999; 340: 920-926.

Sesso HD, Paffenbarger RS Jr, Lee IM. Physical Activity and Coronary Heart Disease in Men: The Harvard Alumni Health Study. *Circulation* 2000; 102: 975-980.

Tanasescu M, Leitzmann MF, Rimm EB, et al. Exercise Type and Intensity in Relation to Coronary Artery Disease in Men. *JAMA* 2002; 288: 194-200.

Yusuf S, Hawken S, Ounpuu S, Dans T, Avezum A, Lanas F, et al INTERHEART Study Investigators. Effect of Potentially Modifiable Risk Factors Associated With Myocardial Infarction in 52 countries (the INTERHEART Study) : Case-Control study. *Lancet* 2004; 364: 937-952.

Yusuf S. Coronary Heart Disease and Its Risk Factors in First Generation Immigrant Asian Indians to the United States of America. *Indian Heart Journal* 1996; 48: 343-353.

Chapter 10

Andreotti F, Marchese N. Women and Coronary Disease. *Heart* 2008; 94: 108-116.

Banerrjee AK. Coronary Artery Disease in Women. *Indian Heart Journal* 2008; 60: 342-345.

Hodis HN, Mack WJ, Azen SP et al. Hormone Therapy and the Progression of Coronary Artery Atherosclerosis in Post-menopausal Women. *New Engl J Med* 2003; 349: 535-545.

Hulley S, Grady D, Bush T et al. Randomized Trial of Estrogen Plus Progestin for Secondary Prevention of Coronary Heart Disease in Post Menopausal Women. Heart and Estrogen/

Progestin Replacement Study (HERS) Research Group. *JAMA* 1998; 280: 605-613.

Mosca L, Appel LJ, Benjamin EJ, et al. Evidence Based Guidelines for Cardiovascular Disease Prevention in Women. *J Am Coll Cardiol* 2004; 43: 900-921.

Chapter 12

Bharucha NE, Kuruvilla T. Hypertension in a Parsi Community of Bombay: A Study on Prevalence, Awareness and Compliance to Treatment. BMC Public Health 2003. January 6;3(1): 1.

Chobanion AV, Bakris GL, Black HR. The Seventh Report of the Joint National Committee on Prevention, Detection, Evaluation and Treatment of High Blood Pressure- The JNC 7 report. *JAMA* 2003; 289: 2560-2572.

Deepa R, Shanthirani CS, Pradeepa R, Mohan V. Is the 'Rule of Halves' in Hypertension Still Valid? Evidence From the Chennai Urban Population Study. *Jour Assoc Physicians India* 2003: 51: 153-157.

He J, Whelton PK, Appel LJ, Charleston J, Klag MJ. Long Term Effects of Weight Loss and Dietary Sodium Reduction on Incidence of Hypertension. Hypertension 2000; 35: 544-549.

Kalavathy MC, Thankappan KR, Sarma PS, Vasan RS. Prevalence, Awareness, Treatment and Control of Hypertension in an Elderly Community--Based Sample in Kerala, India. *National Medical Journal of India* 2000; 13: 9-15.

Victor RG, Kaplan NM. Systemic Hypertension: Mechanisms and Diagnosis. In: Braunwald's Heart Disease: A Textbook of Cardiovascular Medicine. page 1027-1048. Eighth Edition, Elseviers Saunders: 2008.

Kearney PM, Whelton M, Reynolds K, Muntner P, Whelton PK, He Jiang. Global Burden of Hypertension: Analysis of Worldwide Data. *Lancet* 2005; 365: 217-223.

Prakash J, Pandey LK, Singh AK, Kar S. Hypertension in Pregnancy Hospital Based Study. *Jour Assoc Physicians India* 2006; 54: 273-278.

Sacks FM, Svetkey LP, Vollmer WM et al. For the DASH-Sodium Collaborative Research Group. Effects on Blood Pressure of Reduced Dietary Sodium and the Dietary Approaches to Stop Hypertension (DASH) Trial. *New Engl J Med* 2001; 344: 3-10.

Thadhani R, Solomon CG. Pre-eclampsia A Glimpse Into the Future. *New Engl J Med* 2008; 359: 858-860.

Whelton SP, Chin A, Xin X, He J. Effect of Aerobic Exercises on Blood Pressure. *Ann Intern Med* 2002; 136: 493-503.

Xin X, He J, Frontini MG, et al. Effects of Alcohol Reduction on Blood Pressure. *Hypertension* 2001; 38: 1112-1117.

Chapter 13

Deedwania P. Contemporary Approaches for Cardiovascular Risk Reduction in Diabetes. *Indian Heart Journal* 2009; 61: 24-33.

Helmrich SP, Ragland DR, Leung RW, et al. Physical Activity and Reduced Occurrence of Non insulin Dependent Diabetes Mellitus. *N Engl J Med* 1991; 325: 147-152.

Joshi SR. Incidence Data on Diabetes From India. *Jour Assoc Physicians India* 2008; 56: 149-151.

King H, Aubert RE, Hermen WH. Global Burden of Diabetes 995-2005: Prevalence, Numerical Estimates and Projections. *Diabetes Care* 1998; 21: 1114-1131.

Knowler WC, Barrett-Conor E, Fowler SE, et al. Reduction in the Incidence of Type 2 Diabetes with Lifestyle Intervention or Metformin. *N Engl J Med* 2002; 346: 393-403.

Mohan V. Why are Indians More Prone to Diabetes? *Jour Assoc Physicians India* 2004; 52: 468-474.

Pradeepa R, Deepa R, Mohan V. Epidemiology of Diabetes in India--Current Prospective and Future Projections. *J Indian Med Assoc* 2002; 100: 144-148.

Sicree R, Shaw J, Zimmet P. Diabetes and Impaired Glucose Tolerance in India. Diabetes Atlas. Gan D Ed. International Diabetes Federation, 2006: pp 15-103.

Chapter 14

Joshi SR. Metabolic Syndrome--Emerging Clusters of the Indian Phenotype. *Jour Assoc Physicians India* 2003; 51: 445-446.

Misra A, Khurana L. Obesity and the Metabolic Syndrome in Developing Countries. J Clin Endocrinol Metabol 2008; 93: S9-S30.

Misra A, Khurana L, Vikram NK, Goel A, Wasir JS. Metabolic Syndrome in Children: Current Issues and South Asian Perspective. *Nutrition* 2007; 23: 895-910.

Misra A, Chowbey P, Makkar B. Consensus Statement for Diagnosis of Obesity, Abdominal Obesity, and Metabolic Syndrome, for Asian Indians and Recommendations for Physical Activity, Medical and Surgical Management. *Jour Assoc Physicians India* 2009; 57: 163-170.

Chapter 15

National Cholesterol Education Program. Third Report of the National Cholesterol Education Program (NCEP) Expert Panel on Detection, Evaluation, and Treatment of High Blood Cholesterol in Adults (Adult Treatment Panel III): Final Report. *Circulation* 2002; 106: 3143-3421.

Knopp RH. Drug Treatment of Lipid Disorders. *New Engl J Med* 1999; 341: 498-511.

Kris-Etherton PM, Harris WS, Appel LJ. Fish Consumption, Fish Oil, Omega 3 Fatty Acids and Cardiovascular Disease. *Circulation* 2002; 106: 2747-2757.

Durrington P. Dyslipidaemia. *Lancet* 2003; 362: 717-731.

Gotto AM Jr, Brinton EA. Assessing Low Levels of High Density Lipoprotein Cholesterol as a Risk Factor in Coronary Heart Disease. *J Am Coll Cardiol* 2004; 43: 717-724.

Chapter 16

Babu S, Sesikeran B, Bhat RV. Oral Fibrosis Among Teenagers Chewing Tobacco, Areca Nut and Pan Masala. *Lancet* 1999; 348: 692-696.

Gupta BK, Kaushik A, Panwar RB, Chaddha VS et al. Cardiovascular Risk Factors in Tobacco Chewers: A Controlled Study. *Jour Asso Physc India* 2007; 55: 27-31.

Gupta PC. Mouth Cancer in India--A New Epidemic ? *J Indian Med Assoc* 1999; 97: 370-373.

Gupta PC. Tobacco Control in India. *Indian J Med Res* 2006; 123: 579-582.

Jha P, Jacob B, Gajalakshmi V, Gupta PC et al. A Nationally representative Case-Control Study of Smoking and Death in India. *New Engl J Med* 2008; 358: 1137-1147.

Sinha DN, Gupta PC, Pednekar MS, Jones JT, Warren CW. Tobacco Use Among School Personnel in Bihar, India. Tobacco Control 2002; 11: 82-83.

The Global Youth Tobacco Survey Collaborating Group: Tobacco Use Among Youth Across the Country: A Comparison. Tobacco Control 2002; 11 : 252-270.

Chapter 17

Bhardwaj S, Misra A, Khurana L, Gulati S, Shah P, Vikram NK. Childhood Obesity in Asian Indians: A Burgeoning Cause of Insulin Resistance, Diabetes and Subclinical Inflammation. *Asia Pac J Clin Nutr* 2008; 17(S1): 172-175.

Gupta R, Rastogi P, Sarna M, Gupta VP, Sharma SK, Kothari K. Body Mass Index, Waist-Size, Waist-hip Ratio and Cardiovascular Risk Factors in Urban Subjects. *Jour Assoc Physicians India* 2007; 55: 621-627.

Jebb SA, Elia A. Techniques for the Measurement of Body Composition: A Practical Guide. *Int J Obesity* 1993; 41: 810-817.

Misra A, Khurana L. Obesity and Metabolic Syndrome in Developing Countries. *J Clin Endocrinol Metab* 2008; 93: S9-S30.

Misra A, Pandey RM, Devi JR, Sharma R, Vikram NK, Khanna N. High Prevalence of Diabetes, Obesity, Dyslipidemia in Urban Slum Population of Northern India. *Int J Obes Rela Metab Disord* 2001; 25(11): 1722-1729.

Shankuan ZHU. Race-Ethnicity-Specific Waist Circumference Cutoff for Identifying Cardiovascular Disease Risk Factors. *Am J Nutr* 2005; 81: 400-415.

Snehalata C, Viswanathan V, Ramachandran A. Cutoff Values for Normal Anthropometric Variables in Asian Indian Adults. Diabetes Care 2003; 26: 1380-1384.

V Mohan, R Deepa. Obesity and Abdominal Obesity in Asian Indians. *Indian J Med Res*. 2006; 123: 593-596.

Chapter 18

Slattery ML, Jacobs DR Jr, Nichaman MZ. Leisure Time Physical Activity and Coronary Heart Disease Death. The US Railroad Study. *Circulation* 1989; 79: 304-311.

Hakim AA, Curb JD, Petrovitch H, et al. Effects of Walking on Coronary Heart Disease in Elderly Men. The Honolulu Heart Program. *Circulation* 1989; 79: 9-13.

Chapter 19

Jain P. Psychosocial Factors and Cardiovascular Disease. *Indian Heart Journal* 2008; 60: B38-B47.

Kubzansky LD, Kawachi I, Spiro A III et al. Is Worrying Bad for Heart? A Prospective Study of Worry and Coronary Heart Disease in The Normative Aging Study. *Circulation* 1997; 95: 818-824.

Ragland DR, Brand RJ. Type A Behavior and Mortality From Coronary Heart Disease. *N Engl J Med* 1988; 318: 65-69.

Chapter 20

Ornish D, Brown SE, Scherwitz LW, et al. Can Lifestyle Changes Reverse Coronary Heart Disease? The Lifestyle Heart Trial. *Lancet* 1990; 336: 129-133.

Ornish D, Scherwitz LW, Billings JH, et al. Intensive Lifestyle Changes for Reversal of Coronary Heart Diseas. *JAMA* 1998; 280: 2001-2007.

Manchanda SC, Narang R, Reddy KS, et al. Retardation of Coronary Atherosclerosis with Yoga Lifestyle Interventions. *J Assoc Physicians India* 2000; 48: 687-694.

Udupa KN, Singh RH, Settiwar RM. Physiological and Biochemical Studies on the effect of Yogic and Certain Other Exercises. *Indian J Med Res* 1975; 63: 620-624.

Nahin RL, Straus SE. Research into Complementary and Alternative Medicine: Problems and Potentials. *British Medical Journal* 2001: 322: 161-164.

Miller KL, Liebowitz RS, Newby LK. Complementary and Alternative Medicine in Journal Cardiovascular Disease: A Review of Biologically Based Approaches. *American Heart J* 2004; 147: 401-411.

Yeh GY, Davis RB, Phillips RS. Use of Complementary Therapies in Patients with Cardiovascular Disease. *American Heart Journal* 2006; 98: 673-680.

Chapter 21

Burr ML, Frhily AM, Gilbert JF et al. Effects of Changes in Fat, Fish and Fibre Intakes on Death and Myocardial Infarction : Diet and Reinfarction Trial (DART). *Lancet* 1989; 334: 757-761.

C Gopalan, Rama sastri BV, Balasubramanian SC. Nutritive Value of Indian Foods. National Institute of Nutrition, ICMR, Hyderabad 2007.

Enas EA, Senthilkumar A, Chennikkara H, Bjurlin MA. Prudent Diet and Preventive Nutrition From Pediatrics to Geriatrics, Current Knowledge and Practical Recommendations. *Indian Heart Journal* 2003; 55: 310-338.

Etherton PK, Eckel RH, Haward BV, Jeor SS Bazzare TL. Lyon Diet Heart Study. Benefits of Mediterranean-Style Diet, National Cholesterol Education Programme/American Heart association Step I Dietary pattern on cardiovascular Disease. *Circulation* 2001; 103: 1823-1825.

Etherton PK, Eckel RH, Haward BV, Jeor SS Bazzare TL. Lyon Diet Heart Study. Benefits of Mediterranean style Diet, National Cholesterol Education Programme/American Heart Association Step I Dietary Pattern on Cardiovascular Dieases. *Circulation* 2001; 103: 1823-1825.

Ferari R. Florio C. Zappaterra P. The European Cook Book. Healthy Diet, Healthy Heart Arti Grafiche colour Black for European Society of Cardiology. 2010.

Ghafoornisha, Krishnaswamy. Diet and Heart Disease. National Institute of Nutrition, Hyderabad. 2004

Hu FB, Willet WC. Optimal Diets for Prevention of Coronary Heart Disease *JAMA* 2002; 288: 2569-2575.

Manay N S, Shadaksharaswamy. Foods: Facts and Principles. New Age International Publishers, Second edition, 2007.

Rastogi T, Reddy KS, Vaz, M, Spiegelman D, Prabhakaran D, Willett WC, Stampfer MJ, Ascherio A. Diet and Risk of Ischemic Heart Disease in India. *Am J Clinical Nutrition* 2004; 79(4): 582-592.

Tarla Dalal Healthy Cookbook. Sanjay and Company. 2008

Chapter 22

Booyse FM, Parks DA. Moderate Wine and Alcohol Consumption: Beneficial Effects on Cardiovascular Disease. *Thromb Haemost* 2001; 86: 517-528.

Gronbaek M, Becker U, Johansen D, et al. Type of Alcohol Consumed and Mortality from All Cause, Coronary Heart Disease and Cancer. *Ann intern Med* 2000; 133: 411-419.

Mukamal KJ, Conigrave KM, Mittleman MA, et al. Roles of Drinking Patterns and Types of Alcohol Consumed in Coronary Heart Disease in Men. *N Eng J Med* 2003; 348:109-118.

Chapter 23

Diane L Tribble. Antioxidant Consumption and Risk of Coronary Heart Disease: Emphasis on Vitamin C, Vitamin E and Beta-Carotene. *Circulation* 1999; 99: 591-595.

Dwivedi S, Johri R. Beneficial Effects of Terminalia arjuna in Coronary Artery Disease. *Indian Heart Journal* 1997; 49: 507-510.

Dwivedi S. Putative Uses of Indian Cardiovascular Friendly Plants in Preventive Cardiology. *Ann National Med Sci (India).* 1996; 32: 159-175.

Fugh-berman A,. Herb-drug Interactions. *Lancet* 2000; 355: 134-138.

Muller LG. Herbal Medicinal. *Arch Intern Med* 1998; 158: 2200-2211.

Satyawati GV. Gum Guggul (Commiphora mukul): The Success Story of an Ancient Insight Leading to Modern Discovery. *Indian J Med Res* 1988; 87: 327-335.

Stevinson C, Pittler MH, Ernst E. Garlic for Treating Hypercholesterolemia: A Meta-analysis of Randomized Clinical Trials. *Ann Intern Med* 2000; 133: 420-429.

Valli G, Giardina EGV. Benefits, Adverse Effects and Drug Interactions of Herbal Therapies with Cardiovascular Effects. *J Am Coll Cardiol* 2002; 39: 1083-1095.

Vivekananthan DP, Penn MS, Sapp SK, Hsu A, Topol EJ. Use of Antioxidant Vitamins for the Prevention of Cardiovascular Disease: Meta-Analysis of Randomized trials. *Lancet* 2003; 361: 207-2023.

Katan MB, Grundy SM, Jones P et al. Efficacy and Safety of Plant Stanols and Sterols in the Management Blood Cholesterol Levels. *Mayo Clinic Proc* 2003; 78: 498-511.

Chapter 24

Enas EA. Recommendations for The Prevention and Control of Cardiovascular Disease. Second Indo-US Health Summit. New Delhi 2009.

Smith SC Jr, Allen J, Blair SN et al. AHA/ACC Guidelines for Secondary Prevention for Patients with Coronary and other Atherosclerotic Vascular Diseases: 2006 update: Endorsed by the National Heart, Lung and Blood Institute. *Circulation* 2006; 113: 2363-2372.

World Health Organization. European Health Report, 2005.